PET/CT

PET/CT

Essentials for Clinical Practice

Edited by

Ronald B. Workman, Jr., MD

Resident
Department of Radiology
Medical University of South Carolina
Charleston, South Carolina

R. Edward Coleman, MD

Professor
Department of Radiology
Director of Nuclear Medicine
Duke University Medical Center
Durham, North Carolina

Foreword by Martin P. Sandler, MD

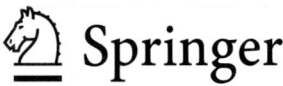 Springer

Ronald B. Workman, Jr., MD
Resident
Department of Radiology
Medical University of South Carolina
Charleston, SC
USA

R. Edward Coleman, MD
Professor
Department of Radiology
Director of Nuclear Medicine
Duke University Medical Center
Durham, NC
USA

Library of Congress Control Number: 2006920601

ISBN-10: 0-387-32166-7
ISBN-13: 978-0387-32166-0

Printed on acid-free paper.

Printed in the United States of America.   (BS/EB)

9 8 7 6 5 4 3 2 1

springer.com

To my loving family.
Ronald Workman, Jr.

To the residents who have taught me what I know.
Ed Coleman

Foreword

PET/CT: Essentials for Clinical Practice, edited by Drs. Workman and Coleman, provides an introductory reference source for physicians who want to learn more about PET/CT, as well as for medical students and residents who are involved in the rapidly growing field of PET/CT.

The first two chapters of the text outline the basic principles involved in patient preparation, imaging interpretation, and reimbursement. The remainder of the text provides information necessary to make a learned and informed decision with regard to the appropriate use of PET/CT in oncologic, cardiac, and neurologic disorders.

An important factor in determining the value of any text is the knowledge and credentials of the editors. Dr. Coleman's background as a leader in the fields of nuclear medicine, PET, PET/CT, and reimbursement places him at the forefront in the knowledge of the subject matter. Dr. Workman, having trained with Dr. Coleman, is eminently suited to co-edit a text of this nature.

PET/CT: Essentials for Clinical Practice is a well-written introductory text, and it provides fundamental information to improve understanding and clinical applications of this rapidly-evolving imaging modality.

The next decade will involve the field of functional/molecular imaging with a variety of innovative instrumentation developments, allowing us to examine smaller components of the human body with greater accuracy.

Martin P. Sandler, MD
Carol D. and Henry P. Pendergrass
Professor and Chairman
Department of Radiology
Vanderbilt University Medical Center
Nashville, TN

Preface

PET and PET/CT have enjoyed tremendous growth in recent years. This growth has been fueled by the well-documented diagnostic accuracy of PET and PET/CT, particularly in oncologic applications. In an effort to mitigate potential growing pains, we have created this guide for you, the clinician, to aid in your understanding of this powerful and increasingly popular imaging modality.

Even at academic medical centers where PET was first introduced and heavily used, there are clinicians who are unfamiliar with the role of PET in their day-to-day practice. As nuclear medicine physicians and diagnostic radiologists who use this technology daily, we see it as our responsibility to educate all of our colleagues involved in patient care about PET and PET/CT. It is not our intention to create a full reference text on PET. Instead, we wish to provide a clinically oriented distillation of high-yield information in a portable and easy-to-use format. That is why we have written *PET/CT: Essentials for Clinical Practice*. We sincerely hope that you find this guide beneficial in your practice.

Ronald B. Workman, Jr., MD
R. Edward Coleman, MD

Acknowledgments

We would like to express our sincere gratitude to our friends and colleagues in the Duke University Department of Radiology and the Duke University PET Facility. We would also like to thank our friends and colleagues at the Medical University of South Carolina and LSU-Health Sciences Center in New Orleans. Without the support of the fine people at these institutions, this book would not have been possible.

Ronald B. Workman, Jr., MD
R. Edward Coleman, MD

Contents

Contributors

Salvador Borges-Neto, MD, FACC
Assistant Professor, Department of Radiology, Division of Nuclear Medicine, Duke University Medical Center, Durham, NC, USA

Bennett B. Chin, MD
Associate Professor, Department of Radiology, Division of Nuclear Medicine, Duke University Medical Center, Durham, NC, USA

R. Edward Coleman, MD
Professor, Department of Radiology, Director of Nuclear Medicine, Duke University Medical Center, Durham, NC, USA

Michael W. Hanson, MD, FACC
Clinical Professor, Department of Radiology, Co-Director of Nuclear Cardiology, Division of Nuclear Medicine, Duke University Medical Center, Durham, NC, USA

Martin J. O'Connell, MD
Professor, Divisions of Nuclear Medicine and Abdominal Imaging, Mater Misericordiae University Hospital, Dublin, Ireland

Nirav P. Shah, MD
Director of PET/CT Imaging, Assistant Professor, Department of Radiology, Boston University School of Medicine, Boston, MA, USA

Terence Z. Wong, MD, PhD
Assistant Professor, Department of Radiology, Division of Nuclear Medicine, Duke University Medical Center, Durham, NC, USA

Ronald B. Workman, Jr., MD
Resident, Department of Radiology, Medical University of South Carolina, Charleston, SC, USA

1. Fundamentals of PET and PET/CT Imaging

Ronald B. Workman, Jr. and R. Edward Coleman

Brief History of Positron Emission Tomography

Positron emission tomography (PET) has been in existence since the 1970s due in large part to the pioneering work of Michael Phelps, PhD, Michel Ter-Pogossian, PhD, and others in the fields of medical physics and nuclear medicine [1]. Although initially a research tool, over the past 10 years PET has become increasingly used in the clinical setting, particularly after CMS (the Centers for Medicare and Medicaid Services, formerly known as the Health Care Financing Administration or HCFA) began reimbursing for PET evaluation of myocardial perfusion in 1995. Clinical utilization rose dramatically in 1998, when CMS began reimbursing for PET evaluation of solitary pulmonary nodules and initial staging of lung cancer. (CMS coverage as it relates to PET is covered in detail in Chapter 2.)

1998 also saw the creation of the first PET/computed tomography (CT) hybrid system, and in 2001, such systems became commercially available. Major manufacturers such as General Electric, Siemens, and Philips are now combining their latest CT technology with their latest PET technology to create very powerful hybrid systems that are the industry mainstay. PET/CT hybrids represent the state of the art in PET scanning, and it is estimated that PET/CT combination systems comprise 90% of sales in the current PET market [2]. The evolution of PET from its beginnings as an instrument of research to its present day wide and growing use in cancer, cardiac, and neurological imaging has resulted in instrumentation that is making a major impact in clinical care.

Before launching an in-depth discussion of the clinical applications of PET, it is important to describe the fundamental basic scientific principles behind nuclear medicine imaging, of which PET is a part.

Basics of Scintigraphy

In diagnostic nuclear medicine, radioactive substances, termed *radiopharmaceuticals*, are administered to patients and an image is obtained by placing the patient under a special scanner called a gamma camera. Such an image is properly termed a *scintigram* (from the Latin *scintilla* meaning spark or glimmer) and is generally referred to as a scan. Bone scans, ventilation/perfusion lung scans, myocardial perfusion scans, thyroid scans, etc., are examples of commonly performed nuclear medicine studies. A radiopharmaceutical is a combination of a radioactive element, or radionuclide, and a pharmaceutical agent. In diagnostic imaging, this pharmaceutical molecule has a negligible pharmacologic effect because very small amounts are administered. Thus, the term *radiotracer* is sometimes used to describe these trace, but detectable, radioactive agents. Once the radiopharmaceutical has been administered, it is distributed within the patient according to its specific pharmacokinetics. Scintigraphic images are obtained by the gamma camera with the patient as the radioactive source.

The nuclear medicine imaging instrument is referred to as a gamma camera because its detection of photons, or gamma rays, generates the images. Gamma photons, sometimes denoted γ, are packets of energy emitted by many radionuclides as they undergo decay. Technetium-99m (^{99m}Tc) is one example of a radionuclide that undergoes gamma decay, and it is the main radionuclide used in conventional nuclear medicine. ^{99m}Tc can be coupled with a variety of pharmaceuticals to generate physiology-based images of many different organs and organ systems. At the heart of the gamma camera is the sodium iodide (NaI) crystal that absorbs the photons emitted by radionuclides such as ^{99m}Tc. The crystal scintillates in response to absorbing a photon, and this scintillation event is converted into an electrical signal that is then processed to ultimately create an image.

The manner by which the gamma camera obtains an image also needs to be discussed. Planar imaging refers to flat, two-dimensional images. To generate a planar image, the gamma camera remains in one plane to collect the emitted photons and does not move, except to shift position as necessary within that same plane to obtain a complete image. An example of a planar image is the anterior view of a whole-body bone scan. Gamma cameras can also rotate around the patient, and with the use of computer-aided image reconstruction, generate tomographic images. This is referred to as SPECT, or single photon emission computed tomography. This technique is used in myocardial perfusion imaging, but can be employed in many other scenarios as well. Figure 1.1 shows a simple graphical representation of various image acquisition methods.

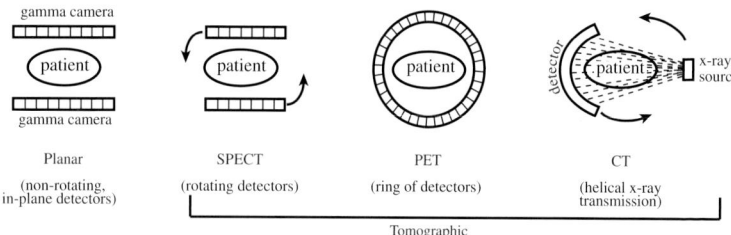

Figure 1.1. Examples of fundamental image acquisition methods. Planar, SPECT, and PET images are generated by emitted photons with the patient as the radiation source following radiopharmaceutical injection. CT images are generated by transmitted x-rays which have passed through the patient from an x-ray source. SPECT, PET, and CT generate tomographic images.

Not all radionuclides decay in the same way, and not all emitted gamma photons have the same energy. Some gamma photons are more energetic than others, and higher energy gamma rays must be imaged by instruments that are appropriately equipped to handle those energies. In addition to isomeric transition that produces gamma rays, there is alpha (α) decay and beta (β) decay in which highly energized particles are emitted from the nuclei of unstable nuclides. Alpha decay is not discussed in this book because it has no use in diagnostic imaging; however, beta decay is at the heart of positron emission tomography and is discussed in detail below.

Fundamentals of Positron Emission Tomography Imaging

PET is based on the physical properties of certain radioactive isotopes known as positron emitters. As their name implies, these radionuclides emit positrons rather than gamma photons when they undergo radioactive decay. Positron decay is a type of beta decay in which a positively charged particle, known as a beta+ particle (denoted $\beta+$), is emitted from a proton-rich nucleus as that nucleus attempts to become more stable. Although simplified, it is convenient and sufficient to think of a $\beta+$ particle as a positively charged electron. This simplification will aid in understanding later discussions concerning how a $\beta+$ interacts with matter. (A negatively charged beta particle, sometimes called a negatron, or $\beta-$ particle, is identical to an electron except that its origin is the nucleus rather than the electron cloud surrounding the nucleus. $\beta-$ particles do not play a role in PET.)

So do PET scanners image positrons? The answer is no. Unlike conventional nuclear medicine imaging with gamma-emitting radionuclides, the photons imaged in PET do not directly come from the nuclei that are undergoing decay. Nor are the positrons being imaged. Because positrons are particles that carry a positive charge, they travel only a very short distance, usually no more than a millimeter or two, before encountering a negatively charged electron. When a positron and electron collide, the particles are annihilated, and according to the conservation of matter and energy, the annihilation of the electron and positron results in the creation of two high energy gamma photons that travel approximately 180 degrees from one another (Figure 1.2). These high energy annihilation photons are not detected efficiently by a conventional gamma camera, and a specialized ring of detectors is used. Their simultaneous detection using short timing intervals is called coincident detection. Photon pairs that do not arrive at opposite points along the PET detector ring at the same time (within a few nanoseconds) are ignored by the PET scanner. This action is called *discrimination* and helps improve localization of true coincident events.

The energy of each coincident photon produced by the annihilation reaction is approximately 511 keV, which is much greater than the less energetic 140 keV photons emitted by ^{99m}Tc. PET detectors are specially engineered to handle these high energy photons, and because there is a ring of detectors, there is no need for the ring to rotate in order to obtain a tomographic image. Instead of

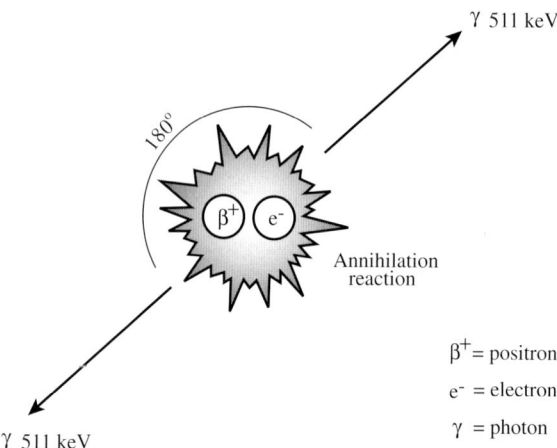

Figure 1.2. Positron–electron annihilation reaction.

traditional sodium iodide (NaI) crystals, PET ring detector crystals are composed of compounds such as bismuth germanate (BGO), lutetium oxyorthosilicate (LSO), or gadolinium oxyorthosilicate (GSO). All of these compounds are used by different PET and PET/CT manufacturers, and they have physical properties which make them well suited to PET imaging. For a comparison of the imaging properties of these compounds, see Table 1.1.[3–5]

Table 1.1. Imaging properties of various PET crystals

Property	Bismuth germanate (BGO)	Lutetium oxyorthosilicate (LSO)	Gadolinium oxyorthosilicate (GSO)
Coincidence efficiency (%)	72	67	56
Energy resolution (%)	15	10	8.5
Decay time (ns)	300	40	60
Image acquisition mode	2D or 3D	3D	3D

Coincidence efficiency is related to count sensitivity and should be as close to 100% as possible.

Energy resolution is related to scatter rejection and the closer it is to 0%, the better it is at rejecting scatter.

Decay time is a measure of how long the scintillation light persists; longer times limit count rate capability.

Attenuation, Absorption, and Scatter

The images generated by PET scanners are accurate representations of the objects being analyzed, but there are several factors that can degrade image quality. Absorption and scatter are two such factors.

In nuclear medicine, attenuation refers to the decrease in intensity of a photon signal as it passes through matter either by absorption or by scatter. Attenuation effects are directly proportional to the density and thickness of the various tissues through which photons travel; that is, the more dense and thick a tissue is, the more it will attenuate. If the matter through which a photon is traveling stops the photon completely, it is called absorption. Scatter refers to the alteration in the direction of a photon's path due to its interaction with matter (e.g. tissues) along that path. These effects are related, and both give rise to image reconstruction errors that can adversely affect the accuracy of a PET scan.

Attenuation correction is a technique in which quantitative methods are used to partially offset the deleterious effects of attenuation on an image. In conventional dedicated PET systems, a transmission image using photons from a germanium-68 (^{68}Ge) source is generated to create what can be conceptualized as an attenuation map of the patient. In this way, the PET system computer obtains data about the attenuation effects of each individual patient's body. The transmission image, together with the emission image, enables the PET scanner to create an "attenuation-corrected" image of the patient. The differences between attenuation-corrected and non-attenuation-corrected images can be seen in many of the PET/CT images presented throughout this book. Non-attenuation-corrected images are denoted NAC.

Instead of using a ^{68}Ge source to create a transmission image, PET/CT systems use a much more diagnostically useful and clinically familiar image – a CT scan. The CT portion of a PET/CT therefore serves two functions: (1) it is a transmission map which is used for attenuation correction of the PET image, and (2) it is an exquisitely detailed anatomic image, familiar to clinicians, which can be used for very precise disease localization. The latest PET/CT systems contain the latest generation of CT technology, and investigations are currently underway at PET centers across the world to adapt existing CT protocols to PET/CT use in various clinical scenarios.

Using CT for attenuation correction is not only more diagnostically beneficial, it also time saving that translates into better patient tolerance and improved throughput. Table 1.2 presents the acquisition and overall scan times for an average adult.

Table 1.2. Average adult PET and PET/CT scan times

	PET	**PET/CT**
Transmission time	18 minutes	20 seconds
Emission time	24 minutes	18 minutes
Overall scan time	42 minutes	18+ minutes

Positron Emission Tomography Radioisotopes and Radiopharmaceuticals

The radioisotopes that are commonly used in PET imaging are detailed in Table 1.3. Notice that these radionuclides have fewer neutrons than their non-radioactive, stable, counterparts; that is, stable carbon has 12 nucleons, stable nitrogen has 14, stable oxygen has 16, and stable fluorine has 19 nucleons. The relative paucity of neutrons within these radionuclides results in protons that are closer together, and repel one another making their nuclei unstable. This repulsion and instability in a proton-rich nucleus is the basis for positron decay, in which a positively charged particle leaves the nucleus and a proton becomes a neutron.

Another characteristic is the short half-life ($t_{1/2}$) of these positron emitters. The short $t_{1/2}$ is one of the main reasons that, until recently, PET imaging was limited to institutions equipped with an on-site circular particle accelerator, called a cyclotron, to make the positron-emitting radioisotopes. Some medical centers without their own cyclotron, or one nearby, were previously unable to acquire the short-lived PET radiotracers needed by a PET facility. However, the recent emergence of companies located throughout the country that specialize in synthesizing and transporting a variety of PET radiopharmaceuticals has enabled many more medical centers, hospitals, and imaging centers to have robust PET practices.

Carbon, nitrogen, and oxygen represent some of the fundamental atomic building blocks of life, and exact radioactive versions of many important biomolecules have been created to further our understanding of biology, physiology, and pathophysiology. Much research has been devoted to fashioning radioactive biomolecules that are labeled with a positron emitter. Radiolabeled versions of amino acids, sugars, and even the nitrogen bases which comprise DNA and RNA have been developed and studied extensively. For some examples of such radiopharmaceuticals, see Table 1.4.

Today, the most widely used PET radiopharmaceutical is ^{18}F-2-fluoro-2-deoxy-D-glucose, also known as fluorodeoxyglucose (FDG). FDG has very similar structure and biochemical behavior to glucose. Note the structural similarity between the FDG and glucose molecules illustrated in Figure 1.3. The dissimilarity, although subtle, between these molecules allows for very powerful information to be obtained from an FDG-PET scan.

Table 1.3. Common PET radioisotopes

Name	Atomic number (protons)	Number of nucleons (protons + neutrons)	Approximate half-life (min)
Carbon-11	6	11	20
Nitrogen-13	7	13	10
Oxygen-15	8	15	2
Fluorine-18	9	18	110

Table 1.4. Examples of PET radiopharmaceuticals

Radiopharmaceutical	Structural analogue	Measured parameter
[^{18}F]Fluorodeoxyglucose (FDG)	Glucose	Glucose metabolism
[^{18}F]Fluoro-DOPA	Dopamine	Amino acid metabolism
[^{18}F]Fluorocholine (FCH)	Choline	Cell membrane synthesis
[^{18}F]Fluorothymidine (FLT)	Thymidine	DNA synthesis
[^{18}F]Fluorestradiol (FES)	Estradiol	Estrogen receptor status
[^{18}F]Sodium fluoride (NaF)	None	Bone formation
[^{13}N]Ammonia	None	Tissue perfusion
[^{11}C]Methionine	Methionine	Amino acid metabolism

Glucose undergoes several chemical reactions within the cells of the body to ultimately produce water, carbon dioxide, and most importantly energy. Glycolysis, the Krebs cycle, and the electron transport chain are all instrumental in generating the energy needed to operate our bodies at the cellular level. While a detailed discussion of these processes is beyond the scope of this book, it is important to review and understand the first few steps of glycolysis as they relate to PET imaging with FDG.

Cancer biologists have known for some time that tumors have a higher glycolytic rate than normal tissue. As a glucose analogue, FDG behaves identically to glucose, but only to a point. Once phosphorylated by hexokinase, FDG-6-phosphate is trapped within cells because it is not a suitable substrate for glucose-6-phosphatase. The disproportionately higher metabolic rate in malignant cells combined with FDG's resemblance to glucose is the basis behind tumor imaging with FDG-PET (Figure 1.4).

There is wide variability of what is considered normal, physiologic distribution of FDG in the body. Normal bowel, heart, skeletal muscle, and even fat can have variable FDG uptake. Consistently high FDG is seen in normal brain and excreted in the urine. For an example of a normal FDG-PET scan, see Figure 1.5.

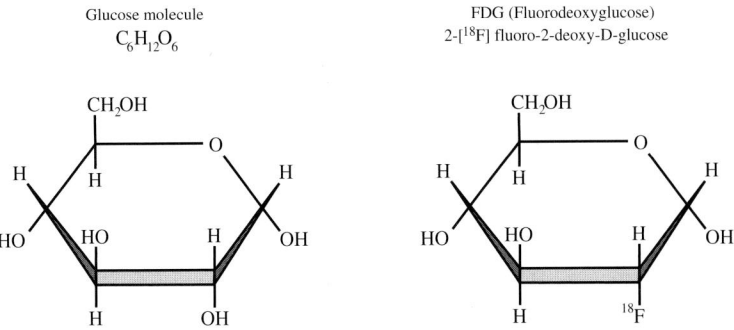

Figure 1.3. Glucose and fluorodeoxyglucose structure.

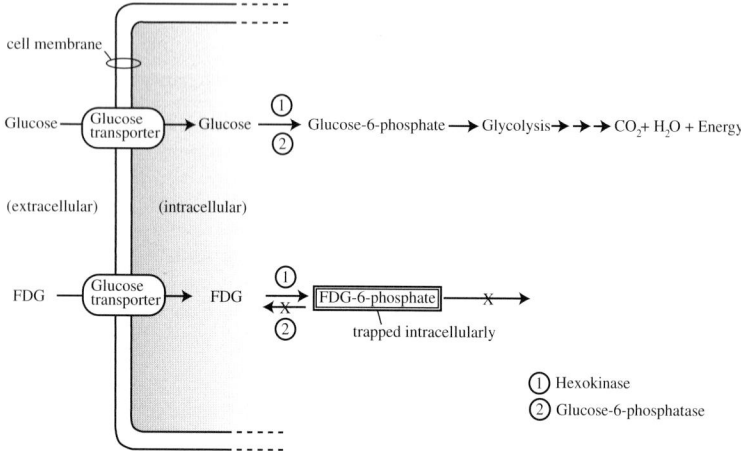

Figure 1.4. Early metabolic paths of glucose and FDG.

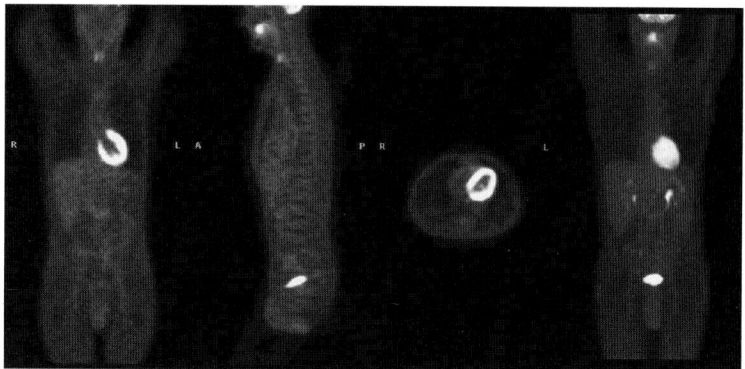

Figure 1.5. Normal FDG-PET whole-body scan. The first three images are tomograms through the body in the coronal, sagittal, and transaxial planes. The image at the far right represents an MIP, or maximum intensity projection image. The MIP image is a summation of all of the slices stacked together, and it is a rapid way to visualize FDG distribution throughout the body. These are grayscale images with whiter regions representing higher amounts of FDG uptake. The normal brain uses large amounts of glucose, which explains its large amount of FDG uptake. Myocardial uptake is variable on FDG scanning with all, some, or none of the myocardium normally visualized on FDG-PET whole-body scanning. FDG primarily undergoes renal excretion, and kidney, ureteral, and bladder activity is normal. There is faint activity in the vocal cords as well as mild activity in the patient's tongue. This represents physiologic muscle uptake in a patient who was likely phonating during the uptake phase. The liver has homogeneous mild uptake, as does non-exerted muscle. Normal lung is relatively photopenic.

Patient Preparation and Radiation Safety

There are a few important points to consider in preparing patients for an FDG-PET scan. Because FDG is a glucose analogue, it is necessary that patients avoid any caloric intake for at least 4–6 hours prior to the study. Typically, patients are asked to fast overnight for morning appointments, and have only a light breakfast for afternoon appointments. Serum glucose is routinely measured prior to FDG injection, and fasting levels are typically 70–110 ng/dl, which are ideal for an FDG-PET scan. Serum glucose levels greater than 200 ng/dl may result in significant changes in FDG distribution, and patients with such levels are usually not scanned until better control is obtained, because hyperglycemia leads to competitive inhibition of FDG uptake into cells. Hyperinsulinemia is also a problem because it results in increased FDG uptake into skeletal muscle. Fasting results in low (basal) insulin levels. Diabetic patients should not have regular insulin administered subcutaneously within 4 hours of having FDG administered.

After administration of FDG, patients must wait a period of at least 40–45 minutes prior to scanning. This period is referred to as the *uptake phase* and is the necessary amount of time for the FDG to be adequately biodistributed and transported into the patient's cells. Patients are asked to rest in a quiet room, devoid of distractions, and they are also asked to keep their movements, including talking, at an absolute minimum. This minimizes physiologic uptake of FDG into skeletal muscle, which can confound interpretation of the scan. Patients should be comfortable and relaxed.

There has never been a documented allergic reaction to FDG, nor has the injection of a glucose analogue such as FDG posed any documented difficulties for diabetic patients. The important consideration with respect to diabetics is that they refrain from insulin administration for at least 4–6 hours for reasons described previously.

In most cases, venous access can be obtained without difficulty by trained technologists or venipuncturists. However, venous access can be quite difficult to obtain in small children, obese patients, the elderly, and patients being treated with chemotherapy, etc. Although not ideal, and to be avoided, rather than cancel an FDG-PET scan for lack of venous access, FDG can be administered orally in liquid form followed by water. If this situation should arise, it is recommended that you discuss options regarding oral FDG administration with your nuclear medicine or radiology specialist [6].

Patients are administered 140 μCi/kg of FDG with a minimum of 10 mCi and a maximum of 20 mCi. Fixed doses of 15 mCi or 20 mCi can also be used. Although the photons created following a positron–electron annihilation are very high energy, the radiation dose from an FDG-PET scan is less than one might expect, for two major reasons. First, the physical half-life for ^{18}F is short at only 110 minutes. Second, the biological half-life of FDG is also relatively short, and it is excreted rapidly by the kidneys and eliminated in the urine. Roughly 50% of the administered dose is present in the urine of those with normally functioning kidneys after about 2 hours. The combination of these two factors results in a relatively low effective $t_{1/2}$. For estimated radiation exposure following intravenous administration of FDG, see Table 1.5. For PET/CT, radiation dose is

Table 1.5. Estimated radiation dose with intravenous administration of FDG in a 70-kg patient

Organ	mGy/185 MBq	rad/5 mCi
Bladder wall	31.45	3.15
Bladder (voided at 1 hour)	11.00	1.10
Bladder (voided at 2 hours)	22.00	2.20
Heart	12.03	1.20
Brain	4.81	0.48
Kidneys	3.88	0.39
Uterus	3.70	0.37
Ovaries	2.78	0.28
Testes	2.78	0.28
Adrenal glands	2.59	0.26
Small intestine	2.40	0.24
Gastric wall	2.22	0.22
Liver	2.22	0.22
Pancreas	2.22	0.22
Spleen	2.22	0.22
Breast	2.04	0.20
Lungs	2.04	0.20
Red bone marrow	2.04	0.20
Other tissues	2.04	0.20
Bone surface	1.85	0.18
Thyroid	1.79	0.18

Source: From Oehr et al. [8], with kind permission of Springer Science and Business Media.

significantly greater than PET alone because of the CT portion of the study, and consideration should be given to overall patient exposure. The typical effective dose can be as much as 1 rad each for a conventional CT scan through the chest, abdomen, or pelvis [7].

FDG-PET can have a significant impact on the treatment plan of a patient with malignancy, and for this reason the relative radiation risk of obtaining the scan is considered negligible. However, pregnant women should avoid undergoing an FDG-PET scan. FDG does cross the placenta, and will be distributed within the fetal brain and be excreted by the fetal kidneys. The mother will also excrete the FDG into her bladder, which increases the radiation dose to the nearby fetus. It is recommended that clinicians consult with their radiologists and nuclear medicine specialists to determine whether another imaging modality may be employed to answer the clinical question in a woman who is pregnant. An FDG-PET scan can certainly be obtained postpartum if necessary. Breast-feeding is not recommended for 10 hours after administration of this FDG.

Some PET centers recommend the use of muscle relaxants, cleansing bowel preparations, and the placement of a Foley catheter in some patients undergoing an FDG-PET scan. Muscle relaxants and anxiolytics (e.g. diazepam) are thought to minimize patient anxiety and lessen potential interference caused by skeletal muscle uptake. Bowel preparations have been employed in the hope of lessening or eliminating physiologic bowel activity which is often seen. Foley catheters, diuretics (e.g. furosemide), and intravenous fluids have been used in various protocols to minimize the interference from excreted activity in the genitourinary tract which could possibly obscure adjacent disease. These steps have met with mixed results, are often unwelcome by patients, and are controversial in some circles. Therefore, many other PET experts believe in a non-invasive, "keep it simple" approach to PET imaging where none of these adjuncts is used. It is the experience of this author that interventions such as those described above are not necessary to render accurate PET interpretations from experienced PET imagers.

Image Acquisition and Interpretation

PET imaging can be obtained in either a two-dimensional (2D) or three-dimensional (3D) manner. In 2D PET, parallel lead septa are extended from the detector array, thereby restricting detection of photons to only those detectors that are in the same or nearby planes. Conversely, in 3D PET the lead septa are not used and photon detection can occur across all detector planes. 2D imaging reduces overall count rate, scatter and random coincidences, and allows for rapid image reconstruction. 3D imaging greatly increases system sensitivity (overall counts), but also increases scatter and random coincidences, and the image reconstruction algorithm takes more time to process. BGO, LSO, and GSO detector crystals have characteristics that are better suited to 2D or 3D, as presented in Table 1.1. For example, LSO and GSO have relatively short decay times and are better at rejecting scatter and random coincidences; therefore, they are better suited for dealing with the high count rates generated with 3D imaging. BGO is better suited to 2D imaging because the count rate burden is less.

For the PET acquisition using a PET/CT scanner, a 2 min/bed position is used for patients 150 lb or less, 3 min/bed position for 151–200 lb, and 4 min/bed position for those greater than 201 lb. Average height adults usually require six bed positions for a scan from the skull base to the mid-thighs. The CT acquisition parameters depend on whether the scan is performed for attenuation correction and anatomic localization or for diagnostic interpretation. A low mA scan is adequate for attenuation correction and anatomic localization, and higher mA is needed for a diagnostic scan. Intravenous contrast material may be used for a diagnostic CT scan, and this scan can be used for attenuation correction also.

Standardized Uptake Value

Although qualitative interpretations of FDG-PET scans are often sufficient, standardized uptake values (SUVs), are sometimes used in FDG-PET reports in order to impart some semi-quantitative measurement of the degree of FDG accumulation to areas of suspicion. The SUV is a unitless ratio that can be understood as the concentration of FDG within a lesion divided by the concentration of radiotracer distributed throughout the body. Mathematically, it can be expressed as follows:

$$SUV = C\ (T)/(dose\ injected/body\ weight)$$

where C is the tissue concentration of FDG at time T.

An SUV is a simplified index of FDG uptake and provides a relative indication of the degree of metabolism within the lesion being evaluated. The SUV measurement is directly proportional to metabolic activity. SUV can be notated as the maximum value within a lesion (SUV_{max}), or the average value within a region of interest drawn around a lesion (SUV_{avg}). The SUV_{max} is more robust because it is more reproducible, being less affected by the size and placement in the region of interest.

Because the SUV is affected by multiple factors and is subject to error, it should be used with caution. These factors include extravasation of radiotracer which alters whole-body distribution, patient obesity (some advocate using lean body mass rather than body weight in SUV determination for this reason), time interval between FDG administration and scanning, size of the region of interest used to make the SUV calculation, and serum glucose level.

SUV is used most frequently when evaluating a solitary pulmonary nodule, where an SUV of 2.5 or greater within that nodule is considered suspicious for malignancy, and an SUV less than 2.5 favors a benign, usually inflammatory condition. Additionally, studies have shown that patients with a solitary pulmonary nodule which has an SUV of 10 or greater have a poor prognosis, even in the absence of metastatic disease. These and other points are discussed further in Chapter 3, PET in Lung Cancer. Another major use of SUV is in the follow-up of cancer after therapy [8]. The SUV provides a semi-quantitative index for determining the effect of therapy.

Artifacts and Limitations of Fluorodeoxyglucose-Positron Emission Tomography

No imaging modality is 100% accurate, and while it has shown great promise, there are significant limitations in PET. One limitation in FDG-PET is the overlap which exists between benign inflammatory disease and malignancy. Inflammatory processes, particularly granulomatous infections and conditions such as sarcoidosis, can have increased FDG uptake that is just as intense as that seen in malignancy. Radiation therapy changes can also have increased FDG uptake that can mimic residual disease. This infection/inflammation accumulation of FDG accounts for many of the false positives in FDG-PET. As discussed previously, in the evaluation of a pulmonary nodule, an SUV of 2.5 is used as the cutoff between a benign and malignant process. While this is true in the majority of cases, overlap does exist. Examples of some commonly encountered artifacts as well as post-surgical, inflammatory, and other non-malignant hypermetabolic conditions are presented in Figures 1.6 through 1.12 and Plate 1.9B in the color insert. Images in the remaining chapters will present additional similar examples.

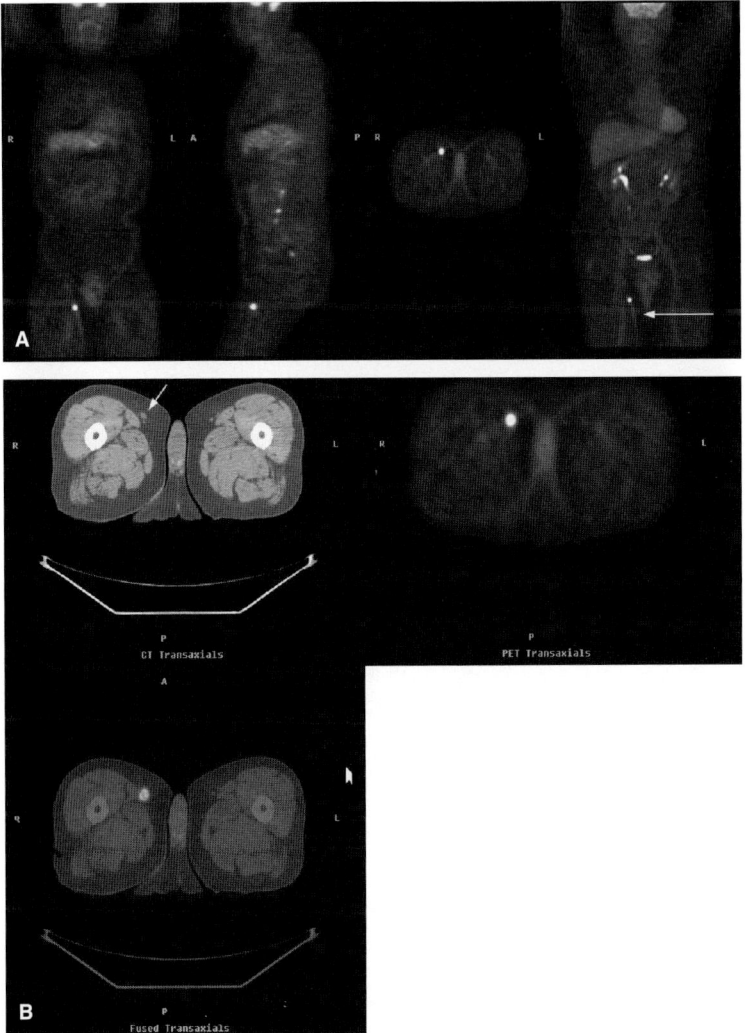

Figure 1.6. Lymphatic tracking of FDG. **(A)** FDG-PET whole-body images following injection in the patient's right foot. There was extravasation of FDG at the injection site, and this resulted in physiologic lymphatic tracking of radiotracer along the medial thigh (white arrow). The patient did not have veins suitable for injection in the upper extremities. **(B)** The lymphatic tracking seen in **(A)** terminates within a normal-sized lymph node in the medial aspect of the proximal right thigh. Because physiologic lymph node uptake of radiotracer is a recognized consequence of extravasation (it follows the same principle as lymphoscintigraphy in breast and melanoma sentinel node identification), it is preferable to inject FDG in a vein of an extremity on the opposite side of any known malignancy.

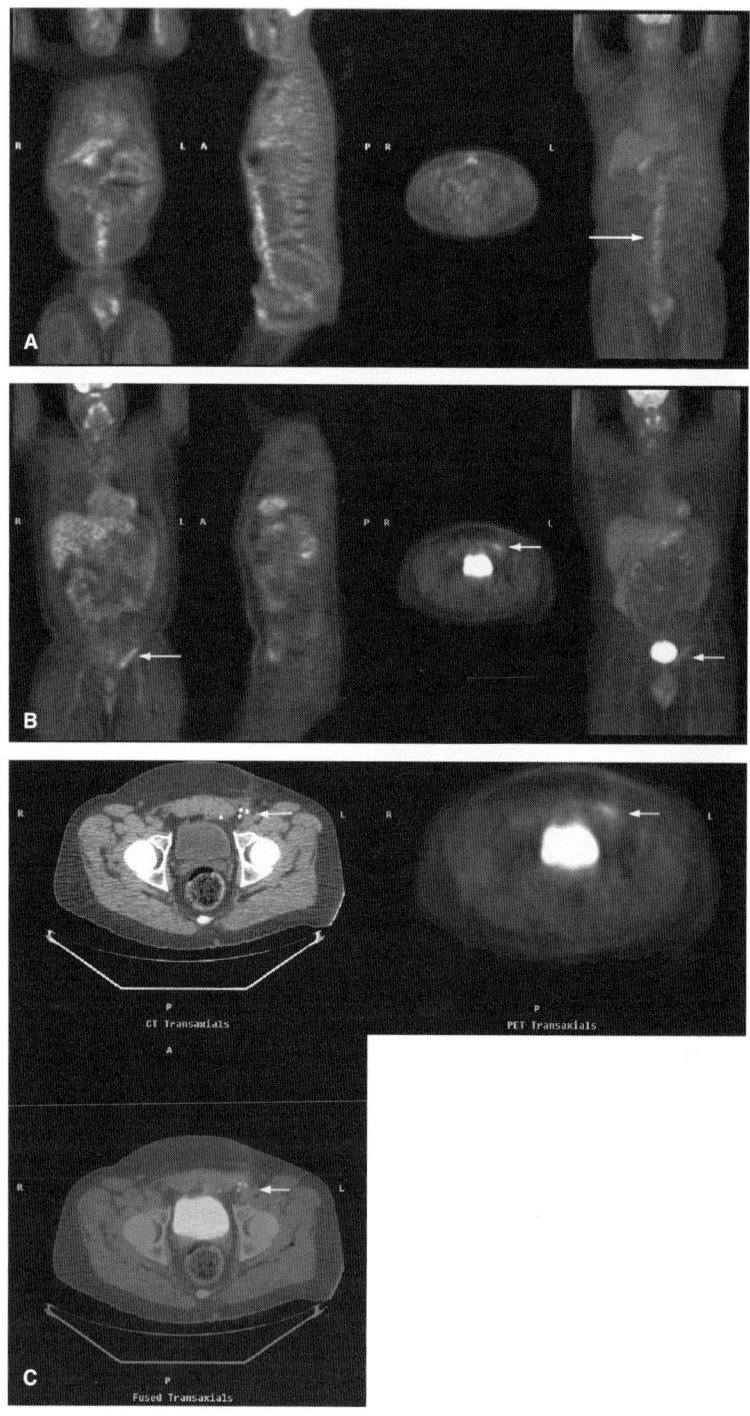

Figure 1.7. **(A)** Healing abdominal wound. This patient is status post bilateral nephrectomies for polycystic kidney disease and also had rejection and removal of a renal transplant. The patient was scanned for fever of unknown origin with clinical concern for lymphoma. There was no evidence of malignancy by FDG-PET; however, scanning did show linear moderate FDG uptake along the patient's healing abdominal midline incision. Also note the lack of excreted FDG within the urinary bladder explained by the patient's history. **(B** and **C)** Healing inguinal hernia repair. FDG-PET whole-body scan for lymphoma restaging. There is no evidence of active disease. There is mild to moderate linear increased activity in the left inguinal region corresponding to the patient's recent left inguinal herniorrhaphy (white arrows).

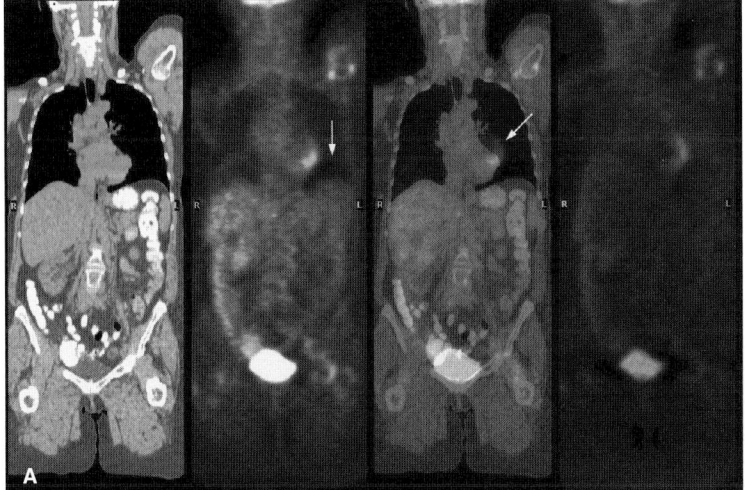

Figure 1.8. Misregistration. **(A** and **B)** FDG-PET/CT images demonstrating severe degenerative changes in the left shoulder joint as well as respiratory motion artifact. Notice the cardiac and left lower lung misregistration due to respiratory motion (white arrows). **(C)** Transaxial FDG-PET/CT images from a patient undergoing restaging of breast cancer. The patient is status post left mastectomy. Notice the cardiac misregistration (white arrow) due to motion. There is also a soft tissue lesion in the right breast which does not demonstrate any FDG uptake, favoring a benign etiology.

Continued.

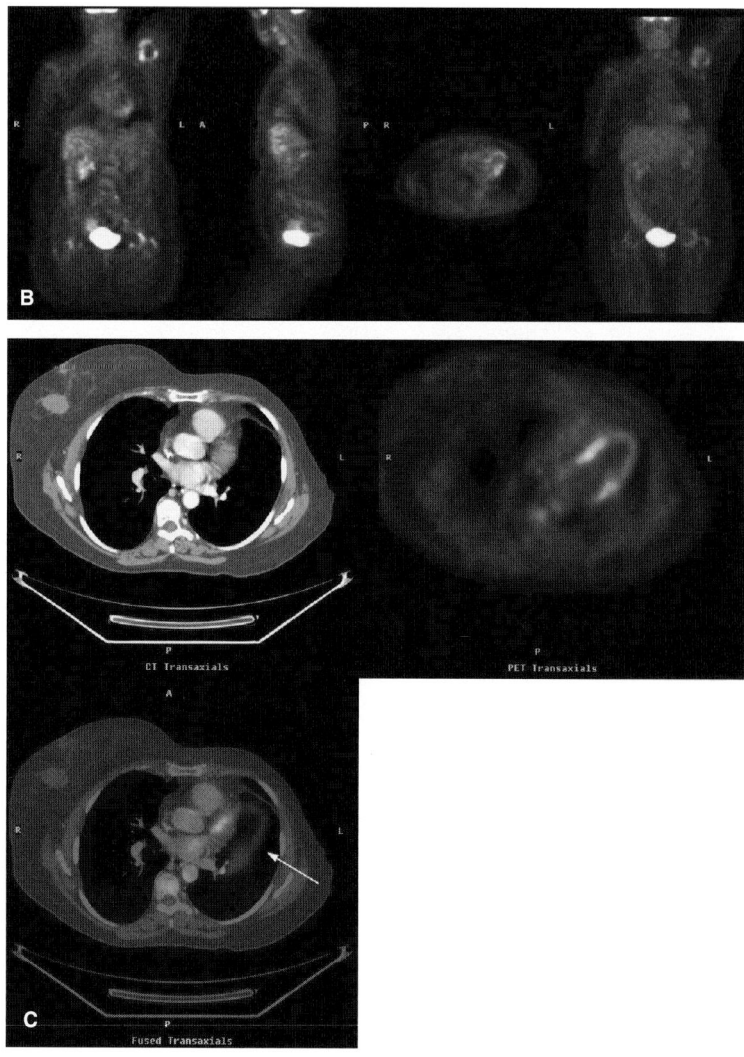

Figure 1.8. *Continued.*

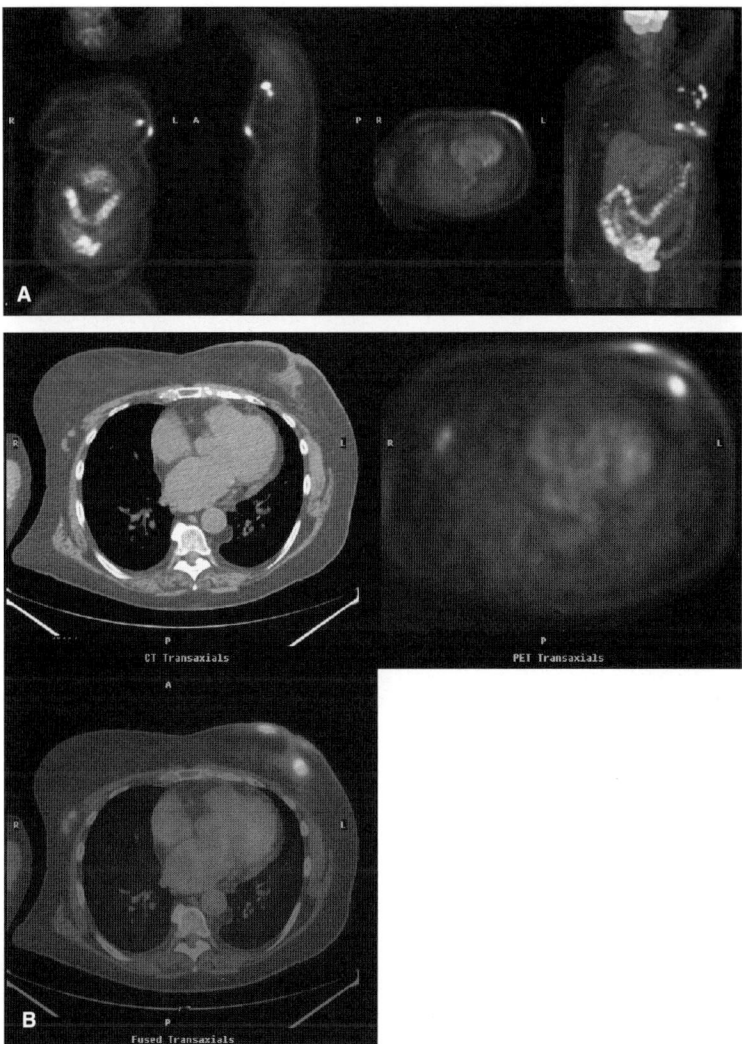

Figure 1.9. **(A)** Bowel uptake. FDG-PET whole-body scan for staging of inflammatory carcinoma of the left breast. Also notice the diffuse increased radiotracer uptake in the colon, which is a normal variant. Suspicion is raised when there is focal bowel activity, although this too can be seen normally. **(B** and **C)** Inflammatory breast cancer. Transaxial images from the same patient demonstrating left breast skin thickening and nodularity with metastatic regional adenopathy. Two smaller hypermetabolic lymph nodes are in the right axilla. Although possibly reactive nodes, in the absence of a regional inflammatory process these are suspicious for metastatic disease. (See part B only in the color insert.)

Continued.

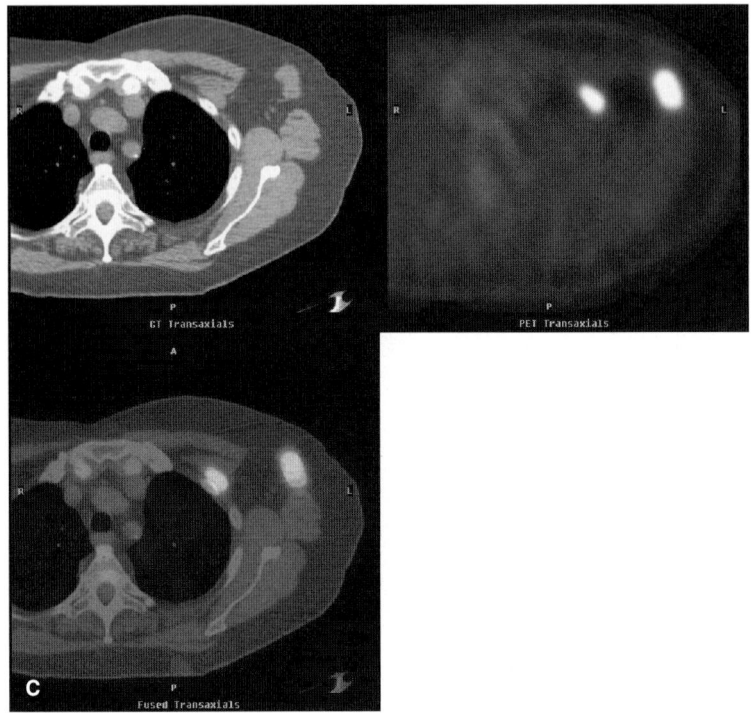

Figure 1.9. *Continued.*

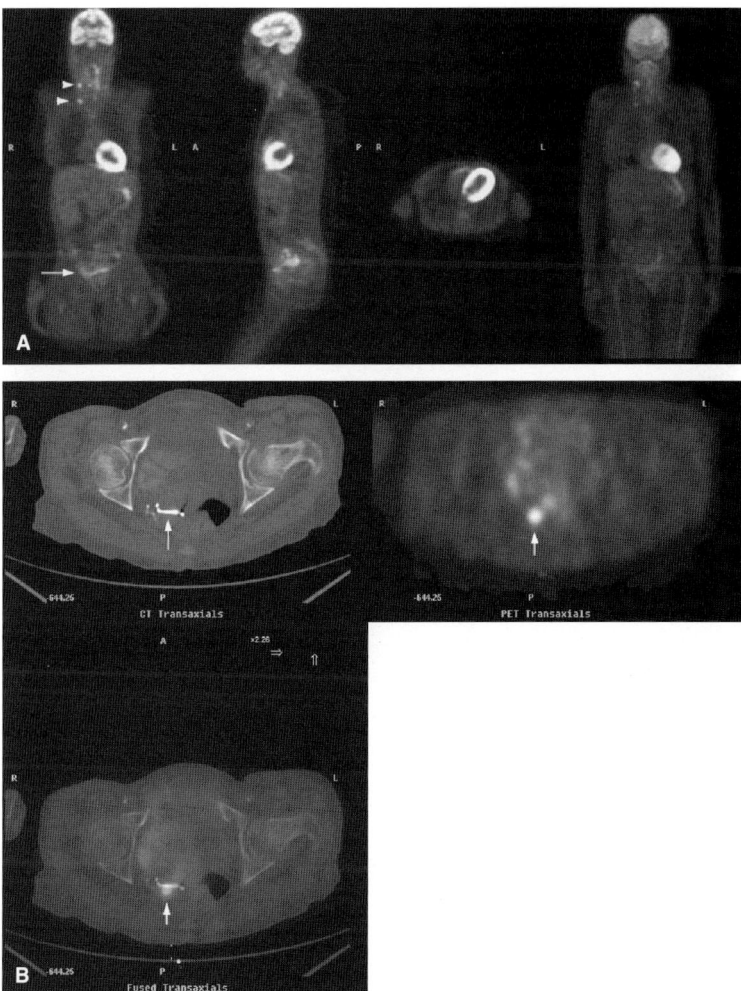

Figure 1.10. Intrauterine device (IUD). **(A)** Whole-body FDG-PET/CT scan in a woman for restaging of head and neck cancer. There is metastatic adenopathy in the low right cervical and right supraclavicular regions (white arrowheads); however, there is also increased activity in the right hemipelvis (white arrow). **(B)** Transaxial images through the pelvis demonstrate increased activity in the uterus adjacent to the patient's IUD consistent with chronic inflammation (white arrows).

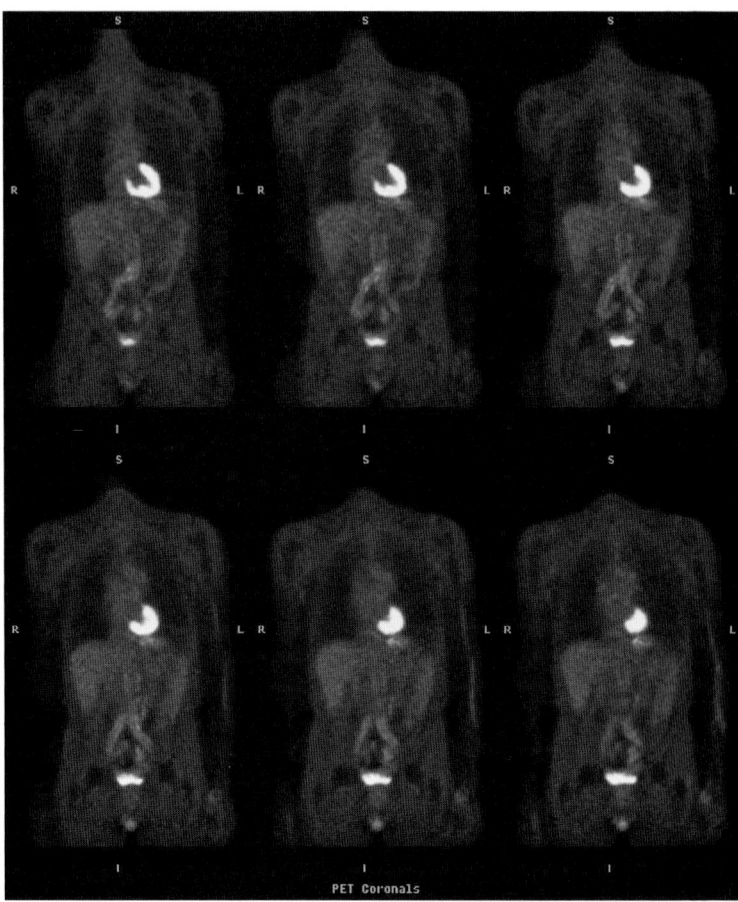

Figure 1.11. Aorto-biiliac graft. FDG-PET coronal images demonstrating mild to moderate increased activity along the patient's aorto-biiliac graft following repair of an aneurysm at that location. The patient was scanned to evaluate a pulmonary nodule which is not seen scintigraphically, consistent with a benign etiology.

Figure 1.12. Brown fat. (A) FDG-PET whole-body maximum intensity projection (MIP) image demonstrates symmetric focal uptake in the lower cervical and supraclavicular regions bilaterally. (B) Transaxial FDG-PET/CT images reveal that the hypermetabolic foci in the lower cervical and supraclavicular regions correlate to fat density on CT. Hypermetabolic brown fat is occasionally encountered and is a normal variant. In addition to its correlation with fat, experienced PET imagers recognize brown fat by its symmetric distribution, usually in the cervical, supraclavicular, and paraspinal regions bilaterally.

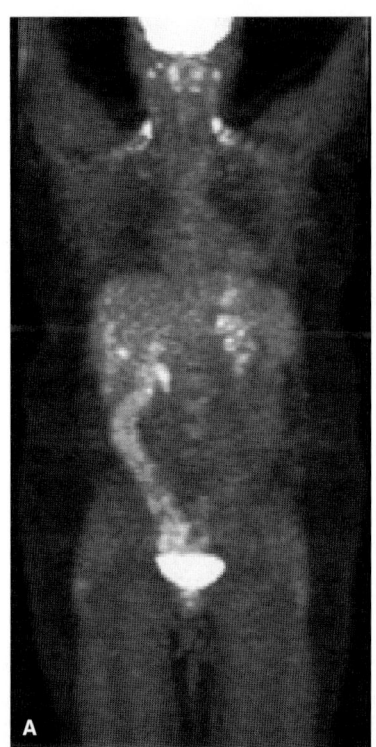

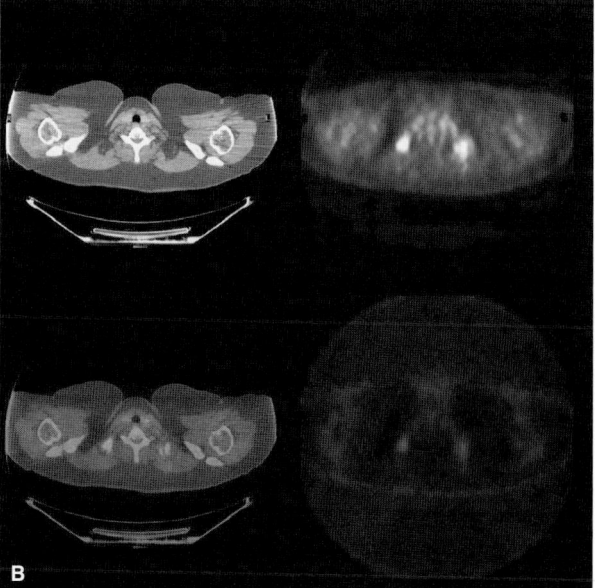

False-negative results also happen in FDG-PET and are typically because of small tumors, low grade malignancies that are not as metabolically active (e.g. bronchioloalveolar carcinoma, bronchial carcinoid, etc.), malignancies that may have increased levels of glucose-6-phosphatase which allow FDG to escape from cells (e.g. hepatocellular carcinoma), or tumors that have large amounts of mucin. A detailed discussion of the false positives and false negatives of PET is presented in the clinical focus chapters.

An important shortcoming of PET imaging technology is the problem of lesion size. Microscopic and small macroscopic disease (i.e., less than 7 or 8 mm) can be missed because of spatial resolution limitations in PET systems. Future technology with improved instrumentation and image processing should allow us to characterize smaller lesions.

References

1. Phelps M, Ter-Pogossian M. A positron-emission transaxial tomograph for nuclear imaging (PETT). Radiology 1975;114:89–98.
2. Harvey D. PET/CT Proving a fruitful union. Radiology Today 2004 September 27,2004: 13.
3. Madsen MT. Selecting a new PET/CT system. Journal of the American College of Radiology 2004;1(5):356–358.
4. Karp JS. Against: Is LSO the future of PET? Eur J Nucl Med Mol Imaging 2002; 29(11):1525–1528.
5. Nutt R. For: Is LSO the future of PET? Eur J Nucl Med Mol Imaging 2002; 29(11):1523–1525.
6. Franc B, Carlisle MR, Segall G. Oral administration of F-18 FDG to evaluate a single pulmonary nodule by positron emission tomography in a patient with poor intravenous access. Clin Nucl Med 2003;28(7):541–544.
7. Wiest PW, Locken JA, Heintz PH, Mettler FA, Jr. CT scanning: a major source of radiation exposure. Semin Ultrasound CT MR 2002;23(5):402–410.
8. Oehr P, Biersack H-J, Coleman RE, editors. PET and PET/CT in Oncology. Berlin: Springer-Verlag; 2004.

2. Reimbursement for PET and PET/CT Imaging

R. Edward Coleman

The utilization of positron emission tomography (PET) and PET/CT is increasing and their major impact is on the management of oncology patients. The utilization of PET and PET/CT scans in oncologic patients is benefiting only a small percentage of patients who could benefit from having these procedures. Since the initial coverage of PET for lung cancer indications by Medicare in January 1998, Medicare and other third-party payers now cover several cancers. The delay in utilization of PET relates to several factors: lack of knowledge about PET by referring physicians; lack of knowledge about PET by patients; limited number of PET scanners available; and limited number of physicians trained to read PET scans. With the recent introduction of combined PET and computed tomography (CT) devices, additional complexity in performing and interpreting PET scans is introduced. Now the decision has to be made concerning the technologist who performs the study (is it a radiologic technologist, a nuclear medicine technologist, or both?) and the physician interpreting the study (is it a diagnostic radiologist alone or a nuclear medicine physician interpreting the PET scan and a diagnostic radiologist interpreting the CT scan?).

This chapter provides a background on the payment for PET and PET/CT in the United States covering the regulatory and reimbursement issues, an overview of the PET and PET/CT market, the costs of doing PET and PET/CT, and a summary of the current status of coverage.

Background

The first PET scans were performed in the United States in the early 1970s, soon after the introduction of CT for brain imaging. The first publications of PET scans and magnetic resonance imaging (MRI) scans occurred at about the same time. MRI developed into a clinical imaging modality much more rapidly than did PET imaging. PET imaging remained as an expensive, difficult research imaging modality at a few academic medical centers. PET was used to provide in vivo studies of blood flow, metabolism, receptor density, etc., primarily of the brain and heart. With the development of fluorodeoxyglucose (FDG) in the late 1970s, the potential clinical applications of PET became apparent in the 1980s.

The initial studies demonstrated clinical utility in the evaluation of disorders of the brain and heart. The role of PET in brain tumors was demonstrated to be the grading of the degree of malignancy and the differentiation of recurrent tumor from necrosis after therapy. The role in refractory seizure disorders was also well documented, and the potential role in evaluation of dementia was demonstrated. FDG-PET myocardial viability studies were demonstrated to be very accurate for determining the patients that would benefit from revascularization procedures. The benefit of PET myocardial perfusion imaging over SPECT myocardial perfusion imaging was demonstrated. The first reimbursement for PET imaging was in 1995 for myocardial perfusion imaging using rubidium-82.

In the 1990s, the PET whole-body techniques for evaluating cancer patients became more widely available and the results were demonstrating clinical utility. At that time, much concern and criticism were occurring related to the rapid increase in utilization of CT and MRI. Healthcare costs were increasing at a rapid rate. The new imaging modalities were seen as a major cause in the increasing cost of medical care, as they are now. Several studies and reports were published during the 1990s that were critical of the approval process for coverage of CT and MRI, and suggested that there was marked over-utilization of these imaging modalities. Thus, as PET was starting to be reviewed as a clinical imaging modality, it came under heightened scrutiny compared to CT and MRI.

An issue for PET imaging was obtaining a New Drug Application (NDA) for FDG. When reimbursement was sought from the Health Care Financing Administration (HCFA), now Centers for Medicare and Medicaid Services (CMS), which administers Medicare, and other third-party payers, the status of approval of FDG by the Food and Drug Administration (FDA) was raised. Because there were essentially no policies for reimbursement at that time, there was no commercial entity interested in producing FDG. The Institute of Clinical PET (ICP) was formed in the early 1990s, and one of its missions was to obtain the appropriate regulatory approval and reimbursement for FDG. Medicare and other third-party payers were not going to provide coverage without an NDA for FDG.

The ICP worked with the FDA in trying to develop a mechanism for approval of FDG. The FDA knew how to regulate large pharmaceutical companies, but they were unable to develop a mechanism for regulating FDG that was produced and used on a local or regional basis. A New Drug Application (NDA) was granted to a hospital in Peoria, Illinois, in 1989 with the indication being refractory seizure disorder being considered for surgical therapy. In 1997, Congress changed the regulation of PET radiopharmaceuticals when it passed the Food and Drug Modernization Act (FDAMA). In that law, PET radiopharmaceuticals that were included in the United States Pharmacopoeia were given the equivalence of FDA approval. The law stated that for the next 2 years, the FDA must work with the PET community to develop a mechanism for regulating PET radiopharmaceuticals and that the PET community would have 2 years to come into compliance. The PET community is continuing to work with the FDA to develop appropriate regulatory guidelines. Thus, the process is many years behind the schedule outlined in the FDAMA.

During 1996 and 1997, representatives of ICP were interacting with representatives of HCFA (now CMS) concerning reimbursement. Medicare provides coverage for persons aged 65 and older as well as certain other specific patient populations. Most third-party payers have policies to cover at least what Medicare covers. The reimbursement by the other third-party payers is determined by a variety of methods including fee for service, discounted rates and capitation. Payment for PET by Medicare was placed under a "National Coverage Determination" that made it unique from CT and MRI because PET would only be covered as a result of a formalized coverage process. There is a statement of "non-coverage" meaning that PET scans would not be paid by Medicare, even if local carriers determined that the indication met medical necessity requirements, unless there was a national coverage policy. The Medicare system pays for PET and other medical procedures by several methods. If the patient is an outpatient seen in the hospital, the payment is made by a special outpatient rate through the Hospital Outpatient Prospective Payment System (HOPPS) under the Ambulatory Payment Classification (APC) at the current rate of $1150 for PET, and $1250 for PET/CT. If the patient is an outpatient seen in an imaging center independent from the hospital, the reimbursement rate is determined by the local carrier and is generally greater than the HOPPS rate. If the patient is an inpatient, procedures performed while in the hospital are paid under one payment for the entire hospitalization under the diagnostic related groups (DRG). The hospital determines how the reimbursement is divided amongst the departments caring for the patients under each DRG.

After FDG received approval through the FDAMA, HCFA announced that it would cover FDG-PET scans for two indications starting January 1, 1998: evaluation of the indeterminate solitary pulmonary nodule and the initial staging of lung cancer. This coverage decision had a major impact on the development of PET. Other third-party payers generally cover indications for coverage developed by Medicare. Several of the large third-party payers have their own technology assessment panels and do their own evaluations. However, most third-party payers cover at least what Medicare does, and many cover indications not approved by Medicare.

The announcement of coverage of PET scans starting in 1998 resulted in an industry developing around the production of FDG and PET scanners. Before that time, a limited number of PET scanners were being sold. With the start of reimbursement, more scanners were sold and more money went into research and development of new scanners. Furthermore, FDG was available commercially at only a very small number of sites in the United States in 1997, and the reimbursement policies resulted in an expansion of the number of commercial entities distributing FDG and the number of sites producing FDG.

Positron Emission Tomography Market

With the development of combined PET/CT devices, the market for PET scanners has decreased as it has increased for PET/CT scanners. The number of commercial facilities providing FDG has increased, and the number of doses of FDG provided per facility has increased. PET/CT scanners continue to improve, and provide better quality images in shorter acquisition times. The PET/CT scanners have resulted in the capability of doing more patients per day than could be done by PET alone devices.

Because of the reimbursement and the rapid expansion of clinical indications, the PET market grew rapidly. The number of clinical PET scans performed in 1998 was estimated at 150,000, the number in 2002 was estimated at 650,000, and the number in 2004 was estimated at more than 1 million. The number of FDG distribution sites in the United States in 1998 was estimated at 10, and the number in 2002 was estimated at 70. Most metropolitan areas have ready access to FDG, and back-up production sites are generally available to provide FDG if a primary site has a problem.

According to National Equipment Manufacturer Association (NEMA) reports, 100 new scanners were sold in 2000, 200 in 2001 and 327 in 2002. PET became a billion dollar industry in 2003. In 2004, the worldwide installed base was 1080 PET scanners and 510 PET/CT scanners. The current new sales were 94% PET/CT, with very few PET alone devices being sold.

The reasons that PET only systems were being bought in recent years are the following: software image fusion can provide registration of the PET with CT or MRI images; CT adds from $600,000 to $1,000,000 to the cost of the device; and PET alone is exempt from the Stark law, thus permitting partnerships with oncology, radiation oncology, and surgery groups. The Stark law is likely to be changed this year to make nuclear medicine, including PET, no longer exempt. The reasons that combined PET/CT devices are being bought are the following: noise-free attenuation correction; short duration transmission scans; shorter duration scans and faster patient throughput; anatomic lesion localization; potential added revenue from CT; competition factor (having the newest and best); adjunct to already established CT service (additional CT access); and improved registration, not only for diagnostic purposes but also for use with radiation oncology for radiation therapy planning and intensity-modulated radiation therapy.

Costs of Positron Emission Tomography and Positron Emission Tomography/Computed Tomography

The costs for doing PET are the capital costs for the scanner, the space for housing the scanner, waiting room, injection room, etc.; staff; ancillary items, such as FDG, contrast, injectors; additional software such as for calcium scoring, lung nodule volume measurement, etc.; and interpretation fees.

The following scenario is presented for a center that has a PET/CT scanner. The cost of a PET/CT scanner is approximately $1.8 million dollars. Assuming that FDG costs $300 per dose, the breakeven point for doing PET if 4 patients per day were scanned would require a reimbursement of approximately $1700 per patient. If more patients are scanned per day, the breakeven point is less. If revenue is generated from the CT scanner, the breakeven point for the PET reimbursement is less.

At reimbursement rates prevalent today in the United States, between 4 and 5 patients per day are needed to break even on purchasing a PET (closer to 4) or PET/CT (closer to 5) scanner. In 2004, the average number of patient studies performed per day on a PET scanner was 3.8. As more patient studies are performed on a scanner each day, the costs per patient decrease.

Current Status of Coverage

After the initial Medicare coverage for evaluation of solitary pulmonary nodules and initial staging of lung cancer became effective in January 1998, the types of cancer and indications have increased. Starting in 1999, Medicare added colorectal cancer with rising carcinoembryonic antigen (CEA), initial staging and restaging of Hodgkin's and non-Hodgkin's lymphoma and initial staging and restaging of melanoma. In 2000, Medicare provided coverage for the diagnosis, staging, and restaging of the following malignancies: lung cancer, colorectal cancer, head and neck cancer, esophageal cancer, melanoma, and Hodgkin's and non-Hodgkin's lymphoma. Brain tumors and thyroid cancer were specifically excluded from coverage in the head and neck cancer category.

In October 2002, Medicare started covering breast cancer for staging, restaging, and monitoring of therapy. This monitoring of therapy for breast cancer was the first time that this indication was approved. In 2003, well-differentiated thyroid cancer that was no longer iodine-131 avid and with a thyroglobulin level greater than 10 was covered. In 2005, the staging of cervical cancer with a negative CT or MRI outside of the pelvis was covered.

In late 2004, CMS announced that it was developing a national registry that would provide coverage with evidence development. In this registry, all cancers and indications not presently covered would be covered except for breast cancer diagnosis, axillary nodal staging of breast cancer, and regional nodal staging of melanoma. The registry is sponsored by the Academy of Molecular Imaging (AMI) and is managed by the American College of Radiology Imaging Network (ACRIN). All PET centers can participate in the registry, and the anticipated fee is $50 per patient. To participate, the PET facility has to register with ACRIN. The referring physician will need to complete a questionnaire before and after the PET scan is performed in order for the facility to be reimbursed for the scan. The registry will assess the change in intended management, and CMS will use this information to determine reimbursement policies. The anticipated start date for the registry was late 2005, and the registry is expected to continue for approximately 2 years.

Positron Emission Tomography/Computed Tomography and Diagnostic Computed Tomography Reimbursement

Medicare covers all of PET and PET/CT imaging with 11 Current Procedure Technology (CPT) codes (Table 2.1). Three codes are for myocardial imaging and two codes are for brain imaging. For oncologic imaging, Medicare

Table 2.1. CPT codes for PET and PET/CT

CPT code	Description
78459	Myocardial imaging, positron emission tomography (PET), metabolic evaluation
78491	Myocardial imaging, positron emission tomography (PET), perfusion, single study at rest or stress
78492	Myocardial imaging, positron emission tomography (PET), perfusion, multiple studies at rest and/or stress
78608	Brain imaging, positron emission tomography (PET); metabolic evaluation
78609	Brain imaging, positron emission tomography (PET); perfusion evaluation
78811	Tumor imaging, positron emission tomography (PET); limited area (e.g. chest, head/neck)
78812	Tumor imaging, positron emission tomography (PET); skull base to mid-thigh
78813	Tumor imaging, positron emission tomography (PET); whole body
78814	Tumor imaging, positron emission tomography (PET) with concurrently acquired computed tomography (CT) for attenuation correction and anatomical localization; limited area (e.g. chest, head/neck)
78815	Tumor imaging, positron emission tomography (PET) with concurrently acquired computed tomography (CT) for attenuation correction and anatomical localization; skull base to mid-thigh
78816	Tumor imaging, positron emission tomography (PET) with concurrently acquired computed tomography (CT) for attenuation correction and anatomical localization; whole body

is now using three CPT codes for PET and three for PET/CT: limited, skull base to mid-thigh, and whole body. Some uncertainty exists concerning the billing for a patient who has a PET/CT and a diagnostic CT (e.g. chest, abdomen, and pelvis) on the same scanner. Increasingly, physicians are ordering PET/CT and diagnostic CT scans on the same patient, and the scans can be performed on the same scanner. Several studies have now shown that the oral and intravenous CT contrast does not cause artifacts on the PET scan. Thus, the diagnostic CT can be used for the attenuation correction scan and for anatomic localization. The American College of Radiology (ACR) is concerned that billing for a PET/CT and the diagnostic CT scan might be considered as billing twice for the CT scans. Thus, ACR recommends billing for a PET scan and for the diagnostic CT scan. Other organizations consider it appropriate to bill for PET/CT and diagnostic CT scans because they were actually performed. CMS has not made any statement concerning their recommendation for this coding conundrum.

Physician Interpretation of Positron Emission Tomography/Computed Tomography

The ACR, Society of Nuclear Medicine, and the Society of Computed Body Tomography and Magnetic Resonance recently published an intersociety dialogue on concurrent PET/CT with a focus on interpreting the studies [1,2]. Many nuclear medicine physicians who have had no training in diagnostic radiology are experts in interpreting PET. Many diagnostic radiologists who have had no training in PET are experts in interpreting CT. Radiology residents completing their training today are trained in both PET and CT, and they have appropriate experience for interpreting PET/CT and diagnostic CT. Nuclear medicine residency training programs are attempting to increase the training in CT so that residents finishing training in the new program will have appropriate experiences for interpretation of PET/CT and diagnostic CT. For nuclear medicine physicians and radiologists already in practice, the number of supervised interpretations and CMS hours needed for supervising and interpreting the studies are discussed in the intersociety dialogue.

References

1. Coleman RE, Delbeke D, Guiberteau MJ, et al. Concurrent PET/CT with an integrated imaging system: intersociety dialogue from the joint working group of the American College of Radiology, the Society of Nuclear Medicine, and the Society of Computed Body Tomography and Magnetic Resonance. J Am Coll Radiol 2005;2:568–584.
2. Coleman RE, Delbeke D, Guiberteau MJ, et al. Concurrent PET/CT with an integrated imaging system: Intersociety dialogue from the joint working group of the American College of Radiology, the Society of Nuclear Medicine, and the Society of Computed Body Tomography and Magnetic Resonance. J Nucl Med 2005;46:1225–1239.

Clinical Chapters

The American Cancer Society estimates that cancer currently accounts for approximately 23% of all deaths in the United States. In 2005, there were an estimated 1,372,910 new cancer cases with approximately 570,280 cancer-related deaths, or about 1500 deaths per day [1]. Clearly, cancer is one of the major foes that physicians and patients face. Fortunately, more battles are being won now than ever before thanks to improvements in public health and education, early detection, and treatment. PET/CT is one such advancement, and it has emerged as a major imaging tool to accurately diagnose, stage, and restage a variety of malignancies. While most PET utilization is in oncology, PET also has a valuable role to play in evaluating heart disease, dementia, and epilepsy. The following chapters discuss the current state and future prospects of PET and PET/CT in oncology, cardiology, and neurology.

There are a few common themes connecting these chapters that should be discussed. First, fluorodeoxyglucose (FDG) is, by far, the most widely used PET radiopharmaceutical. Acting as a glucose analogue, FDG localizes within cells based upon their degree of glycolytic activity. Neoplasms exhibit unregulated growth that must be supported by increased metabolism; thus hypermetabolic foci are a hallmark of malignancy. A second point is that hypermetabolism is not always associated with malignancy, but can be seen with benign physiologic and inflammatory conditions. This limitation should always be kept in mind when considering and interpreting FDG-PET scans. Third, why is PET/CT so attractive? Nuclear medicine imaging with PET offers physicians valuable functional information, and radiographic imaging demonstrates exquisite anatomic detail, particularly with CT and MRI. With PET/CT, function and structure can now be viewed together, providing physicians with impressive insight into human disease. In 1993, while investigating visceral tumors, Wahl et al. described the fusion of FDG-PET images with CT or MRI and coined the resulting image an "anatometabolic" fusion image [2]. Now, use of anatometabolic imaging is entering mainstay medical practice, allowing increased confidence in assessing disease thanks to the merger of these two different, but complementary imaging modalities. Finally, near the end of each clinical chapter, we discuss ongoing work beyond FDG with new and emerging PET radiopharmaceuticals that show tremendous promise in furthering the frontiers of functional imaging.

References

1. Jemal A, Murray T, Ward E, et al. Cancer statistics, 2005. CA Cancer J Clin 2005; 55(1):10–30.
2. Wahl RL, Quint LE, Cieslak RD, Aisen AM, Koeppe RA, Meyer CR. "Anatometabolic" tumor imaging: fusion of FDG PET with CT or MRI to localize foci of increased activity. J Nucl Med 1993;34(7):1190–1197.

3. PET in Lung Cancer

Ronald B. Workman, Jr. and R. Edward Coleman

Epidemiology

During 2005, there were approximately 172,570 new cases of lung cancer diagnosed in the United States. Although lung cancer accounts for about 13% of all new cancer cases, it is responsible for almost 28% of all cancer deaths and is the leading cause of cancer mortality for both men and women. An estimated 163,510 deaths were from lung cancer alone in 2005. Approximately 60% of those diagnosed with lung cancer die within 1 year, 75% die within 2 years, and the combined 5-year survival rate for all stages of lung cancer is only 15%. These figures have not changed substantially in almost a decade [1]. These statistics reflect the fact that the majority of cases are advanced at presentation; however, if caught early, various series have shown that surgical resection of a solitary lung cancer carries a 5-year survival rate of 40–80% [2,3].

The two main histopathologic categories for lung malignancy are small cell lung cancer (SCLC) and non-small cell lung cancer (NSCLC). In both its clinical behavior and treatment, SCLC is distinct from NSCLC. SCLC accounts for the minority (about 14%) of all lung cancer cases and is composed of poorly differentiated, rapidly growing cells with disease usually occurring centrally rather than peripherally. It metastasizes early. Management for SCLC is nonsurgical, and therapy is via chemotherapy alone or in combination with radiotherapy. The majority of lung cancers are non-small cell in origin. While their classification is complex, it can be broadly broken down into the most common cell types: squamous, adenocarcinoma, and large cell. Table 3.1 provides a detailed outline of non-small cell cancer types [4].

Like most cancers, treatment for limited disease is usually surgical, with combination therapy reserved for more advanced cases depending on tumor site and patient performance status. Lung cancer is currently staged via the Tumor, Node, Metastasis (TNM) scheme devised by the American Joint Committee on Cancer. Table 3.2 provides the TNM staging classification of lung cancer. Curative surgery alone is the treatment of choice for patients with stage IA and IB disease, although inoperable early stage patients can undergo an attempt at curative radiotherapy. Surgery in combination with chemoradiation can be performed up to stage IIIA disease. For stages IIIB and IV, treatment is non-surgical and aimed more at palliation [5].

As with the other malignancies discussed in this book, there are PET reimbursement codes that have been established by the Centers for Medicare and Medicaid Services (CMS) for various covered indications [6]. In practical terms,

Table 3.1. The new World Health Organization/International Association for the Study of Lung Cancer histologic classification of non-small cell lung cancers

---

1. Squamous cell carcinoma
    Papillary
    Clear cell
    Small cell
    Basaloid
2. Adenocarcinoma
    Acinar
    Papillary
    Bronchioloalveolar carcinoma
        Non-mucinous
        Mucinous
        Mixed mucinous and non-mucinous or indeterminate cell type
    Solid adenocarcinoma with mucin
    Adenocarcinoma with mixed subtypes
    Variants
        Well-differentiated fetal adenocarcinoma
        Mucinous ("colloid") adenocarcinoma
        Mucinous cystadenocarcinoma
        Signet ring adenocarcinoma
        Clear cell adenocarcinoma
3. Large cell carcinoma
    Variants
        Large cell neuroendocrine carcinoma
        Combined large cell neuroendocrine carcinoma
        Basaloid carcinoma
        Lymphoepithelioma-like carcinoma
        Clear cell carcinoma
        Large cell carcinoma with rhabdoid phenotype
4. Adenosquamous carcinoma
5. Carcinomas with pleomorphic, sarcomatoid or sarcomatous elements
    Carcinomas with spindle and/or giant cells
    Spindle cell carcinoma
    Giant cell carcinoma
    Carcinosarcoma
    Pulmonary blastoma
6. Carcinoid tumor
    Typical carcinoid
    Atypical carcinoid
7. Carcinomas of salivary-gland type
    Mucoepidermoid carcinoma
    Adenoid cystic carcinoma
    Others
8. Unclassified carcinoma

Source: Non-small cell lung cancer cellular classification. National Cancer Institute (www.cancer.gov); 2005 Accessed April 2005.

Table 3.2. TNM staging for lung cancer

Primary tumor (T)

TX   Primary tumor cannot be assessed, or tumor proven by the presence of
         malignant cells in sputum or bronchial washings but not visualized
         by imaging or bronchoscopy

T0   No evidence of primary tumor

Tis   Carcinoma in situ

T1   Tumor 3 cm or less in greatest dimension, surrounded by lung or
         visceral pleura, without bronchoscopic evidence of invasion more
         proximal than the lobar bronchus* (i.e., not in the main bronchus)

T2   Tumor with any of the following features of size or extent:
         More than 3 cm in greatest dimension
         Involves main bronchus, 2 cm or more distal to the carina
         Invades the visceral pleura
         Associated with atelectasis or obstructive pneumonitis that extends to
         the hilar region but does not involve the entire lung

T3   Tumor of any size that directly invades any of the following: chest wall
         (including superior sulcus tumors), diaphragm, mediastinal pleura,
         parietal pericardium; or tumor in the main bronchus less than 2 cm
         distal to the carina, but without involvement of the carina; or
         associated atelectasis or obstructive pneumonitis of the entire lung

T4   Tumor of any size that invades any of the following: mediastinum,
         heart, great vessels, trachea, esophagus, vertebral body, carina; or
         separate tumor nodules in the same lobe; or tumor with a malignant
         pleural effusion†

Regional lymph nodes (N)

NX   Regional lymph nodes cannot be assessed

N0   No regional lymph node metastasis

N1   Metastasis to ipsilateral peribronchial and/or ipsilateral hilar lymph
         nodes, and intrapulmonary nodes including involvement by direct
         extension of the primary tumor

N2   Metastasis to ipsilateral mediastinal and/or subcarinal lymph nodes

N3   Metastasis to contralateral mediastinal, contralateral hilar, ipsilateral or
         contralateral scalene, or supraclavicular lymph nodes

Distant metastasis (M)

MX   Distant metastasis cannot be assessed

M0   No distant metastasis

M1   Distant metastasis present (includes separate tumor nodule(s) in a
         different lobe, ipsilateral or contralateral)

Stage grouping			
Occult carcinoma	TX	N0	M0
Stage 0	Tis	N0	M0
Stage IA	T1	N0	M0
Stage IB	T2	N0	M0
Stage IIA	T1	N1	M0

Continued.

Table 3.2. *Continued.* TNM staging for lung cancer

Stage IIB	T2	N1	M0
	T3	N0	M0
Stage IIIA	T1	N2	M0
	T2	N2	M0
	T3	N1	M0
	T3	N2	M0
Stage IIIB	Any T	N3	M0
	T4	Any N	M0
Stage IV	Any T	Any N	M1

* *Note*: the uncommon superficial tumor of any size with its invasive component limited to the bronchial wall, which may extend proximal to the main bronchus, is also classified T1.

† *Note*: Most pleural effusions associated with lung cancer are due to tumor. However, there are a few patients in whom multiple cytopathologic examinations of pleural fluid are negative for tumor. In these cases, fluid is non-bloody and is not an exudate. Such patients may be further evaluated by videothoracoscopy (VATS) and direct pleural biopsies. When these elements and clinical judgment dictate that the effusion is not related to the tumor, the effusion should be excluded as a staging element and the patient should be staged T1, T2, or T3.

Source: Used with permission of the American Joint Committee on Cancer (AJCC), Chicago, Illinois. The original source for this material is the *AJCC Cancer Staging Manual*, Sixth Edition (2002), published by Springer-Verlag, New York, www.springeronline.com.

these indications are as follows: (1) Diagnosis: Is the lesion benign or malignant? (2) Initial staging: What is the extent of disease? (3) Restaging: Is disease present after treatment? CMS was covering these indications under specific G-codes but is now using CPT codes (see Chapter 2: Reimbursement for PET and PET/CT Imaging).

Diagnosis – Fluorodeoxyglucose-Positron Emission Tomography and Evaluation of the Solitary Pulmonary Nodule

A solitary pulmonary nodule (SPN) has been defined as a single intra-parenchymal opacity completely surrounded by lung without any associated atelectasis or lymph node enlargement and with a diameter less than or equal to 3 cm [7,8]. If a lesion is larger than 3 cm, it is termed a mass rather than a nodule. Such masses are almost always malignant.

The solitary pulmonary nodule is a common finding, with an estimated 130,000 nodules identified each year in the United States by plain chest radiograph. Most SPNs are benign entities such as granulomas or hamartomas. But, in patient populations at high risk for developing a primary lung cancer (e.g.

history of smoking, radon or asbestos exposure), and with nodules growing or becoming symptomatic, they are especially worrisome for malignancy. While most malignant SPNs are bronchogenic carcinomas, extrapulmonary metastatic disease accounts for 10–30% of all malignant SPNs.

Twenty to thirty percent of lung cancer patients have an SPN as their initial presentation of disease [9]. Proponents of early detection of lung cancer claim that it offers the best chance for cure [10]. Therefore, accurate and timely assessment of the SPN may be important in successful patient management.

The goal of radiologic evaluation of the SPN is to accurately differentiate benign from malignant lesions. Size, contour, margin, and calcification pattern are some of the morphologic characteristics employed in conventional radiologic analysis. Table 3.3 provides a more detailed list of the radiologic features a lesion may possess that can aid in assessing whether it is benign or malignant. Although the information gained with conventional radiography is invaluable, the vast majority of SPNs are indeterminate by plain film chest radiography and computed tomography [11–13]. In many cases, a tissue diagnosis must be obtained under imaging guidance. In cases where suspicious nodules are technically

Table 3.3. Solitary pulmonary nodule (SPN) imaging characteristics favoring benignancy or malignancy

Findings favoring a benign lesion	Findings favoring a malignant lesion
Conventional imaging with chest radiograph and/or CT	
Size less than 2 cm	Size greater than 3 cm
Stable appearance (especially for >2 years)	Interval change
Smooth margin	Spiculated, irregular, or lobulated margin
Diffuse calcification (lamellated or central calcification is typical for granulomas; "popcorn" calcification is typical for hamartomas)	Stippled or eccentric calcification
Satellite nodules (when seen at the periphery of a dominant smooth nodule this suggests an infectious granuloma)	
If cavitation is present, smooth, thin walls (i.e., 4 mm or less) favor a benign process [12]	If cavitation is present, irregular, thick walls (i.e., greater than 15 mm) favor malignancy [12]
Nodule enhancement <15 Hounsfield Units (HU) [13]	Malignant lesions are relatively hypervascular
Imaging with FDG-PET	
SUV <2.5, or visually less metabolically active than mediastinal blood pool (for nodules >1.0 cm)	SUV >2.5, or visually more metabolically active than mediastinal blood pool (for nodules >1.0 cm)

difficult to biopsy, co-morbidities make biopsy too risky, prior biopsy has been non-diagnostic or prior biopsy was negative because of sampling error and concern remains for a false-negative biopsy in a high-risk patient, FDG-PET can be used to assess the character of a pulmonary lesion without intervention. For this reason, an FDG-PET scan can be thought of as a non-invasive metabolic biopsy. For examples of FDG-PET/CT scans for evaluation of SPN, see Figures 3.1 and 3.2.

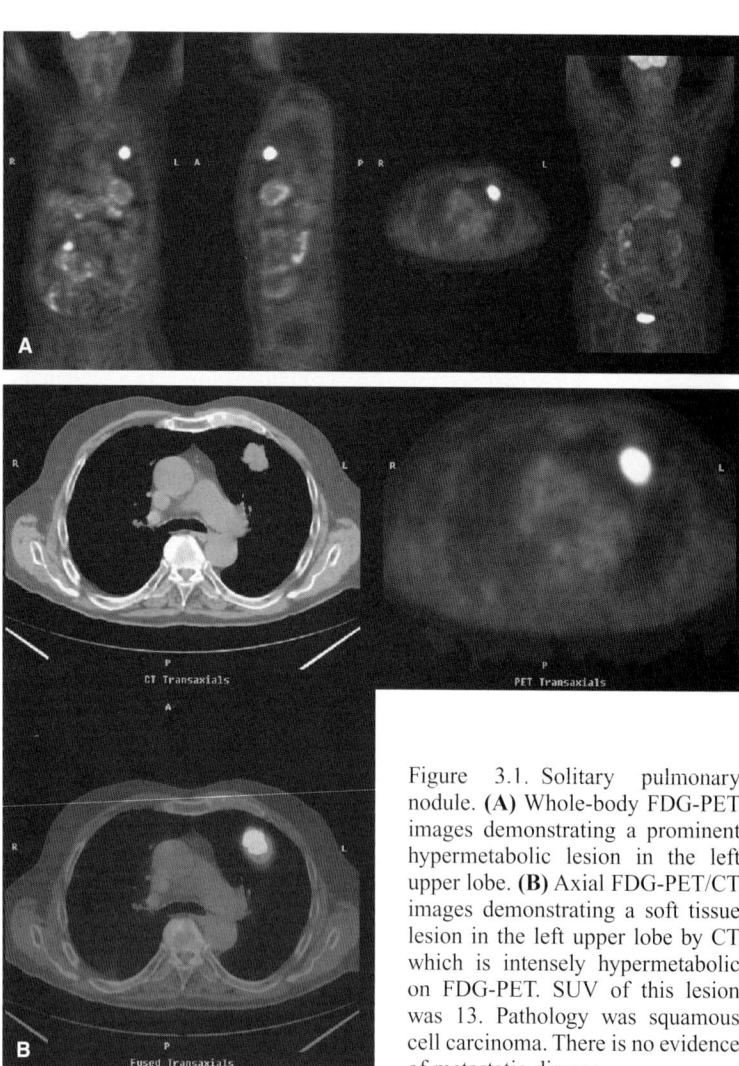

Figure 3.1. Solitary pulmonary nodule. **(A)** Whole-body FDG-PET images demonstrating a prominent hypermetabolic lesion in the left upper lobe. **(B)** Axial FDG-PET/CT images demonstrating a soft tissue lesion in the left upper lobe by CT which is intensely hypermetabolic on FDG-PET. SUV of this lesion was 13. Pathology was squamous cell carcinoma. There is no evidence of metastatic disease.

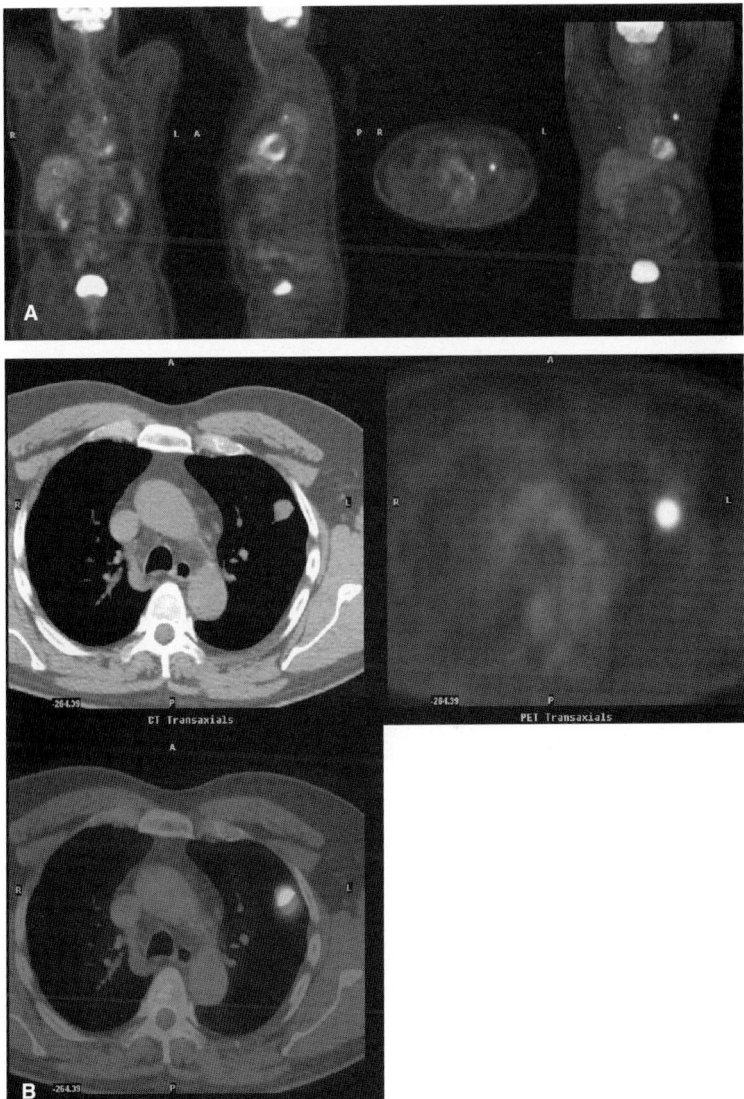

Figure 3.2. Solitary pulmonary nodule with ipsilateral hilar metastasis. **(A)** FDG-PET whole-body scan of another patient with a suspicious left upper lobe nodule which is hypermetabolic (SUV = 6) and highly suspicious for malignancy. A faint focus of increased activity is seen in the left hilar region. **(B)** Axial FDG-PET/CT images through the left upper lobe lesion demonstrate hypermetabolism consistent with malignancy.

Continued.

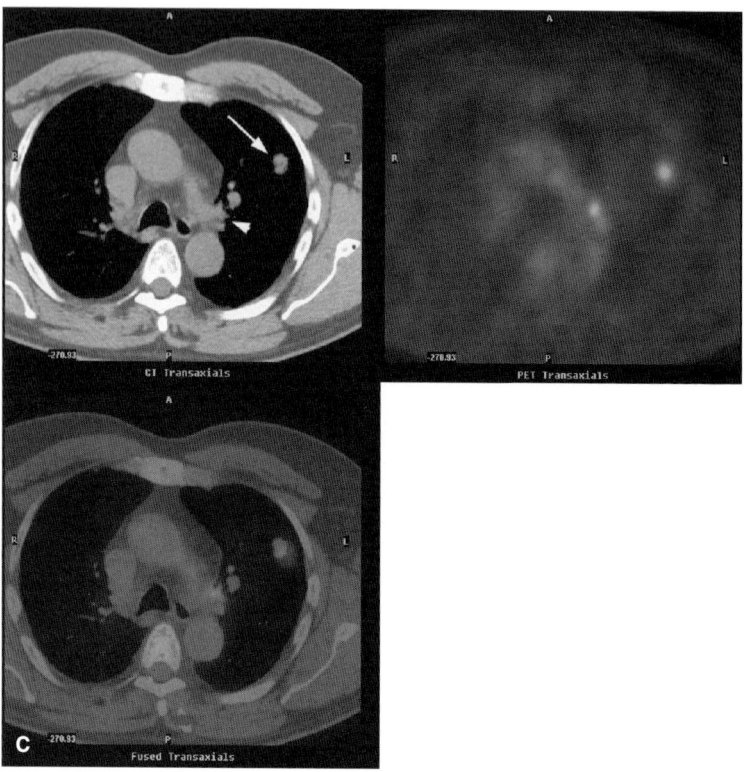

Figure 3.2. *Continued.* **(C)** Additional axial images slightly more inferiorly again demonstrate the hypermetabolic left upper lobe lesion (white arrow). There is increased focal uptake in the left hilar region consistent with metastatic adenopathy (white arrowhead).

Standardized Uptake Value and the Solitary Pulmonary Nodule

Since the 1920s, biochemists have demonstrated that cancers are more meta-bolically active than normal tissue. To support this hypermetabolism, cancer cells have increased uptake and utilization of glucose. As discussed in Chapter 1, the standardized uptake value (SUV) is a semi-quantitative measure of the relative degree of FDG metabolism within a lesion of interest. While there are certain important limitations that will be addressed later in this chapter, in general, an SUV greater than 2.5 is an indicator of malignancy [14–16]. Visually, when the metabolic activity of the lesion is greater than that seen within the mediastinum (often called mediastinal blood pool activity) it is also considered malignant.

The degree of FDG accumulation within a primary lesion has been shown to have prognostic value. The SUV within an SPN inversely correlates with the lesion's doubling time (i.e., the time required for a tumor to double in volume). The higher the SUV, the shorter the doubling time. For lesions that have an SUV less than 10, median patient survival is approximately 24 months. In lesions with an SUV greater than 10, median survival is only about 11 months. If a nodule is greater than 3 cm in diameter and the SUV is greater than 10, median survival is 6 months. Several studies have reported similar results [17].

Accuracy of Fluorodeoxyglucose-Positron Emission Tomography in Lung Cancer Diagnosis

In 2001, the *Journal of the American Medical Association* published a comprehensive meta-analysis of the accuracy of FDG-PET in diagnosing pulmonary nodules and mass lesions. The authors compiled data from the previous 4 years of work, and selected 40 studies for inclusion. Based on their analysis of almost 1500 total focal pulmonary lesions, FDG-PET scanning had a sensitivity of 96.8% and a specificity of 77.8% [18].

Fluorodeoxyglucose-Positron Emission Tomography in Lung Cancer Staging

FDG-PET and FDG-PET/CT are whole-body scans. In patients with biopsy-proven, non-small cell lung cancer, FDG-PET is the most accurate, non-invasive method for staging the entire body with the exception of the brain. (For an in-depth discussion of FDG-PET in evaluating intracranial metastatic disease, see Chapter 13, PET in Neurology.) In one study, investigators took 100 patients with newly diagnosed bronchogenic carcinoma and compared FDG-PET staging with that of chest CT, bone scan, and contrast-enhanced CT or magnetic resonance imaging (MRI) of the brain [19]. Radiologic staging with FDG-PET and conventional imaging using chest CT, bone scintigraphy with ^{99m}Tc methylene diphosphonate (MDP), and brain CT or MRI were compared with pathologic stage. In overall staging, FDG-PET was accurate in 83%, compared to 65% for conventional imaging ($P < 0.005$). Staging of mediastinal lymph nodes was accurate in 85%, compared to 58% with conventional imaging ($P < 0.001$). Nine percent of patients had metastases detected with FDG-PET that were not identified by conventional imaging, and conversely 10% of patients suspected of having metastatic disease by conventional imaging were correctly shown by FDG-PET to be free of metastatic disease. In unresectable (N3) disease the sensitivity and specificity of FDG-PET were 92% and 93%, respectively, compared to sensitivity and specificity of 25% and 98% for CT. FDG-PET was also superior in correctly identifying those patients with metastatic (i.e., M1) disease in 91% versus 80% for conventional imaging.

FDG-PET is superior to bone scintigraphy for detecting osseous metastatic disease from bronchogenic carcinoma, with a sensitivity and specificity of 92% and 99%, respectively, compared to a sensitivity and specificity of 50% and 92%, respectively, with bone scan [19]. More recent research comparing bone scintigraphy using ^{99m}Tc MDP and FDG-PET in retrospective staging of newly diagnosed lung cancer patients has echoed these earlier results and further suggests that bone scintigraphy can be eliminated from the initial work-up since it provides redundant and less accurate information compared to FDG-PET [20]. In practice, bone scintigraphy is likely to remain commonplace in oncologic imaging for the foreseeable future because of its long record of high accuracy as well as its ready availability, and familiarity compared to FDG-PET, especially in communities that may not be able to support PET equipment and personnel.

Once whole-body scanning with FDG-PET has excluded distant metastatic disease, staging of the mediastinum is critical to determine lesion resectability thereby maximizing the chance for cure. Although the gold standard for staging the mediastinum remains mediastinoscopy, FDG-PET offers vital information. In a report published in 2003, researchers retrospectively studied 400 patients with NSCLC. Each patient underwent a CT scan of the chest and upper abdomen as well as an FDG-PET scan 1 month before planned surgery. All suspicious N2 lymph nodes by either chest CT or FDG-PET scan were biopsied. Patients without malignant involvement of mediastinal or distant nodes and without metastasis underwent pulmonary resection and complete thoracic lymphadenectomy. Results demonstrated that FDG-PET had a higher sensitivity (71% vs. 43%, $P < 0.001$), positive predictive value (44% vs. 31%, $P < 0.001$), negative predictive value (91% vs. 84%, $P = 0.006$), and accuracy (76% vs. 68%, $P = 0.037$) than CT scan for N2 lymph nodes. Similarly, FDG-PET had a higher sensitivity (67% vs. 41%, $P < 0.001$), but lower specificity (78% vs. 88%, $P = 0.009$) than CT scan for N1 lymph nodes. FDG-PET led to unnecessary mediastinoscopy in 38 patients (10%). FDG-PET was most commonly falsely negative for nodes located in the subcarinal region and the aortopulmonary window. It accurately upstaged 28 patients (7%) with unsuspected metastasis and accurately downstaged 23 patients (6%) [21]. A meta-analysis conducted in 1999 of 14 FDG-PET studies and 29 CT studies demonstrated an overall diagnostic accuracy of 92% for FDG-PET and 75% for CT in staging the mediastinum [22].

FDG-PET is more accurate than CT alone in staging the mediastinum. A positive finding in the mediastinum on FDG-PET warrants mediastinoscopy with tissue biopsy at that location. Also, the use of FDG-PET in initial staging improves patient selection by eliminating those with unsuspected metastatic or unresectable disease from undergoing futile therapy. A recent meta-analysis concluded that unexpected extrathoracic metastatic disease is seen in as many as 12% of patients undergoing FDG-PET [23]. However, an FDG-PET scan that is positive for distant metastatic disease should be confirmed by undergoing directed biopsy of the probable metastasis in order to avoid excluding a patient from potentially curative therapy. See Figures 3.3, 3.4 and 3.5 for examples of staging FDG-PET/CT scans.

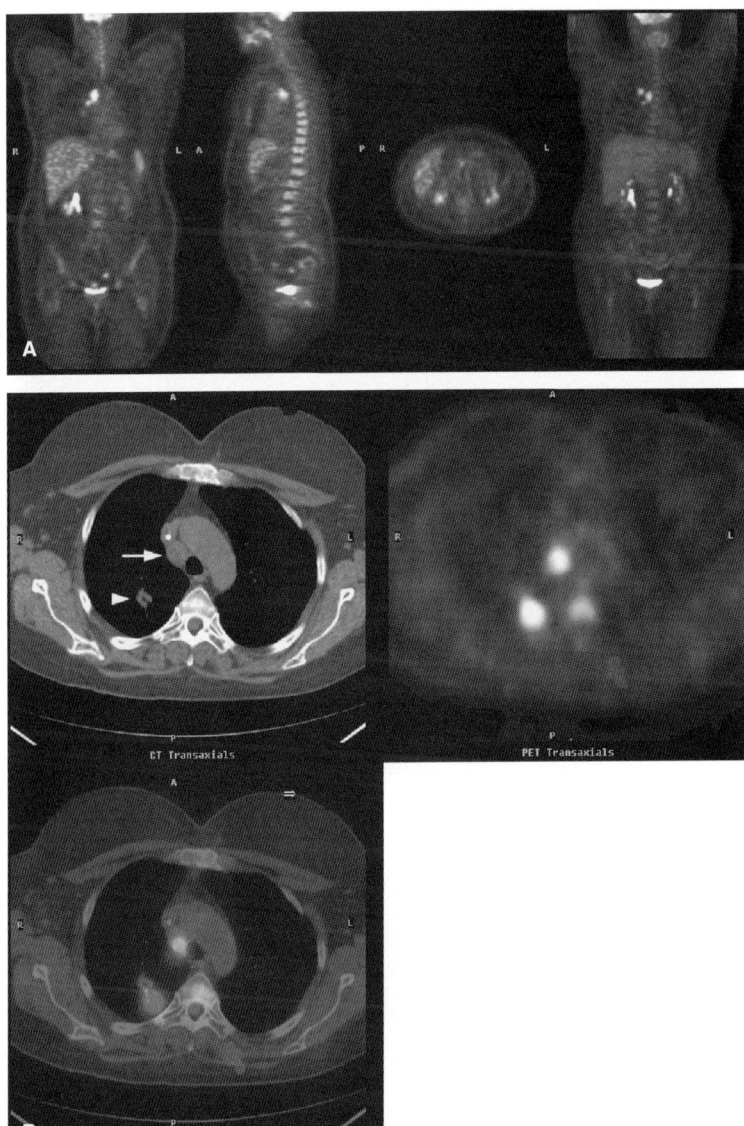

Figure 3.3. Right upper lobe NSCLC with ipsilateral metastatic adenopathy and a benign left adrenal adenoma. **(A)** FDG-PET whole-body scan demonstrating a right hilar malignancy with ipsilateral metastatic adenopathy. No evidence of distant disease is seen. **(B)** Axial FDG-PET/CT image through the right upper lobe lesion (white arrowhead) and the right paratracheal nodal metastasis (white arrow). Also notice the slight image misregistration.

Continued.

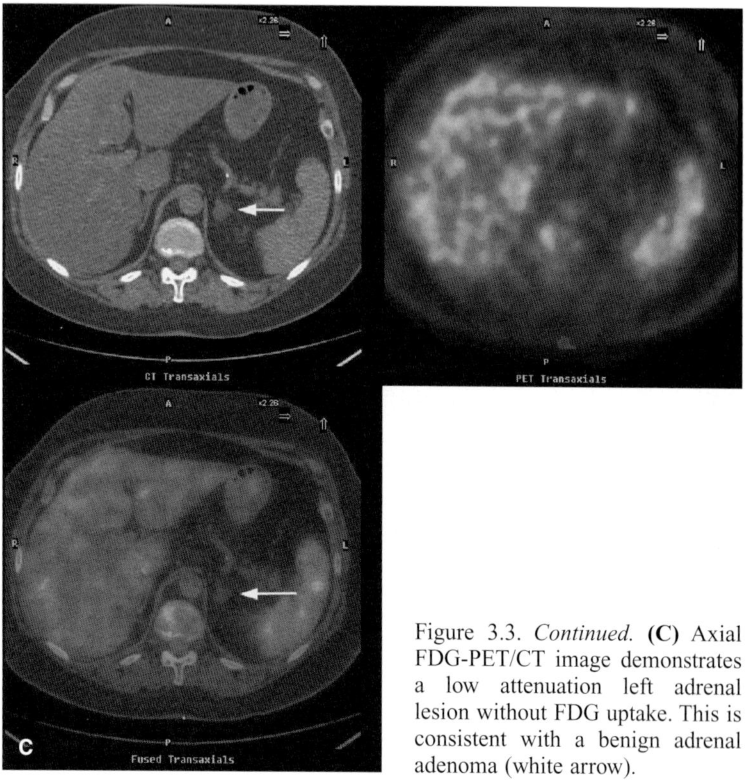

Figure 3.3. *Continued.* **(C)** Axial FDG-PET/CT image demonstrates a low attenuation left adrenal lesion without FDG uptake. This is consistent with a benign adrenal adenoma (white arrow).

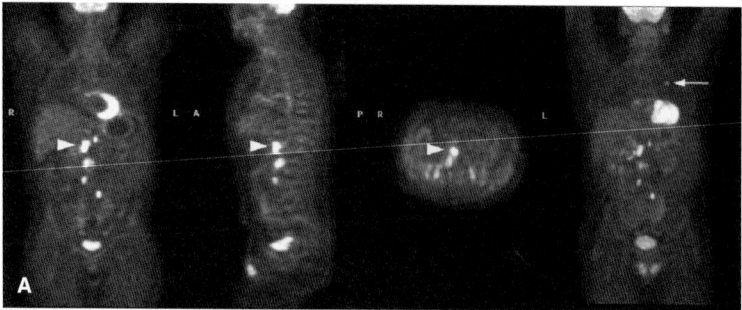

Figure 3.4. Left upper lobe NSCLC with distant metastases. **(A)** FDG-PET whole-body image demonstrating a left upper lobe malignancy (white arrow) with right adrenal metastasis (white arrowhead). Additional metastases are seen in the retroperitoneum.

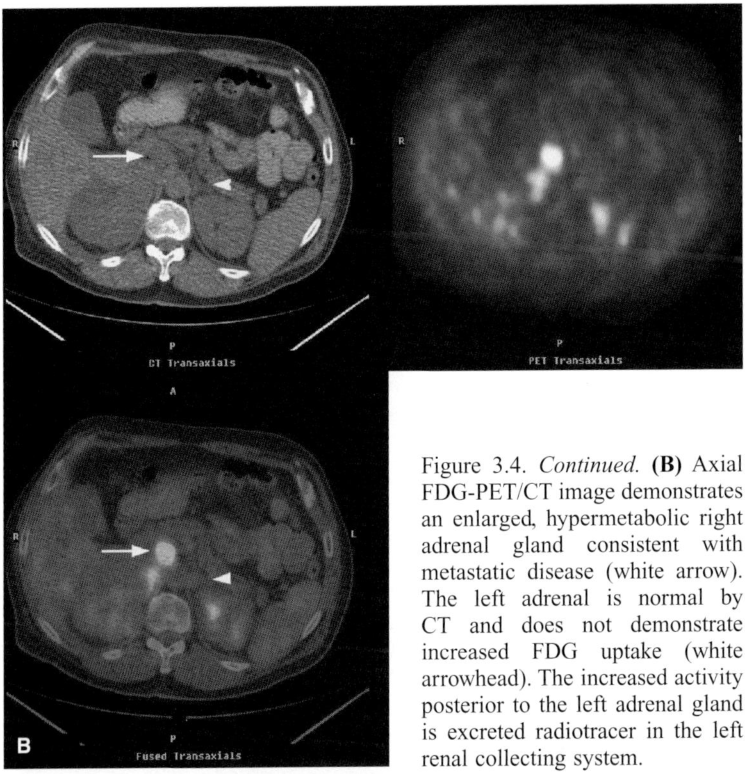

Figure 3.4. *Continued.* (**B**) Axial FDG-PET/CT image demonstrates an enlarged, hypermetabolic right adrenal gland consistent with metastatic disease (white arrow). The left adrenal is normal by CT and does not demonstrate increased FDG uptake (white arrowhead). The increased activity posterior to the left adrenal gland is excreted radiotracer in the left renal collecting system.

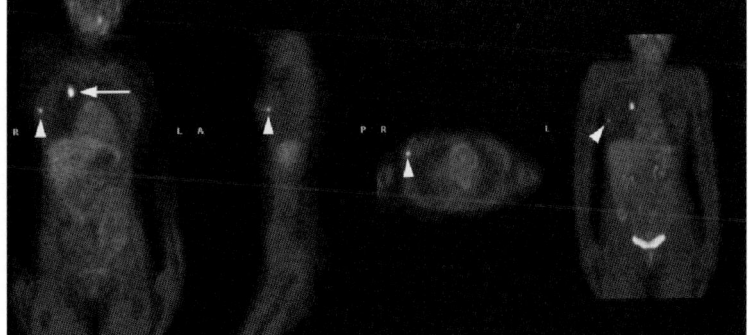

Figure 3.5. Lung cancer staging scan with incidental second primary. FDG-PET whole-body scan of a patient with NSCLC of the right mid lung (white arrow). In this case, an additional hypermetabolic lesion was detected in the lower outer quadrant of the right breast (white arrowhead). Subsequent biopsy confirmed the lesion to be a breast primary.

Fluorodeoxyglucose-Positron Emission Tomography in Lung Cancer Restaging

FDG-PET has an important role in monitoring for recurrence and in evaluating the effects of treatment. Because FDG-PET gauges metabolic activity, treated disease can be evaluated on the basis of its physiology in addition to the morphologic assessment provided by CT. FDG-PET is more accurate than CT in differentiating between post-therapy change and residual or recurrent disease. In one study of 126 patients with stage I–IIIB disease treated with radiation therapy, FDG-PET had a sensitivity and specificity of 100% and 92%, respectively, in detecting active disease. Positive and negative predictive values were 92% and 100%, respectively. By comparison, CT had a sensitivity and specificity of 72% and 95%, respectively, and positive and negative predictive values of 93% and 79%, respectively [24].

FDG-PET scanning following therapy also has prognostic value. The response to therapy can be classified as complete remission, partial remission, no response, or progression of disease. In 2003, MacManus et al. examined 73 patients who underwent radical radiotherapy or chemoradiotherapy followed by FDG-PET at 10 weeks. Each patient had a determination made as to response to therapy based on both CT and FDG-PET, and these responses were then correlated with survival. The response to therapy determined by FDG-PET was found to be superior to CT in predicting survival duration [25]. In another recent study of 56 patients, the change in the maximum SUV (SUV_{max}) within a lesion on FDG-PET scan after neoadjuvant therapy was found to hold a near linear relationship with pathologic response and was a more accurate predictor than was the change in lesion size on CT scan. This study found that when the SUV_{max} decreases by 80% or more there is a high likelihood (with 96% accuracy), that the patient is a complete responder irrespective of cell type, neoadjuvant treatment, or the final absolute SUV_{max} [26]. See Figures 3.6 and 3.7 for examples of restaging studies (see also Plate 3.6B, in the color insert).

Figure 3.6. Recurrence adjacent to radiation therapy field. **(A)** FDG-PET whole-body images from a patient with a history of metastatic lung cancer. The patient is status post radiation therapy to the left upper lobe. Multiple metastatic foci are seen in distant sites including the axial and proximal appendicular skeleton. **(B)** Axial images demonstrate intense FDG uptake at the anterior margin of the radiation therapy field consistent with tumor recurrence (white arrow). Notice the less intense diffuse uptake in the remainder of the treated lung consistent with inflammatory post-therapy changes (white arrowhead). (See part B only in the color insert.)

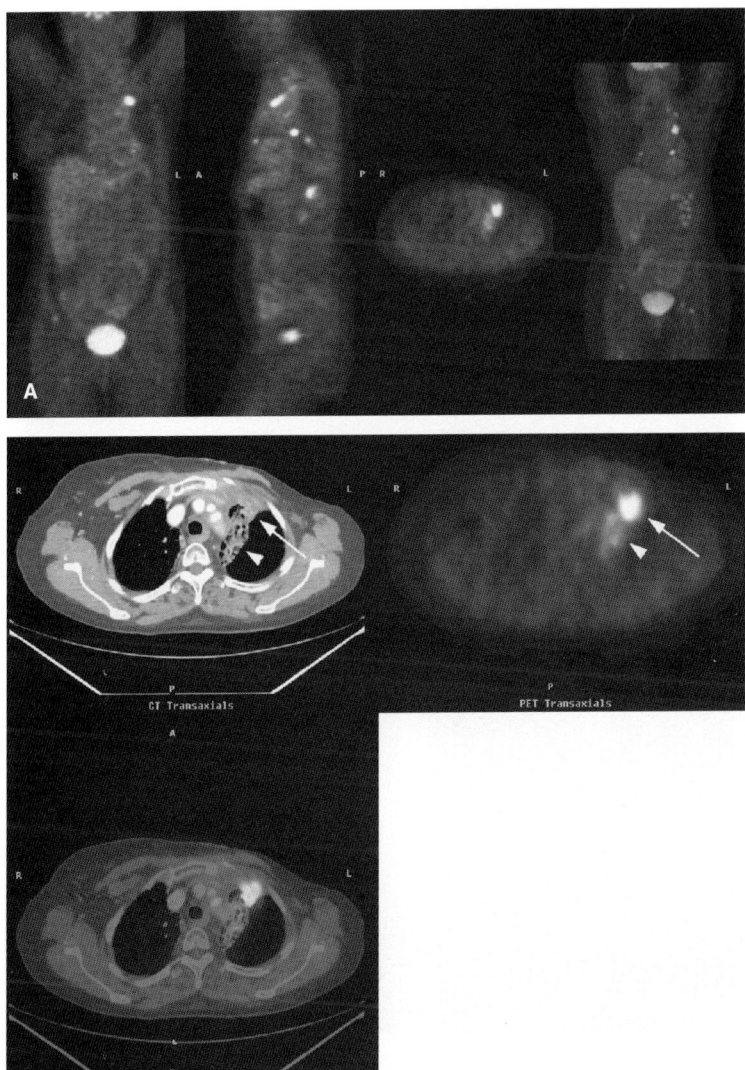

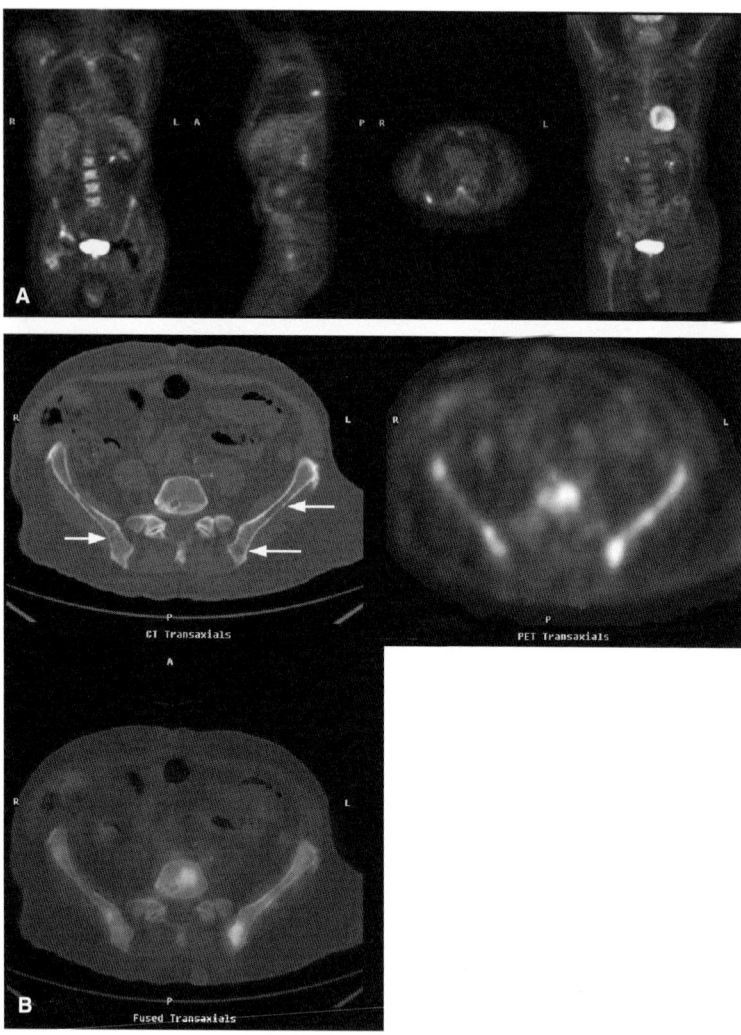

Figure 3.7. Skeletal metastatic disease in the setting of reactive marrow. **(A)** FDG-PET whole-body images demonstrate moderate diffuse FDG uptake in the bone marrow. This can be seen in patients undergoing chemotherapy, as a response to anemia, or following colony-stimulating factors. In this patient, however, there are foci of increased activity best seen in a right rib and within the pelvis consistent with skeletal metastatic disease. Also notice the photopenic left hip prosthesis on the coronal image. **(B)** Axial images demonstrate several lytic lesions in the bony pelvis (white arrows) with corresponding hypermetabolism. Notice the diffuse, less intense FDG uptake elsewhere in bones likely represents physiologic marrow recruitment changes.

Fluorodeoxyglucose-Positron Emission Tomography/Computed Tomography in Lung Cancer

With the increasing prevalence of hybrid FDG-PET/CT systems, imaging specialists can offer clinicians more accurate information than can be obtained by either PET or CT alone. In 2003, Lardinois et al. prospectively looked at 50 patients with proven or suspected NSCLC and compared the accuracy of PET/CT with that of PET alone, CT alone, and with visually correlated PET and CT scans obtained separately (i.e., not obtained simultaneously with an integrated PET/CT system). Imaging stage was then compared with pathologic stage. Their results, published in the *New England Journal of Medicine*, demonstrated that integrated PET/CT provided additional information in 20 of 49 patients (41%), beyond that provided by conventional visual correlation of PET and CT. Furthermore, integrated PET/CT had better diagnostic accuracy than the other imaging methods. Tumor staging was significantly more accurate with integrated PET/CT than with CT alone ($P = 0.001$), PET alone ($P < 0.001$), or visual correlation of PET and CT ($P = 0.013$); node staging was also significantly more accurate with integrated PET/CT than with PET alone ($P = 0.013$). In evaluating for metastasis, integrated PET/CT increased the diagnostic certainty in two of eight patients [27].

Specifically, integrated PET/CT was helpful in clarifying the extent of the primary tumor (i.e., T stage), particularly in determining whether there was chest wall invasion. PET/CT was also helpful in clarifying mediastinal invasion and pinpointing nodal involvement within the mediastinum, hila, and supraclavicular regions because precise node localization is not possible with PET alone. In this study, software fusion of PET with CT (as opposed to integrated PET/CT) was no better than PET alone. FDG-PET/CT is poised to be the single most powerful radiologic examination in evaluating the lung cancer patient. New advances in hybrid scanner technology, PET scanner resolution, and intravenous contrast protocols for the CT portion of the study should further improve diagnostic accuracy and patient care.

Not only does FDG-PET/CT improve diagnostic accuracy, it also improves the ability of radiation oncologists to more accurately target diseased tissue in their planning. In those patients who are to undergo preoperative radiation therapy or palliation radiotherapy, FDG-PET/CT allows for much more precise delineation of tumor target volumes with the use of the fused (i.e., registered) PET and CT images. Use of PET/CT fusion images has the potential to reduce irradiation of non-diseased, non-target organs, to reduce the incidence of geographic misses, and to improve the radiation oncologist's understanding of tumor metabolism and biology [28].

Some institutions do not use intravenous or oral contrast for the CT scans performed in the evaluation of suspected or documented lung cancer. For these patients, the CT scan performed with the PET/CT can be obtained as a diagnostic CT scan if ordered by the referring clinician. Furthermore, several centers are now performing contrast-enhanced CT scans when ordered with the PET/CT scan, and these can be obtained sequentially on the PET/CT scanner.

Limitations

Lesion size is an important factor when a patient is undergoing FDG-PET evaluation for lung cancer. The threshold for lesion detection for most FDG-PET scanners currently in use is between 6 and 8 mm. As a rule, for lesions that are greater than 1 cm, an SUV greater than or equal to 2.5 or a visual intensity greater than that within the mediastinal blood pool are accepted criteria for malignancy. Any activity seen within a nodule less than 1 cm is suspicious. The smaller the lesion, the greater is the likelihood of a false-negative scan because of volume averaging with surrounding normal tissue. Other important causes of a false-negative FDG-PET scan are well-differentiated cancers such as bronchioloalveolar carcinoma (BAC), slow growing neuroendocrine tumors such as bronchial carcinoid (Figure 3.8), and mucinous neoplasms.

As discussed throughout this book and throughout the FDG-PET literature, not all that is hypermetabolic is cancer. Infectious and inflammatory processes aggregate metabolically active macrophages which also have increased glucose demand and can cause false-positive results on an FDG-PET scan. Some examples of false positives include cases of granulomatous infection, fungal infection, sarcoidosis, radiation-induced lung injury, pneumonitis/pneumonia, talc pleurodesis, and recent surgery/trauma. For an example of a patient who has had talc pleurodesis, see Figure 3.9. To offset some of these limitations, several

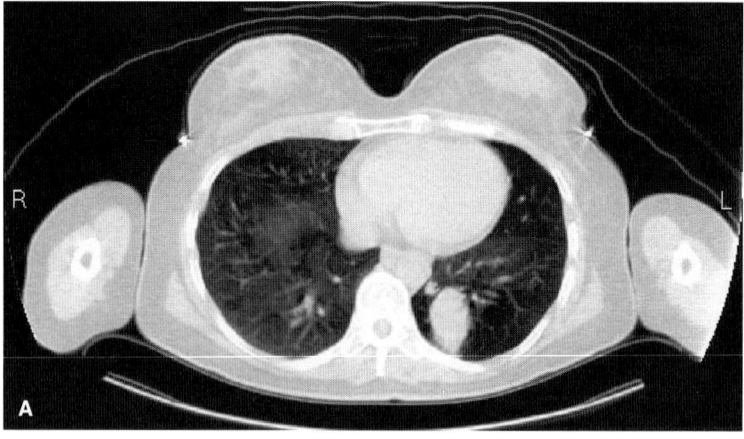

Figure 3.8. Bronchial carcinoid (**A** and **B**). FDG-PET/CT images demonstrate a mass measuring 3.5 × 2.7 cm in the left lower lobe. The mass has an SUV of 2.1 and is similar in intensity to the activity of the mediastinal blood pool. This degree of activity, although non-specific, suggests a benign inflammatory etiology. The patient subsequently underwent resection and surgical pathology revealed well-differentiated neuroendocrine carcinoma with endobronchial extension. (Case courtesy of Ronald B. Workman, Sr., MD.)

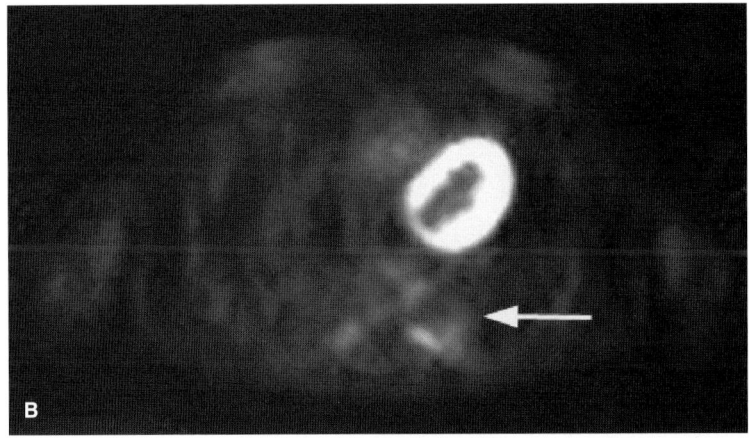

Figure 3.8. *Continued.*

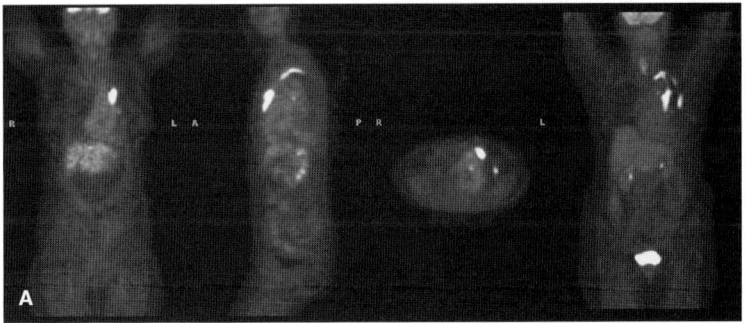

Figure 3.9. Intense FDG uptake associated with talc pleurodesis. **(A)** Whole-body FDG-PET images demonstrate intense focal uptake along the margin of the left upper lung. By PET alone, and without important history, this would be consistent with malignancy. Incidentally noted is diffuse activity in the right lobe of the thyroid (in the maximum intensity projection image on the right). This was stable compared to the patient's prior scans and was felt to represent chronic thyroiditis. **(B)** Axial FDG-PET/CT images reveal high attenuation pleural thickening with corresponding intense hypermetabolism along the anterior and anterolateral surface of the left lung (white arrows). This is consistent with chronic pleural inflammation following talc pleurodesis. Surgical clips from left upper lobectomy are also seen in the left hilum. The low level uptake in the left hilum likely represents reaction to chronic pleural inflammation.

Continued.

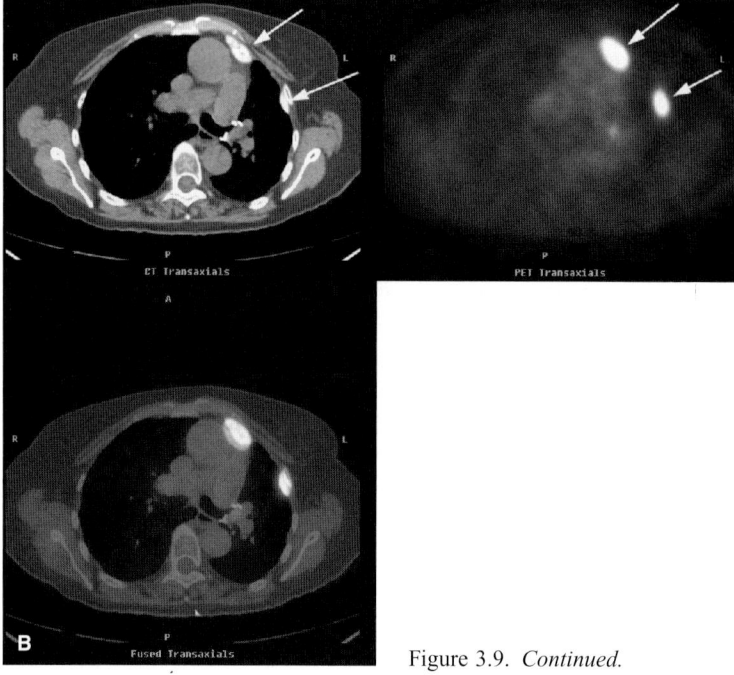

Figure 3.9. *Continued.*

researchers have conducted studies based on the observation that as a rule, malignancies demonstrate a continually increasing uptake of FDG whereas inflammatory lesions do not [29,30]. So-called dual-time point FDG-PET scanning at 1 and 2 hours after FDG administration can be performed with excellent sensitivity and specificity in the detection of malignant pulmonary nodules [31]. The advantage of dual-time point imaging over that of first imaging at 2 hours after FDG administration has not been demonstrated.

References

1. What are the key statistics for lung cancer? American Cancer Society (www.cancer.org); 2005 Accessed March 2005.
2. Mountain CF. Revisions in the International System for Staging Lung Cancer. Chest 1997;111(6):1710–1717.
3. Suzuki K, Nagai K, Yoshida J, et al. Prognostic factors in clinical stage I non-small cell lung cancer. Ann Thorac Surg 1999;67(4):927–932.
4. Non-small cell lung cancer cellular classification. National Cancer Institute (www.cancer.gov); 2005 Accessed April 2005.

5. Greene FL, Page DL, Fleming ID, et al. AJCC Cancer Staging Manual, sixth edition. New York: Springer-Verlag; 2002.

6. Medicare Coverage Homepage. Centers for Medicare and Medicaid Services (www.cms.hhs.gov/coverage/); 2005 Accessed April 2005.

7. Leef JL, 3rd, Klein JS. The solitary pulmonary nodule. Radiol Clin North Am 2002; 40(1):123–143, ix.

8. Midthun DE, Swensen SJ, Jett JR. Approach to the solitary pulmonary nodule. Mayo Clin Proc 1993;68(4):378–385.

9. Viggiano RW, Swensen SJ, Rosenow EC, 3rd. Evaluation and management of solitary and multiple pulmonary nodules. Clin Chest Med 1992;13(1):83–95.

10. Henschke CI, Yankelevitz DF, Kostis WJ. CT screening for lung cancer. Semin Ultrasound CT MR 2003;24(1):23–32.

11. Gurney JW, Lyddon DM, McKay JA. Determining the likelihood of malignancy in solitary pulmonary nodules with Bayesian analysis. Part II. Application. Radiology 1993;186(2):415–422.

12. Woodring JH, Fried AM, Chuang VP. Solitary cavities of the lung: diagnostic implications of cavity wall thickness. AJR Am J Roentgenol 1980;135(6):1269–1271.

13. Swensen SJ, Viggiano RW, Midthun DE, et al. Lung nodule enhancement at CT: multicenter study. Radiology 2000;214(1):73–80.

14. Lowe VJ, Hoffman JM, DeLong DM, Patz EF, Coleman RE. Semiquantitative and visual analysis of FDG-PET images in pulmonary abnormalities. J Nucl Med 1994; 35(11):1771–1776.

15. Lowe VJ, Fletcher JW, Gobar L, et al. Prospective investigation of positron emission tomography in lung nodules. J Clin Oncol 1998;16(3):1075–1084.

16. Goldsmith SJ, Kostakoglu L. Role of nuclear medicine in the evaluation of the solitary pulmonary nodule. Semin Ultrasound CT MR 2000;21(2):129–138.

17. Ahuja V, Coleman RE, Herndon J, Patz EF, Jr. The prognostic significance of fluorodeoxyglucose positron emission tomography imaging for patients with nonsmall cell lung carcinoma. Cancer 1998;83(5):918–924.

18. Gould MK, Maclean CC, Kuschner WG, Rydzak CE, Owens DK. Accuracy of positron emission tomography for diagnosis of pulmonary nodules and mass lesions: a meta-analysis. JAMA 2001;285(7):914–924.

19. Marom EM, McAdams HP, Erasmus JJ, et al. Staging non-small cell lung cancer with whole-body PET. Radiology 1999;212(3):803–809.

20. Cheran SK, Herndon JE, 2nd, Patz EF, Jr. Comparison of whole-body FDG-PET to bone scan for detection of bone metastases in patients with a new diagnosis of lung cancer. Lung Cancer 2004;44(3):317–325.

21. Cerfolio RJ, Ojha B, Bryant AS, Bass CS, Bartalucci AA, Mountz JM. The role of FDG-PET scan in staging patients with nonsmall cell carcinoma. Ann Thorac Surg 2003;76(3):861–866.

22. Dwamena BA, Sonnad SS, Angobaldo JO, Wahl RL. Metastases from non-small cell lung cancer: mediastinal staging in the 1990s – meta-analytic comparison of PET and CT. Radiology 1999;213(2):530–536.

23. Hellwig D, Ukena D, Paulsen F, Bamberg M, Kirsch CM. [Meta-analysis of the efficacy of positron emission tomography with F-18-fluorodeoxyglucose in lung tumors.

Basis for discussion of the German Consensus Conference on PET in Oncology 2000]. Pneumologie 2001;55(8):367–377.

24. Bury T, Corhay JL, Duysinx B, et al. Value of FDG-PET in detecting residual or recurrent nonsmall cell lung cancer. Eur Respir J 1999;14(6):1376–1380.

25. MacManus MP, Hicks RJ, Matthews JP, et al. Positron emission tomography is superior to computed tomography scanning for response-assessment after radical radiotherapy or chemoradiotherapy in patients with non-small-cell lung cancer. J Clin Oncol 2003;21(7):1285–1292.

26. Cerfolio RJ, Bryant AS, Winokur TS, Ohja B, Bartolucci AA. Repeat FDG-PET after neoadjuvant therapy is a predictor of pathologic response in patients with non-small cell lung cancer. Ann Thorac Surg 2004;78(6):1903–1909; discussion 1909.

27. Lardinois D, Weder W, Hany TF, et al. Staging of non-small-cell lung cancer with integrated positron-emission tomography and computed tomography. N Engl J Med 2003;348(25):2500–2507.

28. Ciernik IF, Dizendorf E, Baumert BG, et al. Radiation treatment planning with an integrated positron emission and computer tomography (PET/CT): a feasibility study. Int J Radiat Oncol Biol Phys 2003;57(3):853–863.

29. Gupta N, Gill H, Graeber G, Bishop H, Hurst J, Stephens T. Dynamic positron emission tomography with F-18 fluorodeoxyglucose imaging in differentiation of benign from malignant lung/mediastinal lesions. Chest 1998;114(4):1105–1111.

30. Zhuang H, Pourdehnad M, Lambright ES, et al. Dual time point 18F-FDG PET imaging for differentiating malignant from inflammatory processes. J Nucl Med 2001; 42(9):1412–1417.

31. Matthies A, Hickeson M, Cuchiara A, Alavi A. Dual time point 18F-FDG PET for the evaluation of pulmonary nodules. J Nucl Med 2002;43(7):871–875.

4. PET in Lymphoma

Ronald B. Workman, Jr. and R. Edward Coleman

Epidemiology

Lymphoid neoplasms are broadly divided into Hodgkin's disease (HD) and non-Hodgkin's lymphoma (NHL). NHL is the fifth most common cancer in the United States, and the American Cancer Society estimated that 56,390 people would be diagnosed in 2005. HD is less common than NHL, and an estimated 7350 cases were diagnosed in 2005 [1].

While the causes behind most cases of lymphoma are unknown, there are recognized associations and risk factors. Slightly more men than women are afflicted, and incidence is higher in the white population. B-cell lymphomas are more common in adults, and T-cell lymphomas are more common in children. Lymphoma can be associated with Epstein–Barr virus (EBV), human T-cell leukemia/lymphoma virus (HTLV-1), and human immunodeficiency virus (HIV) infection. Lifestyle factors such as tobacco and alcohol use do not appear to elevate risk; however, environmental exposures to radiation and certain chemicals such as benzene have been associated with higher incidence. Those who are immunocompromised as a result of infection, immunosuppressive medication, or genetic immunodeficiency also have an increased risk of developing lymphoma.

Although outcomes vary by cell type, grade, and stage at diagnosis, overall NHL survival rates are 59% at 5 years and 42% at 10 years. HD survival rates are 85% at 5 years and 77% at 10 years. Approximately 21,000 people in the United States died of lymphoma in 2005 [1]. In recent decades, mortality has improved significantly, in part due to imaging advances which have aided clinicians in accurately staging and planning treatment.

Histopathologic Classification and Therapy

Lymphoma, especially NHL, is a very heterogeneous group of tumors. The World Health Organization (WHO) classification of lymphoid neoplasms formulated in 1999 provides a solid foundation to establish an internationally recognized nomenclature for these diseases. See Table 4.1 for details [2].

Unlike most cancers where both surgical and medical treatments are utilized, lymphoma is a non-surgical disease. The mainstays of treatment include chemotherapy, radiation therapy, immunotherapy, and bone marrow or peripheral blood stem cell transplant. For HD, current standard chemotherapy usually follows the ABVD (Adriamycin (doxorubicin), bleomycin, vinblastine, and dacarbazine) protocol. NHL treatment relies mainly on the CHOP (cyclophosphamide,

Table 4.1. WHO classification of lymphoid neoplasms

Non-Hodgkin's lymphoma
B-cell neoplasms
Precursor B-cell neoplasms
Precursor B-lymphoblastic leukemia/lymphoma (precursor B-cell acute
   lymphoblastic leukemia)

Mature (peripheral) B-cell neoplasms
B-cell chronic lymphocytic leukemia/small lymphocytic lymphoma
B-cell prolymphocytic leukemia
Lymphoplasmacytic lymphoma
Splenic marginal zone B-cell lymphoma (with/without villous lymphocytes)
Hairy cell leukemia
Plasma cell myeloma/plasmacytoma
Extranodal marginal zone B-cell lymphoma of mucosa-associated lymphoid
   tissue (MALT) type
Nodal marginal zone B-cell lymphoma (with or without monocytoid B-cells)
Follicular lymphoma
Mantle-cell lymphoma
Diffuse large B-cell lymphoma
Burkitt's lymphoma/Burkitt's cell leukemia

T-cell and NK-cell neoplasms
Precursor T-cell neoplasm
Precursor T-lymphoblastic lymphoma/leukemia (precursor T-cell acute
   lymphoblastic leukemia)

Mature (peripheral) T-cell neoplasms
T-cell prolymphocytic leukemia
T-cell granular lymphocytic leukemia
Aggressive natural killer (NK)-cell leukemia
Adult T-cell lymphoma/leukemia (HTLV-1 positive)
Extranodal NK/T-cell lymphoma, nasal type
Enteropathy-type T-cell lymphoma
Hepatosplenic gamma-delta T-cell lymphoma
Subcutaneous panniculitis-like T-cell lymphoma
Mycosis fungoides/Sézary syndrome
Anaplastic large cell lymphoma, T/null cell, primary cutaneous type
Peripheral T-cell lymphoma, not otherwise characterized
Angioimmunoblastic T-cell lymphoma
Anaplastic large cell lymphoma, T/null cell, primary systemic type

Hodgkin's lymphoma (Hodgkin's disease)
Nodular lymphocyte-predominant Hodgkin's lymphoma
Nodular sclerosing Hodgkin's lymphoma (most common type)
Classic, lymphocyte-rich Hodgkin's lymphoma
Mixed cellularity Hodgkin's lymphoma
Lymphocyte-depleted Hodgkin's lymphoma

Source: from Jaffe et al. [2], by permission of the *American Journal of Clinical Pathology*.

hydroxydaunorubicin, Oncovin (vincristine), and prednisone) protocol. Therapy advances including new chemotherapy drugs, drug combinations, and innovative protocols have improved treatment efficacy. Furthermore, molecular biology and therapeutic nuclear medicine innovations have resulted in the addition of immunotherapeutic and radioimmunotherapeutic agents to the clinical armamentarium to better combat more indolent and resistant variants of the disease (e.g. Rituxan, Bexxar, and Zevalin).

Therapy regimen is based on the cell type, grade, and stage of disease. The American Joint Committee on Cancer (AJCC) has adopted the Ann Arbor classification staging scheme for lymphoma based on the number of nodal regions involved, their extent, and the presence of extralymphatic involvement. This applies to lymphoid neoplasms, both NHL and HD. See Table 4.2 for lymphoma staging as outlined by the AJCC [3].

Table 4.2. Staging of lymphoma

Stage I	Involvement of a single lymph node region (I); or localized involvement of a single extralymphatic* organ or site in the absence of any lymph node involvement (IE) (rare in Hodgkin's lymphoma)
Stage II	Involvement of two or more lymph node regions on the same side of the diaphragm (II); or localized involvement of a single extralymphatic organ or site in association with regional lymph node involvement with or without involvement of other lymph node regions on the same side of the diaphragm (IIE). The number of regions involved may be indicated by a subscript, as in $II_{\#}$
Stage III	Involvement of lymph node regions on both sides of the diaphragm (III), which also may be accompanied by extralymphatic extension in association with adjacent lymph node involvement (IIIE) or by involvement of the spleen (IIIS) or both (IIIE, S)
Stage IV	Diffuse or disseminated involvement of one or more extralymphatic organs, with or without associated lymph node involvement; or isolated extralymphatic organ involvement in the absence of adjacent regional lymph node involvement, but in conjunction with disease in distant site(s). Any involvement of the liver or bone marrow, or nodular involvement of the lung(s). The location of stage IV disease is identified further by specifying the site with an abbreviation†

* For the purposes of staging, lymph nodes, Waldeyer's ring, and spleen are considered *nodal* or *lymphatic* sites. *Extranodal* or *extralymphatic* sites include the bone marrow, the gastrointestinal tract, skin, bone, central nervous system, lungs, gonads, ocular adnexae, liver, kidneys, and uterus, etc.
† Spleen (S), pulmonary (L), bone marrow (M), hepatic (H), pericardium (Pcard), pleura (P), Waldeyer's ring (W), osseous (O), gastrointestinal (GI), skin (D), soft tissue (Softis), thyroid (Thy)
Source: Used with permission of the American Joint Committee on Cancer (AJCC), Chicago, Illinois. The original source for this material is the *AJCC Cancer Staging Manual*, Sixth Edition (2002), published by Springer-Verlag, New York, www.springeronline.com.

In HD, the most important distinction to be made is between low/interme-
diate stage disease (stages I and II) and advanced stage disease (stages III and
IV). HD is usually more limited at diagnosis, confined to a few contiguous lymph
node regions, without initial evidence of extralymphatic involvement. NHL, on
the other hand, is usually more disseminated at diagnosis, involving multiple
nodal regions frequently with extralymphatic involvement. NHL is divided into
low, intermediate, and high grade. Low-grade NHL is characterized by slow,
steady disease progression and is considered non-curable. High-grade lymphoma
is more aggressive, but responds more favorably to therapy, with long-term
remission or cure common.

Fluorodeoxyglucose-Positron Emission Tomography versus Conventional Imaging in Lymphoma

Whole-body imaging using CT has been the cornerstone of staging and
restaging lymphoma patients. While CT provides excellent anatomic detail and
can be used to measure response based on lymph node size criteria, it does not
provide information regarding the functional status of tumor masses. Normal-
sized lymph nodes can contain tumor, and enlarged lymph nodes can be benign.
In monitoring treatment response, the viability of a treated lymph node con-
glomeration or tumor mass cannot be adequately characterized by CT alone.
In such a case, a residual soft tissue mass on CT can represent fibrosis consistent with treated inactive disease, or it can represent persistent viable
tumor.

Nuclear medicine imaging allows physicians to better assess the functional
status of lymphoma within the body. Scanning with gallium-67 citrate (gallium)
is one such technique, but it is limited by low resolution and lack of specificity,
particularly in the abdomen. FDG-PET has become routine in evaluating patients
with lymphoma, and gallium scintigraphy is largely being replaced by PET at
imaging centers with readily available PET capability. Prior to FDG-PET, whole-
body gallium scanning was the primary nuclear medicine technique to assess for
residual active disease. Although less sensitive, gallium scintigraphy remains an
option in evaluating patients with lymphoma at institutions which do not have
access to PET.

FDG-PET has many advantages over gallium scintigraphy. An FDG-PET
scan is more sensitive in assessing for viable tumor in both nodal and extranodal sites, with sensitivities ranging from 72% to 100% as opposed to 63–83%
for gallium [4–6]. Gallium SPECT is less sensitive than FDG-PET when disease
is small or involves extranodal sites such as the skeleton or the spleen. From a
practical standpoint, FDG-PET scanning can be done in 1 day instead of the
2–7 days required for gallium imaging. Radiation dose is also significantly less
for FDG-PET – roughly one fourth – compared to gallium studies [7]. For
an example of a false-negative gallium scan demonstrated by FDG-PET, see
Figure 4.1.

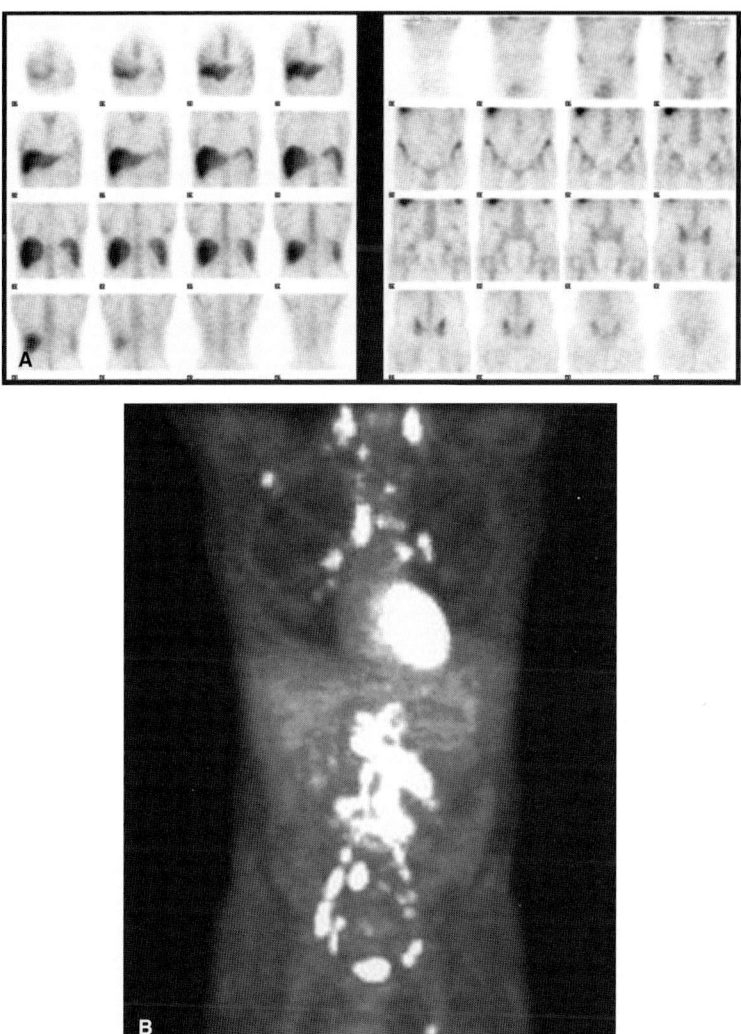

Figure 4.1. Coronal images from a gallium scan demonstrate normal radiotracer distribution in this patient with HD **(A)**. FDG-PET maximum intensity projection (MIP) image from the same patient reveals widespread lymphoma above and below the diaphragm **(B)**. (Courtesy of Barry A. Siegel, MD.)

Diagnosis and Staging

The accuracy of FDG-PET in initial staging of lymphoma is well established in the literature. PET is rarely used for diagnosis of lymphoma because suspicious lesions usually proceed directly to diagnostic biopsy. Initial staging of biopsy proven disease, response to therapy, and restaging are the common indications.

In a recent review, Friedberg and Chengazi summarized data from a variety of studies on the sensitivity of FDG-PET in detecting lymphoma based on histopathology according to the WHO classification of lymphoid neoplasms. One of the major studies reviewed was a retrospective evaluation of FDG-PET scans in 172 patients from the University of Pennsylvania [8]. They reported that FDG-PET has excellent accuracy (greater than 90%) in detecting disease in cases of diffuse large B-cell NHL, classical HD, follicular NHL, and mantle cell NHL. FDG-PET was less reliable (50–90%) in evaluating marginal zone/mucosa-associated lymphoma tissue (MALT), small lymphocytic NHL, and peripheral T-cell lymphoma [9]. Data on other subtypes are limited.

CT is readily accessible, familiar to most clinicians, and has an extensive proven history as an effective modality in the staging of lymphoma. With CT scanning, radiologists can precisely measure and localize tumor masses – something that cannot be done consistently and reliably with PET. FDG-PET does not replace CT, but is a powerful complementary technique. In 2001, Reske and Kotzerke compiled data from 11 studies including over 500 patients with lymphoma and determined that FDG-PET demonstrated a 10% increased sensitivity compared to CT alone [10]. Another recent study in the journal *Cancer* compared CT and PET in 81 patients with HD. In a patient-to-patient comparison of PET and CT, both modalities were positive in 24 of 25 cases (96%). However, in a lesion-to-lesion analysis for determination of initial stage, PET

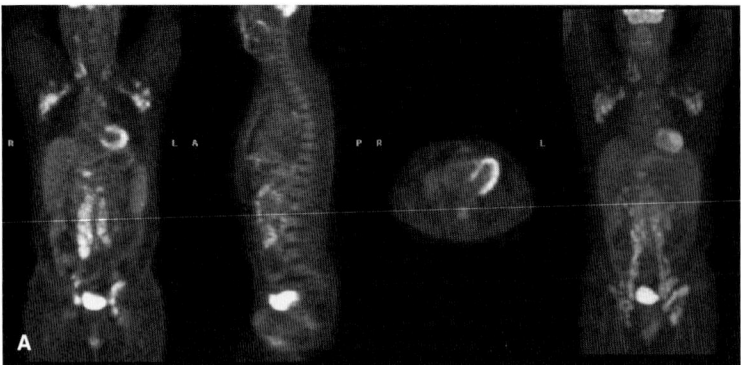

Figure 4.2. FDG-PET/CT whole-body images **(A)** demonstrate widespread hypermetabolic lymphadenopathy within virtually all lymph node chains in this patient with stage IV, grade I NHL. The spleen is also enlarged with slightly increased hypermetabolism diffusely, suspicious for lymphomatous involvement.

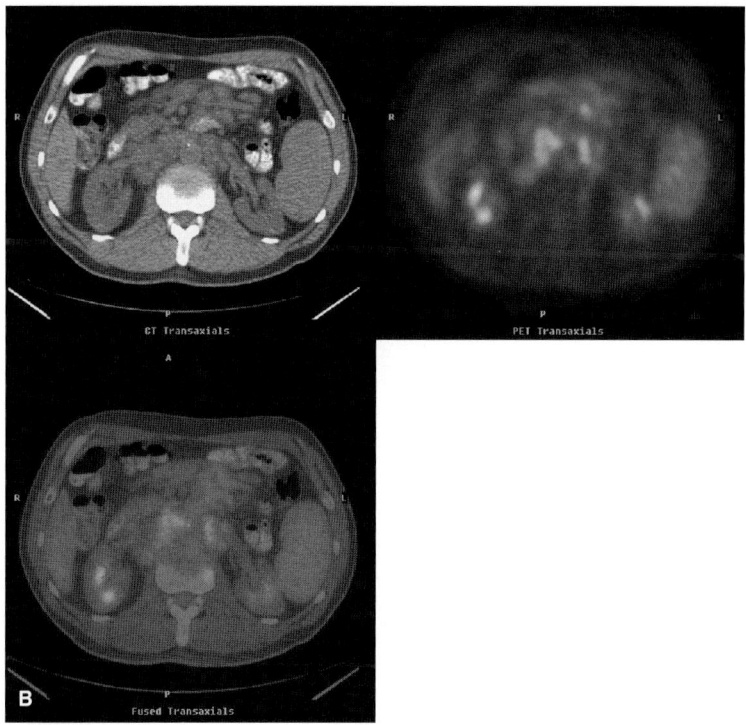

Figure 4.2. *Continued.* PET-CT images **(B)** through the level of the kidneys demonstrate hypermetabolic retroperitoneal adenopathy.

demonstrated 96% accuracy versus 56% for conventional imaging with CT [11]. For an example of widespread lymphoma, see Figure 4.2.

Work is ongoing to develop comprehensive PET/CT protocols, and FDG-PET/CT is likely to gain acceptance as a replacement to separate diagnostic CT and FDG-PET scans in many lymphoma indications. In one recent study, researchers looked at the incremental benefit of FDG-PET/CT compared to FDG-PET alone. Seventy-three patients were evaluated, and results showed an overall accuracy of 93% with PET/CT compared to 84% with PET. There was 10% discordance between PET/CT and PET, with PET/CT correctly upstaging 2 patients and downstaging 5 [12]. Image findings were verified by clinical follow-up, additional imaging, and histology. For an example of the added benefit of CT, see Figure 4.3 (and also Plate 4.3B in the color insert).

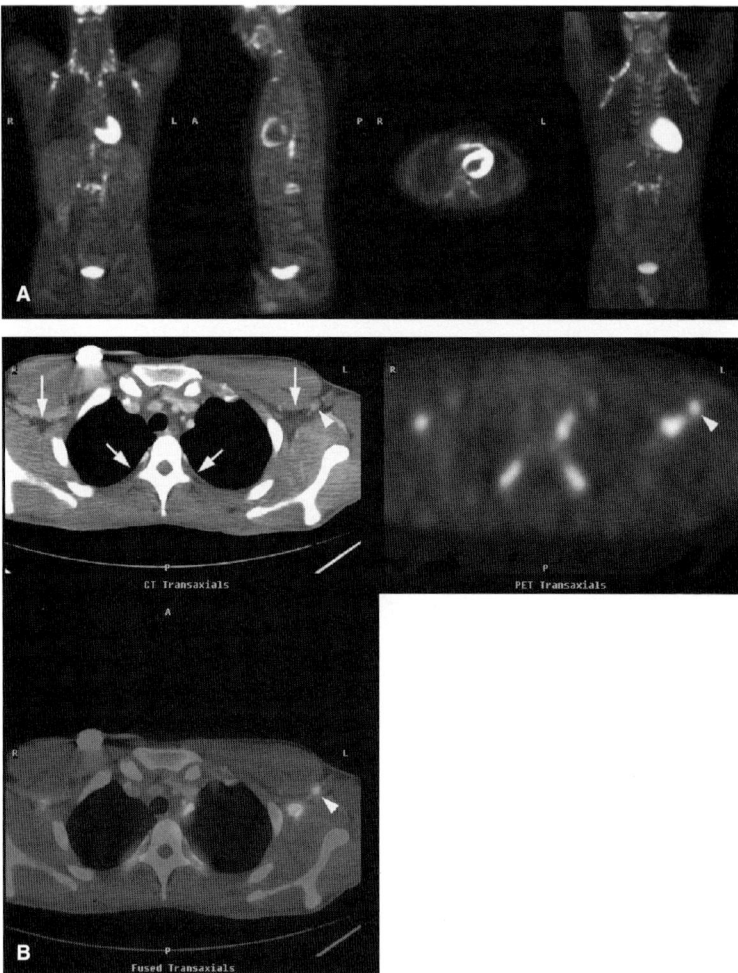

Figure 4.3. FDG-PET/CT images (**A** and **B**) of an adolescent with nodular scle-rosing HD demonstrate extensive FDG uptake within brown fat (white arrows), as well as hypermetabolism within a left axillary node (white arrowhead). This is an example of the benefit of CT. Image (**C**) demonstrates destruction of the L2 vertebra with surrounding abnormal hypermetabolic soft tissue in the same patient which is consistent with lymphomatous involvement. This was later con-firmed by biopsy. (See part B only in the color insert.)

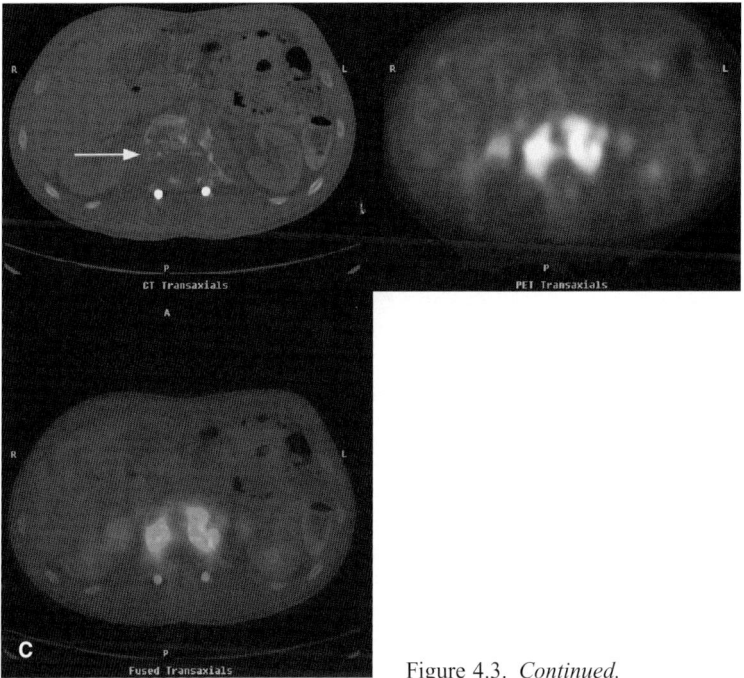

Figure 4.3. *Continued.*

Restaging and Monitoring Therapy Response

FDG-PET/CT provides powerful information on tumor characteristics – both morphologic and functional. As mentioned above, patients who have undergone therapy often have residual tissue at sites of previously active disease. The viability of this residual tissue cannot be assessed by CT alone. In such cases, FDG-PET complements CT by determining whether treated tissue is active disease or inactive fibrosis/scar. A recent large meta-analysis of 723 patients from 15 studies examined the accuracy of FDG-PET in differentiating viable lymphoma from non-viable scar tissue following chemotherapy. The sensitivity of FDG-PET for detection of active disease was 71–100%, and the specificity was 69–100%. CT demonstrated specificity and positive predictive value of 4–31% and 19–60%, respectively. FDG-PET had a high negative predictive value of 80–100%, and the 1-year progression-free survival in those patients was 86–100%. Conversely, those with residual FDG-avid disease had a much worse prognosis, with 1-year progression-free survival of only 0–40% [13]. FDG-PET/CT can be used to guide biopsy for confirmation of imaging findings in cases where residual tissue is suspicious for active lymphoma. For several examples of staging and restaging, see Figures 4.4–4.6 (and also Plate 4.4B in the color insert).

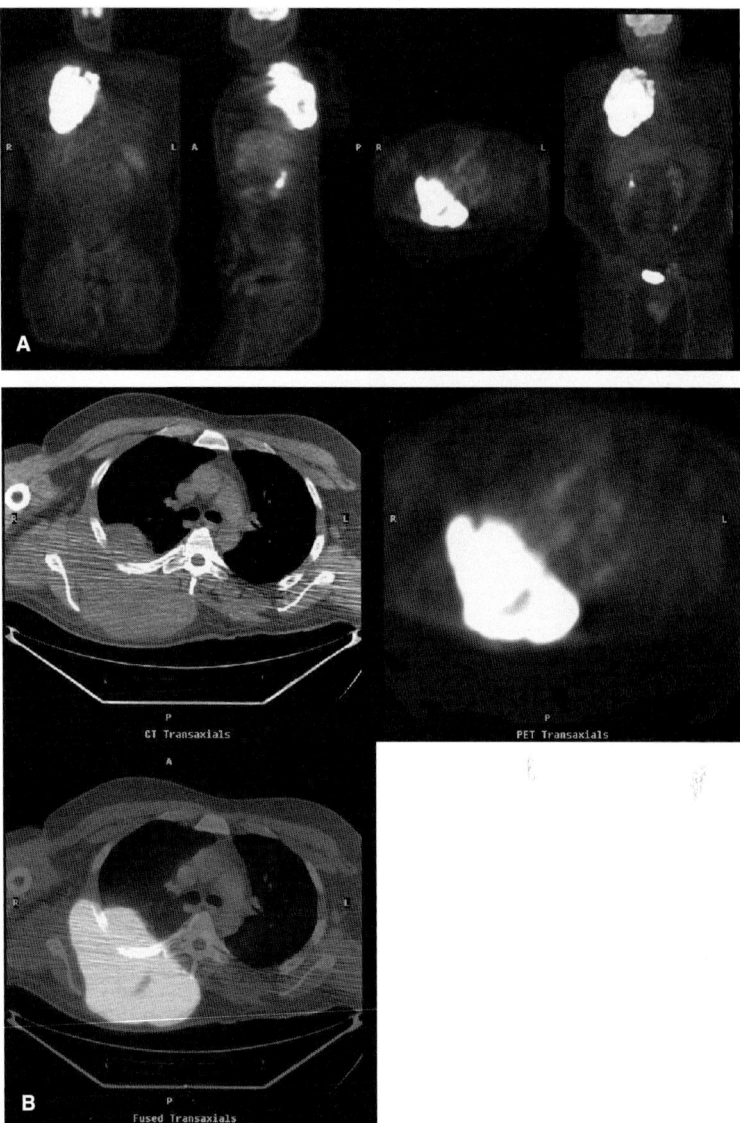

Figure 4.4. FDG-PET/CT images (**A** and **B**) of a patient who has a large hyper-metabolic mass in the right posterior thoracic wall with partial destruction of the rib at that location. There is central decreased FDG uptake within the mass consistent with necrosis. Biopsy was positive for B-cell lymphoma.

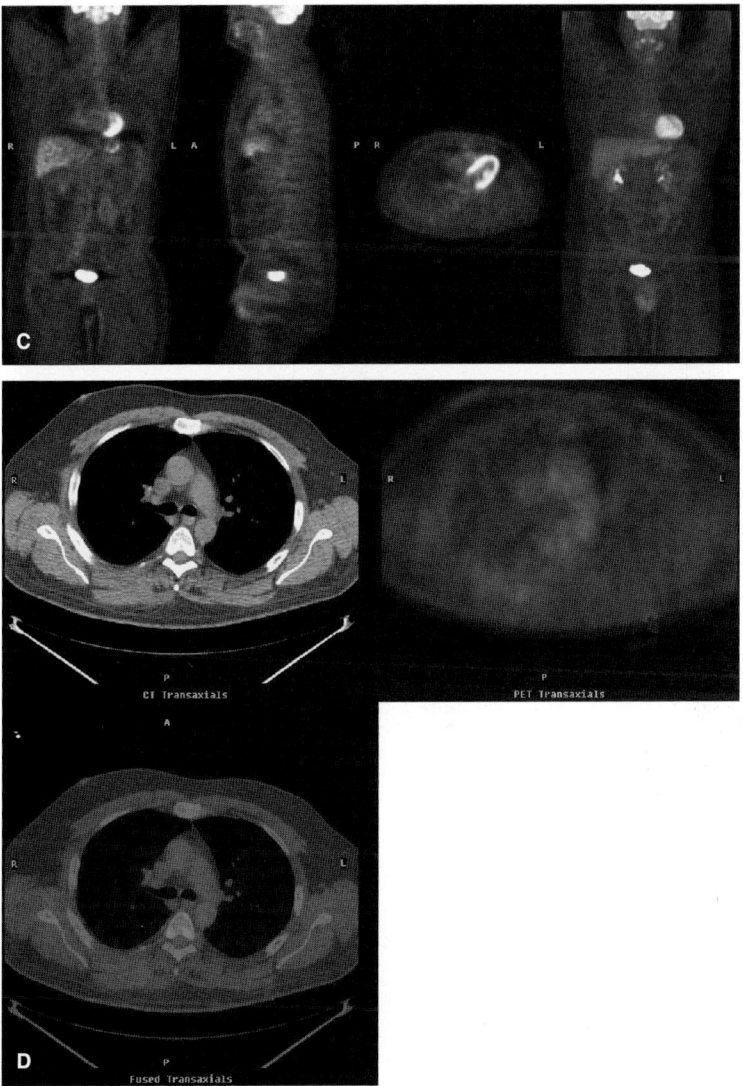

Figure 4.4. *Continued.* Three months following six cycles of R-CHOP chemotherapy, there was marked interval improvement as seen in images **(C)** and **(D)** with no evidence of disease. Also note the normal variability in myocardial uptake on the pre- and post-therapy whole-body images. (See part B only in the color insert.)

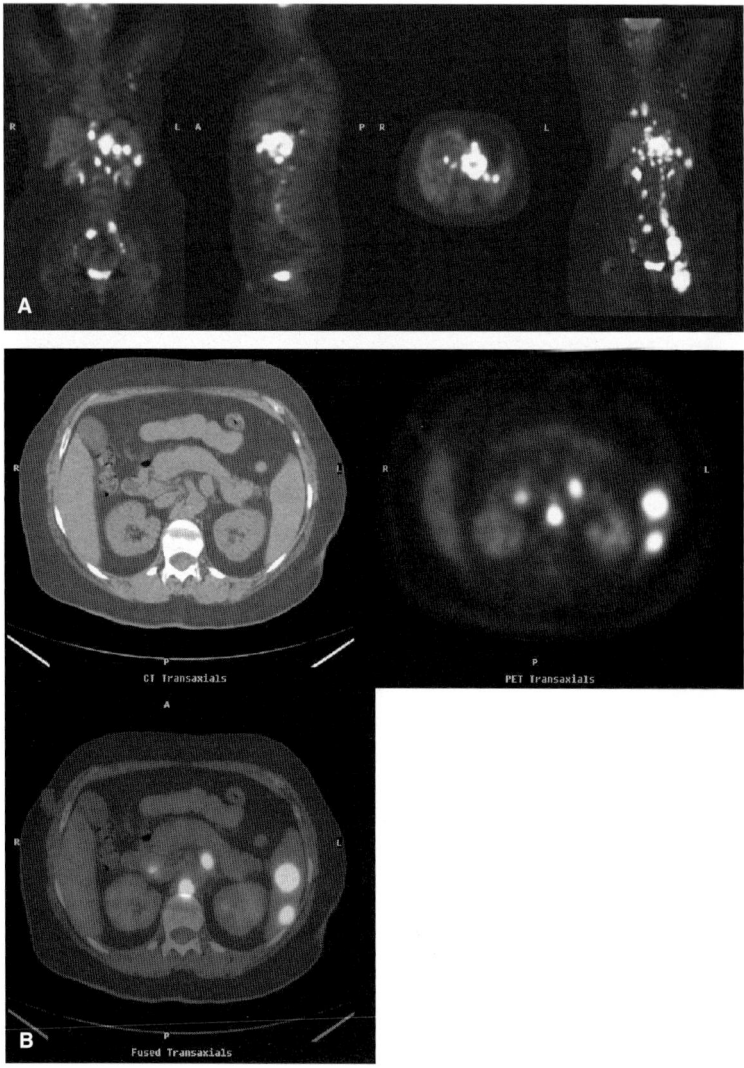

Figure 4.5. Initial staging FDG-PET/CT scans for large cell lymphoma (A and B) demonstrate diffuse bulky hypermetabolic lymphadenopathy above and below the diaphragm. Additional extranodal focal disease is seen within the spleen and within the spine. Post-therapy scan (C) 5 months later demonstrates interval resolution. Note the diffuse moderate increased activity within the bone marrow which is frequently seen in patients who have recently received or are currently receiving chemotherapy. Hypermetabolic marrow recruitment is also seen in response to anemia and in patients receiving colony-stimulating factors.

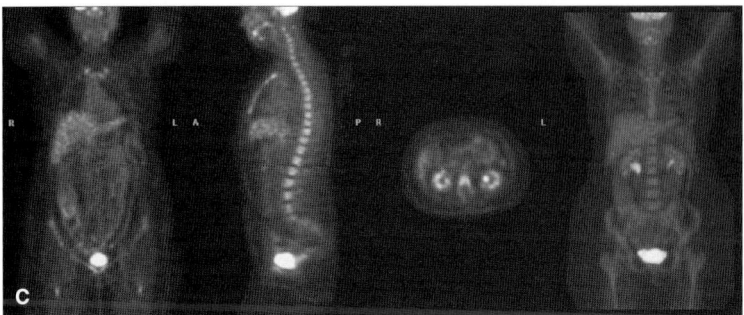

Figure 4.5. *Continued.*

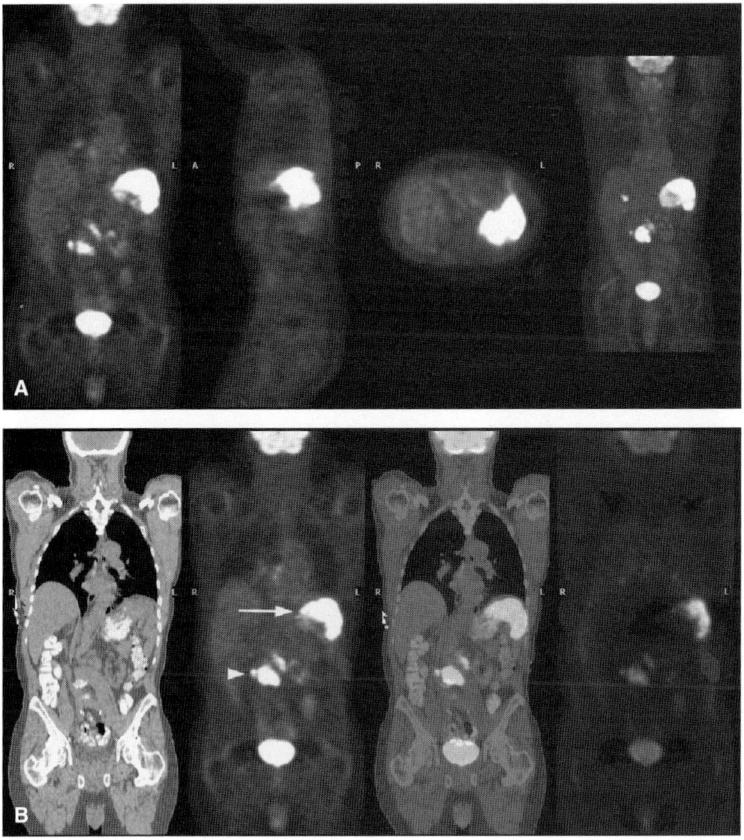

Figure 4.6. Staging **(A** and **B)** and restaging **(C)** FDG-PET/CT scans of a patient with large cell NHL. This patient had extensive involvement of the spleen (white arrow) as well as bulky lymphadenopathy in the retroperitoneum (white arrowhead). Following therapy, the previously seen abnormalities have resolved. Also, note the variable myocardial activity.

Continued.

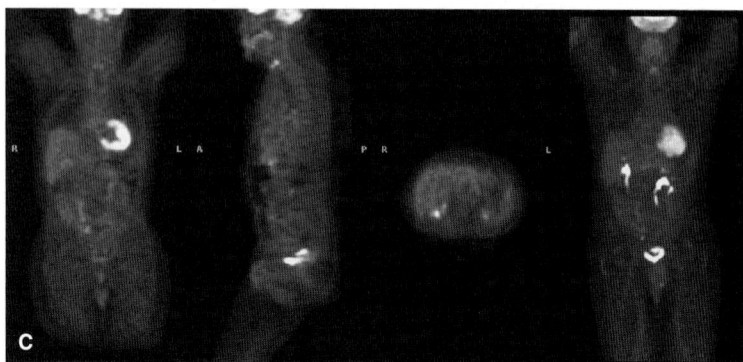

Figure 4.6. *Continued.*

The prognostic value of FDG-PET has also been demonstrated early in the course of therapy. Several studies have shown that FDG-PET obtained after only a few cycles is a strong predictor of subsequent outcome. In one such study, researchers concluded that FDG-PET scan after one cycle of chemotherapy is predictive of 18-month outcome in patients with aggressive NHL and HD [14]. Early FDG-PET scanning in these cases can help identify non-responders, thus allowing early treatment modification (Figure 4.7).

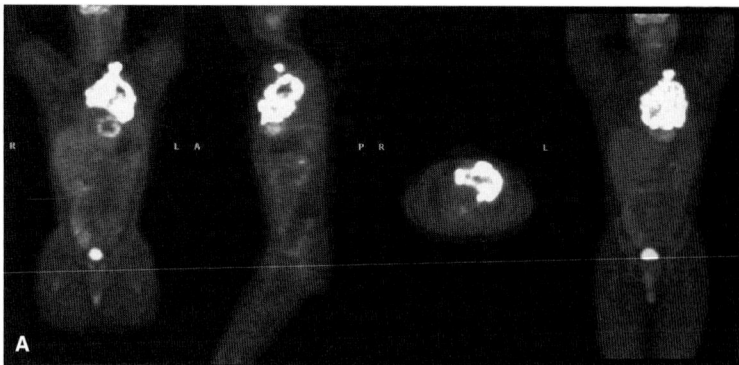

Figure 4.7. This is a patient with B-cell lymphoma arising in the anterior mediastinum. The mass seen on initial staging FDG-PET/CT is markedly hypermetabolic and demonstrates central hypometabolism consistent with necrosis (**A** and **B**). Restaging scans (**C** and **D**), following two cycles of R-CHOP, demonstrate significant improvement; however, there is persistent activity within the treated tumor mass (white arrow).

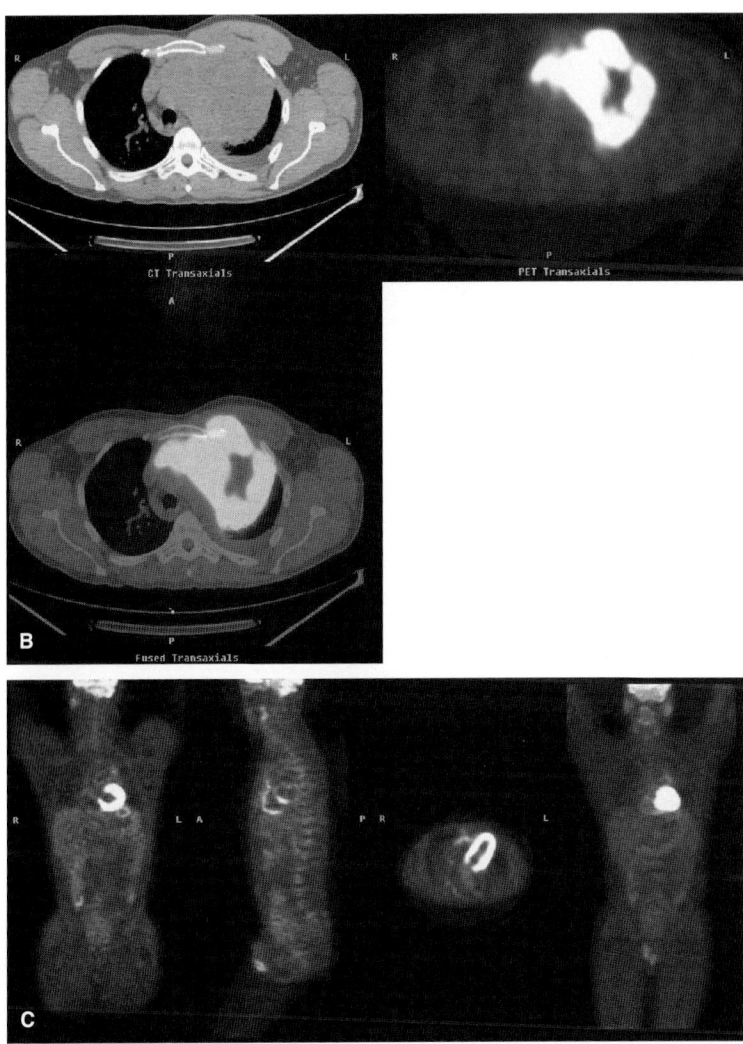

Figure 4.7. *Continued.*

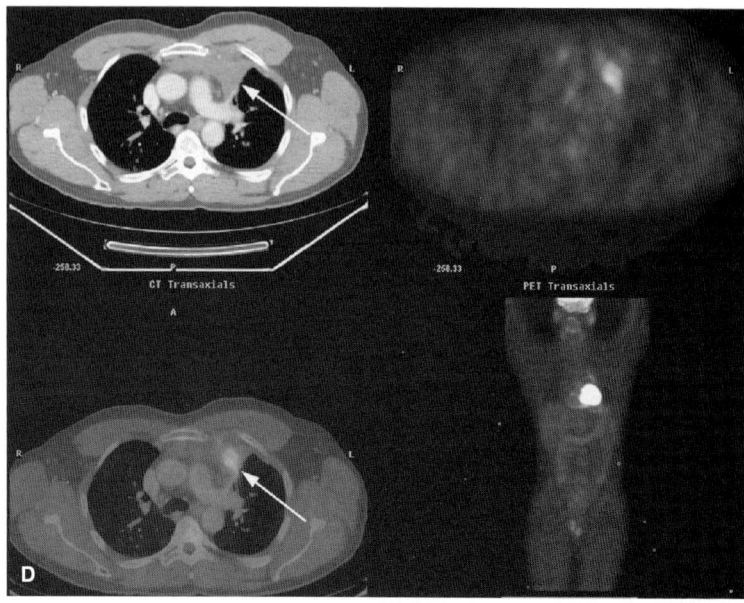

Figure 4.7. *Continued.*

Limitations

Although highly accurate, FDG-PET in lymphoma does have several limitations. As with other malignancies, FDG-PET is unable to detect microscopic and small macroscopic disease. FDG-PET may also fail to identify indolent, low-grade lymphomas as well as missing marrow involvement in patients with a low tumor cell fraction in the marrow [15]. Although some studies have demonstrated that FDG-PET is equivalent to or slightly superior to bone marrow biopsy, others have indicated that it is unreliable in the detection of bone marrow involvement regardless of lymphoma subtype [8]. It is our opinion that FDG-PET does not replace bone marrow biopsy.

Potential causes for a false-positive FDG-PET study in lymphoma include brown fat activity, reactive marrow due to chemotherapy or colony-stimulating factors, and thymic hyperplasia following chemotherapy (Figure 4.8). Infectious, inflammatory, and post-surgical conditions can also mimic malignancy on FDG-PET (Figure 4.9). While all of these entities can be confused with active disease, the experienced radiologist and nuclear medicine physician are aware of such pitfalls. Also, the anatomic correlation afforded by PET/CT has resulted in improved specificity in many such cases.

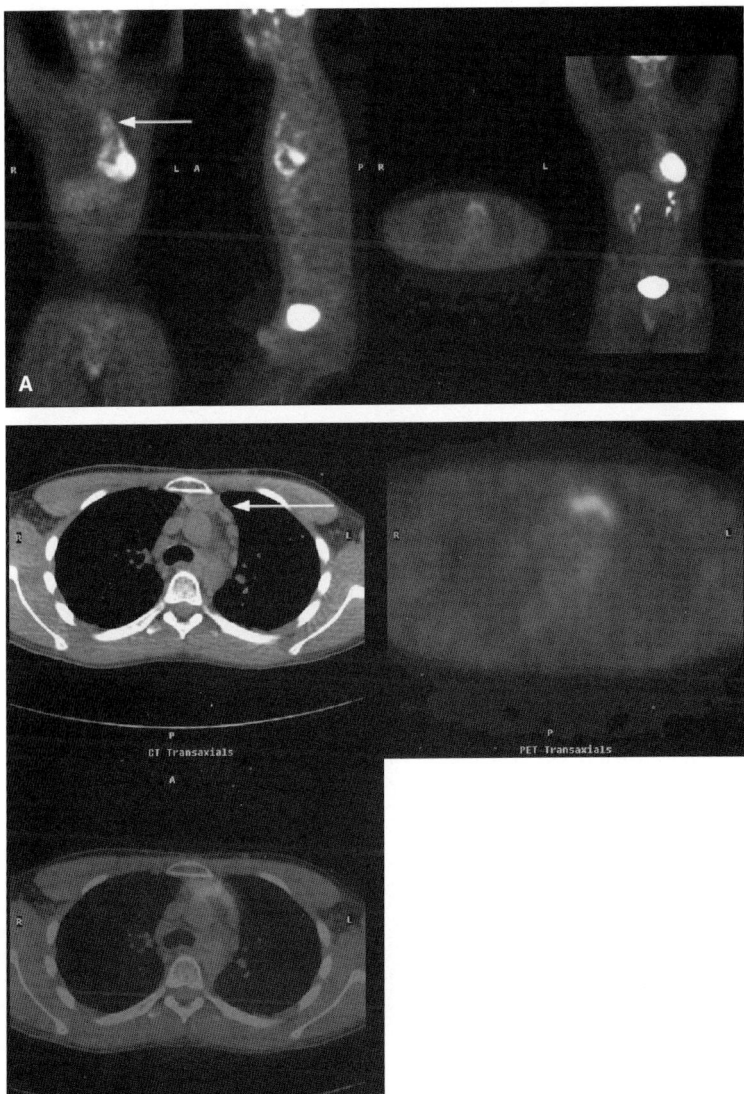

Figure 4.8. FDG-PET whole-body **(A)** and PET-CT images **(B)** from a patient with HD following completion of chemotherapy. There is physiologic distribution of FDG. Note the increased activity within the anterior mediastinum corresponding to the thymus gland (white arrow). Thymic hyperplasia in this setting, also known as thymic rebound, can be seen after cessation of chemotherapy typically in younger patients.

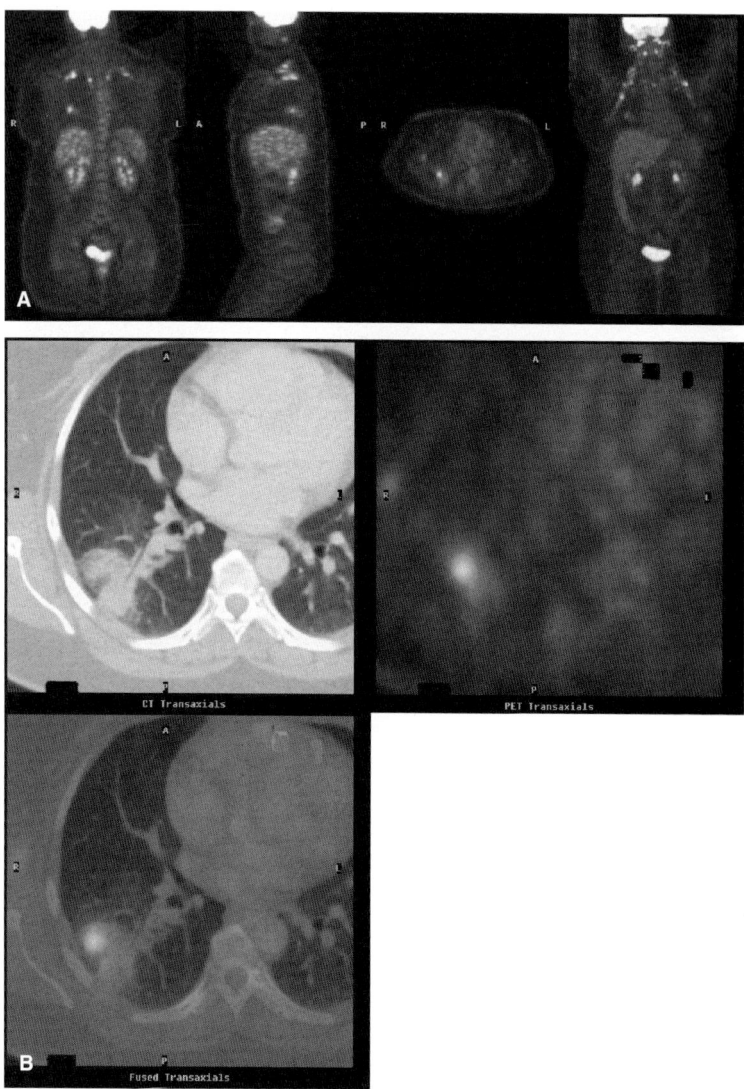

Figure 4.9. This patient with HD originally had disease in the left neck. The patient was subsequently treated and responded well. The patient later developed an opacity in the right lung on chest radiograph. Restaging FDG-PET (A) demonstrates hypermetabolic foci in the lower right hemithorax as well as symmetric activity in the infra- and supraclavicular regions. PET-CT images (B) reveal an opacity in the right lower lobe with air bronchograms and mild-to-moderate FDG uptake. This was felt to represent infection, and the patient subsequently cleared the opacity on follow-up chest radiograph. In (C), the infra- and supraclavicular FDG uptake corresponds to metabolically active brown fat. There is no definite evidence of active lymphoma by FDG-PET/CT.

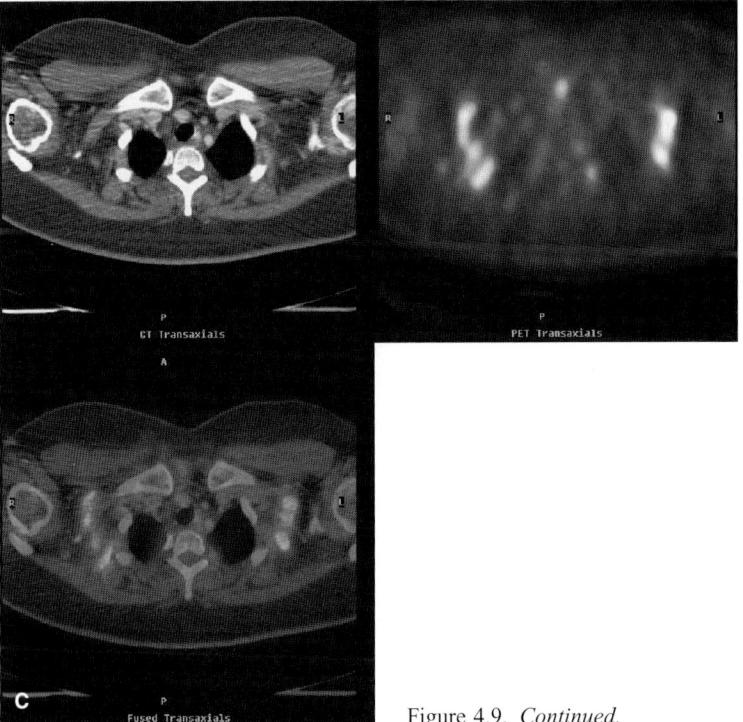

Figure 4.9. *Continued.*

References

1. What are the key statistics for Hodgkin's disease and non-Hodgkin's lymphoma? American Cancer Society (www.cancer.org); 2005 Accessed June 2005.
2. Jaffe ES, Harris NL, Diebold J, Muller-Hermelink HK. World Health Organization classification of neoplastic diseases of the hematopoietic and lymphoid tissues. A progress report. Am J Clin Pathol 1999;111(1 Suppl 1):S8–S12.
3. Greene FL, Page DL, Fleming ID, et al. AJCC Cancer Staging Manual, sixth edition. New York: Springer-Verlag; 2002.
4. Kostakoglu L, Leonard JP, Kuji I, Coleman M, Vallabhajosula S, Goldsmith SJ. Comparison of fluorine-18 fluorodeoxyglucose positron emission tomography and Ga-67 scintigraphy in evaluation of lymphoma. Cancer 2002;94(4):879–888.
5. Shen YY, Kao A, Yen RF. Comparison of ^{18}F-fluoro-2-deoxyglucose positron emission tomography and gallium-67 citrate scintigraphy for detecting malignant lymphoma. Oncol Rep 2002;9(2):321–325.

6. Bar-Shalom R, Yefremov N, Haim N, et al. Camera-based FDG PET and ^{67}Ga SPECT in evaluation of lymphoma: comparative study. Radiology 2003;227(2):353–360.

7. Spaepen K, Stroobants S, Verhoef G, Mortelmans L. Positron emission tomography with [(18)F]FDG for therapy response monitoring in lymphoma patients. Eur J Nucl Med Mol Imaging 2003;30 Suppl 1:S97–S105.

8. Elstrom R, Guan L, Baker G, et al. Utility of FDG-PET scanning in lymphoma by WHO classification. Blood 2003;101(10):3875–3876.

9. Friedberg JW, Chengazi V. PET scans in the staging of lymphoma: current status. Oncologist 2003;8(5):438–747.

10. Reske SN, Kotzerke J. FDG-PET for clinical use. Results of the 3rd German Inter-disciplinary Consensus Conference, "Onko-PET III", 21 July and 19 September 2000. Eur J Nucl Med 2001;28(11):1707–1723.

11. Hueltenschmidt B, Sautter-Bihl ML, Lang O, et al. Whole body positron emission tomography in the treatment of Hodgkin disease. Cancer 2001;91(2):302–310.

12. Macapinlac HA. The utility of 2-deoxy-2-[^{18}F]fluoro-D-glucose-positron emission tomography and combined positron emission tomography and computed tomography in lymphoma and melanoma. Mol Imaging Biol 2004;6(4):200–207.

13. Reske SN. PET and restaging of malignant lymphoma including residual masses and relapse. Eur J Nucl Med Mol Imaging 2003;30(Suppl 1):S89–S96.

14. Kostakoglu L, Coleman M, Leonard JP, Kuji I, Zoe H, Goldsmith SJ. PET predicts prognosis after 1 cycle of chemotherapy in aggressive lymphoma and Hodgkin's disease. J Nucl Med 2002;43(8):1018–1027.

15. Najjar F, Hustinx R, Jerusalem G, Fillet G, Rigo P. Positron emission tomography (PET) for staging low-grade non-Hodgkin's lymphomas (NHL). Cancer Biother Radiopharm 2001;16(4):297–304.

5. PET in Melanoma

Terence Z. Wong, Ronald B. Workman, Jr., and R. Edward Coleman

Epidemiology

Well over one million cases of skin cancer are diagnosed annually in the United States with the vast majority of these being basal cell and squamous skin cancers. Melanoma, although much less common, is the most aggressive skin malignancy, and it is the dominant cause of morbidity and mortality from skin cancer. The prognosis is very good in patients with early disease, but advanced metastatic melanoma is associated with poor survival rates. In the United States, approximately 59,580 new cases of melanoma were diagnosed in 2005 and approximately 7770 people died from this malignancy. There is a slight male predominance for melanoma, with males accounting for 56% of newly diagnosed melanoma [1]. Light pigmentation of the skin increases the susceptibility to melanoma, and the incidence and mortality from melanoma is a growing health concern among fair-skinned populations. Worldwide, the number of melanoma cases is increasing more rapidly than any other cancer [2]. The major environmental risk factor for development of cutaneous malignant melanoma is sun exposure, although the type of sun exposure appears to be an important consideration. Sunburn history, particularly during childhood, is a significant risk factor. There is evidence that intermittent sun exposure is a much stronger risk factor than chronic or occupational sun exposure [3]. Family history is another risk factor for melanoma. Although genetic mutations (i.e., CDKN2A) have been associated with melanoma, the role of genetic testing has not been established. No definitive associations have been established between melanoma and other environmental factors such as smoking, diet, fluorescent light exposure, or hormonal therapy [2].

Diagnosis

Melanomas can occur anywhere on the body. Women most commonly have the melanomas located on the lower extremities whereas men most commonly have the lesions on the upper back. These lesions are usually detected by the individual or physician because of variability in color, irregular surface, irregular perimeter or ulceration. A pigmented lesion that is undergoing a change is suspicious for melanoma and a biopsy should be performed. Imaging does not play a role in the diagnosis of this superficial lesion.

Table 5.1. TNM staging for melanoma

Primary tumor (T)	
TX	Primary tumor cannot be assessed (e.g. shave biopsy or regressed melanoma)
T0	No evidence of primary tumor
Tis	Melanoma in situ
T1	Melanoma ≤1.0 mm in thickness with or without ulceration
T1a	Melanoma ≤1.0 mm thickness and level II or III, no ulceration
T1b	Melanoma ≤1 mm thickness and level IV or V or with ulceration
T2	Melanoma 1.01–2.0 mm in thickness with or without ulceration
T2a	Melanoma 1.01–2.0 mm thickness, no ulceration
T2b	Melanoma 1.01–2.0 mm thickness, with ulceration
T3	Melanoma 2.01–4.0 mm in thickness with or without ulceration
T3a	Melanoma 2.01–4.0 mm thickness, no ulceration
T3b	Melanoma 2.01–4.0 mm thickness, with ulceration
T4	Melanoma >4.0 mm in thickness, with or without ulceration
T4a	Melanoma >4.0 mm thickness, no ulceration
T4b	Melanoma >4.0 mm thickness, with ulceration

Regional lymph nodes (N)	
NX	Regional lymph nodes cannot be assessed
N0	No regional lymph node metastasis
N1	Metastasis in one lymph node
N1a	Clinically occult (microscopic metastasis)
N1b	Clinically apparent (macroscopic) metastasis
N2	Metastasis in two to three regional nodes or intralymphatic regional metastasis without nodal metastases

Staging

Disease stratification plays an extremely important role in melanoma. Patients with localized disease have a 98% 5-year survival rate, while patients with regional and distant metastatic disease have significantly poorer prognosis, with 5-year survival rates of 60% and 16%, respectively [1]. The original American Joint Committee on Cancer (AJCC) staging system for melanoma took into account major factors which influenced prognosis, including the depth of the primary lesion (such as Clark level and Breslow measurement), lymph node involvement, and the presence of distant metastatic disease. A revised staging system for melanoma was approved by the AJCC in 2001 which accounts for additional factors that were found to have a significant impact on prognosis, including the presence or absence of ulceration in the primary lesion, the number of lymph nodes involved, serum lactate dehydrogenase (LDH) level, and sites of distant metastases. The newer staging system also accounts for the presence of microscopic lymph node involvement in sentinel lymph nodes, as determined through lymphoscintigraphy. The revised staging system has been validated through a study of 17,600 melanoma patients in the AJCC database [4]. The new TNM staging criteria and staging classifications are summarized in Tables 5.1 and 5.2.

Table 5.1. *Continued.*

N2a	Clinically occult (microscopic metastasis)
N2b	Clinically apparent (macroscopic) metastasis
N2c	Satellite or in-transit metastasis without nodal metastasis
N3	Metastasis in four or more regional nodes, or matted metastatic nodes, or in-transit metastasis or satellite(s) with metastasis in regional node(s)

Distant metastasis (M)

MX	Distant metastasis cannot be assessed
M0	No distant metastasis
M1	Distant metastasis
M1a	Metastasis to skin, subcutaneous tissues, or distant lymph nodes
M1b	Metastasis to lung
M1c	Metastasis to all other visceral sites or distant metastasis at any site associated with an elevated serum lactic dehydrogenase (LDH)

Source: Used with permission of the American Joint Committee on Cancer (AJCC), Chicago, Illinois. The original source for this material is the *AJCC Cancer Staging Manual*, Sixth Edition (2002), published by Springer-Verlag, New York, www.springeronline.com.

Table 5.2. TNM stage groupings for cutaneous melanoma

	Clinical staging			Pathologic staging		
	T	N	M	T	N	M
0	Tis	N0	M0	Tis	N0	M0
IA	T1a	N0	M0	T1a	N0	M0
IB	T1b	N0	M0	T1b	N0	M0
	T2a	N0	M0	T2a	N0	M0
IIA	T2b	N0	M0	T2b	N0	M0
	T3a	N0	M0	T3a	N0	M0
IIB	T3b	N0	M0	T3b	N0	M0
	T4a	N0	M0	T4a	N0	M0
IIC	T4b	N0	M0	T4b	N0	M0
III	Any T	N1	M0			
		N2				
		N3				
IIIA				T1–4a	N1a	M0
				T1–4a	N2a	M0
IIIB				T1–4b	N1a	M0
				T1–4b	N2a	M0
				T1–4a	N1b	M0
				T1–4a	N2b	M0
				T1–4a/b	N2c	M0
IIIC				T1–4b	N1b	M0
				T1–4b	N2b	M0
				Any T	N3	M0
IV	Any T	Any N	Any M1	Any T	Any N	Any M1

Source: Used with permission of the American Joint Committee on Cancer (AJCC), Chicago, Illinois. The original source for this material is the *AJCC Cancer Staging Manual*, Sixth Edition (2002), published by Springer-Verlag, New York, www.springeronline.com.

Fluorodeoxyglucose-Positron Emission Tomography for Imaging Melanoma

In general, malignant melanoma cells avidly accumulate fluorodeoxyglucose (FDG) (2-deoxy-2-[^{18}F]-fluoro-D-glucose), and macroscopic melanoma foci are readily revealed on PET scans. The degree of FDG uptake in melanoma cells correlates with viability and proliferation rate [5]. Multiple studies have demonstrated that FDG-PET imaging is more accurate than conventional anatomic imaging (CT or MRI) for staging melanoma; consequently, PET has been reported to alter clinical management in a significant proportion (15–49%) of cases [6–10]. The metastatic spread of melanoma can be highly unpredictable, and a significant advantage that PET has over routine CT imaging is the ability to evaluate the whole body from head to toe. Imaging of the extremities for superficial and deep lesions can be particularly important for evaluating in-transit disease and surveying for metastatic disease.

FDG-PET imaging was approved for Medicare reimbursement in 2000 for diagnosis, staging, and restaging of melanoma. At that time, it was recognized that PET imaging was not as sensitive as sentinel node lymphoscintigraphy for detecting early regional involvement (see below), and reimbursement was specifically not provided for PET evaluation of the regional lymph node basin in the initial staging of melanoma. Lymphoscintigraphy with sentinel lymph node biopsy remains the most sensitive technique for detecting metastatic disease in these patients.

FDG-PET is most accurate for evaluating stage III and stage IV disease, and has much less sensitivity for detecting primary stage I and II lesions. Early stage melanoma is frequently difficult to detect on PET imaging because of the superficial nature of the tumor and the background activity normally present in the skin. Specificity of PET findings in the skin is also an issue, as inflammatory lesions, post-surgical changes, injection sites, and urinary contamination can give false-positive results. Realizing these limitations, it is still important to carefully survey the skin for additional cutaneous lesions when interpreting PET scans in melanoma patients.

In a recent review by Friedman and Wahl [11], FDG-PET is the imaging modality of choice in melanoma for four major indications:

1. Patients with high risk for distant metastases based on extent of locoregional disease.
2. Patients with findings suspicious for distant metastases.
3. Patients with known distant metastatic disease who may benefit from therapies if new lesions are discovered or treated lesions regress.
4. Patients at high risk for systemic relapse who are considering aggressive medical therapy.

Sentinel lymph node (SLN) biopsy has dramatically changed the surgical staging and management of patients with melanoma. SLN biopsy is recommended for patients with primary melanoma >1 mm thick or at high risk for locoregional disease. Completion lymph node dissection is recommended for patients in whom nodal metastases are found [12].

The major advantages that PET provides for melanoma patients are more accurate staging and more accurate assessment of recurrent disease [13]. This improved accuracy has implications in terms of both treatment options and prognosis, and the value of PET has been demonstrated in multiple studies. In a retrospective study of 126 scans in 92 patients (84 patients with stage III or IV disease), Harris et al. [9] found that FDG-PET impacted the clinical decision-making in 43 of 126 patient studies (32%). They concluded that PET was especially valuable for determining whether or not patients were suitable for surgical intervention. Notably, PET did not have any impact on management in patients with stage I or II disease. In another prospective study of 106 patients with stage III disease [8], PET scanning discovered unsuspected disease in 19.7% of cases and altered clinical management in 15.1% of the patients. Gulec et al. [10] studied a group of 49 patients who underwent conventional imaging (chest, abdomen, pelvis CT; brain MRI), followed by PET imaging. Treatment plans were formulated prior to and following the PET studies for comparison. PET identified additional metastatic sites in 55% of the patients, and changed clinical management in 49% of the cases.

An example of a patient with melanoma is illustrated in Figure 5.1. This man presented with right inguinal adenopathy, which proved to be melanoma on biopsy. He also had palpable disease in the right popliteal region. PET/CT imaging confirmed the known disease, along with a questionable focus of FDG accumulation which localized to the small bowel (Figure 5.2). The primary

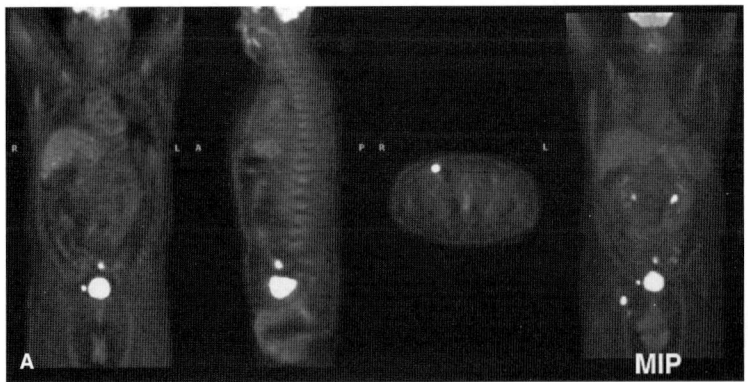

Figure 5.1. Coronal, sagittal, axial, and maximum intensity projection (MIP) FDG-PET images of a man who presented with right inguinal adenopathy, biopsy proven to be melanoma. Attenuation-corrected images of the body (**A**) and lower extremities (**B**) are shown. The primary melanoma site was never discovered. Images of the legs demonstrate post-surgical changes in the foot from removal of a plantar wart, and metastatic disease in the popliteal region, right inguinal region, and pelvis (see Figure 5.2).

Continued.

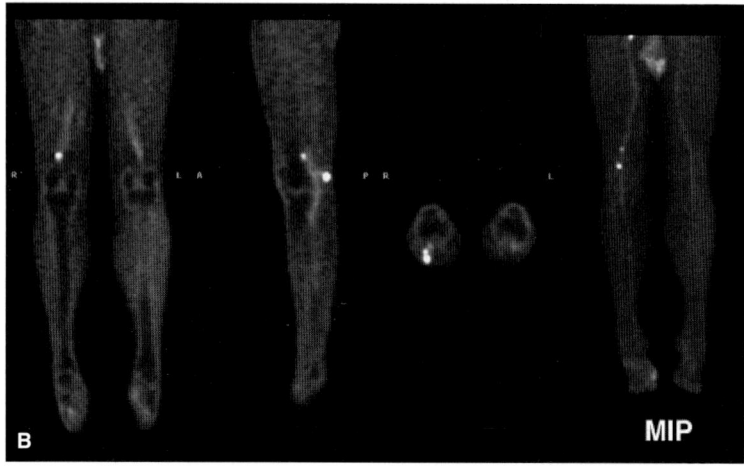

Figure 5.1. *Continued.*

cutaneous lesion was not identified either clinically or by PET/CT. Following this scan, the patient underwent lymphadenectomy and exploratory laparotomy, at which time the small bowel examination was negative. Follow-up CT scan 1 year later demonstrated markedly progressive disease, including an intraluminal mass within the small bowel.

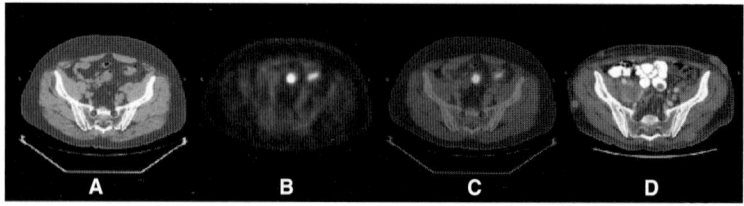

Figure 5.2. Same patient as in Figure 5.1. Axial **(A)** CT, **(B)** attenuation-corrected PET, and **(C)** fused PET/CT images demonstrate intense focal activity in the pelvis which is suspicious for small bowel metastasis on PET, although lack of oral contrast makes evaluation of the CT scan difficult. Follow-up CT scan 1 year later **(D)** demonstrates new and progressive disease, with subcutaneous metastases, external iliac adenopathy, as well as an intraluminal small bowel mass.

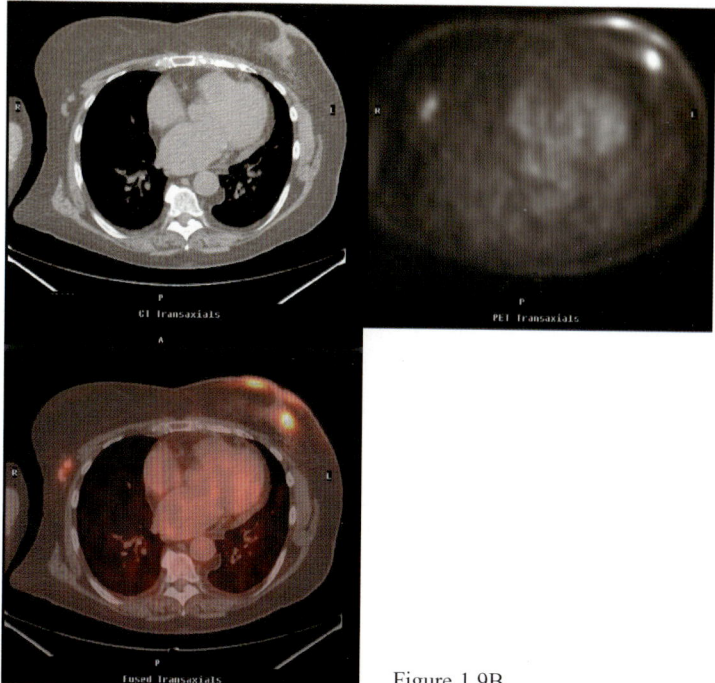

Figure 1.9B.

Figure 3.6B.

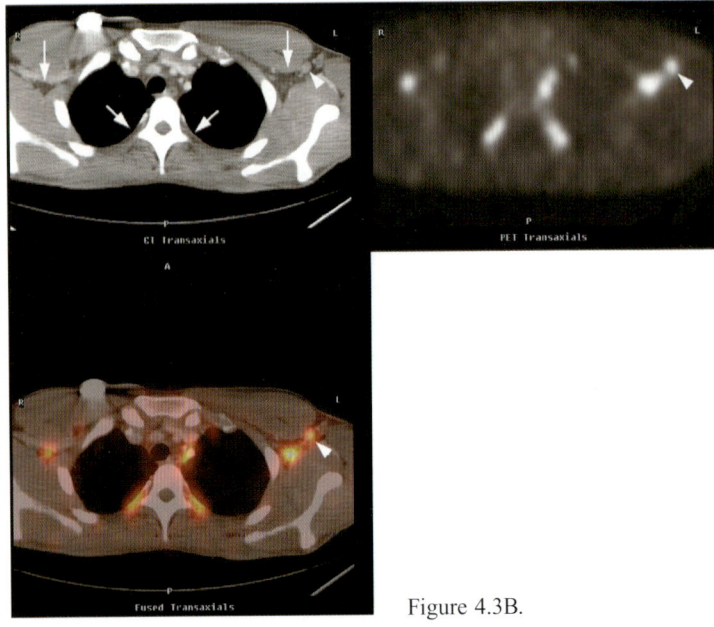

Figure 4.3B.

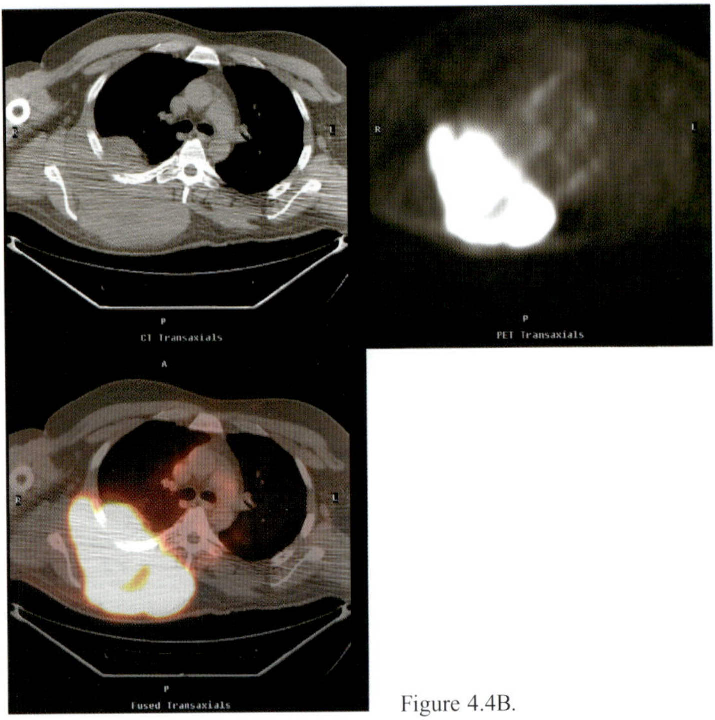

Figure 4.4B.

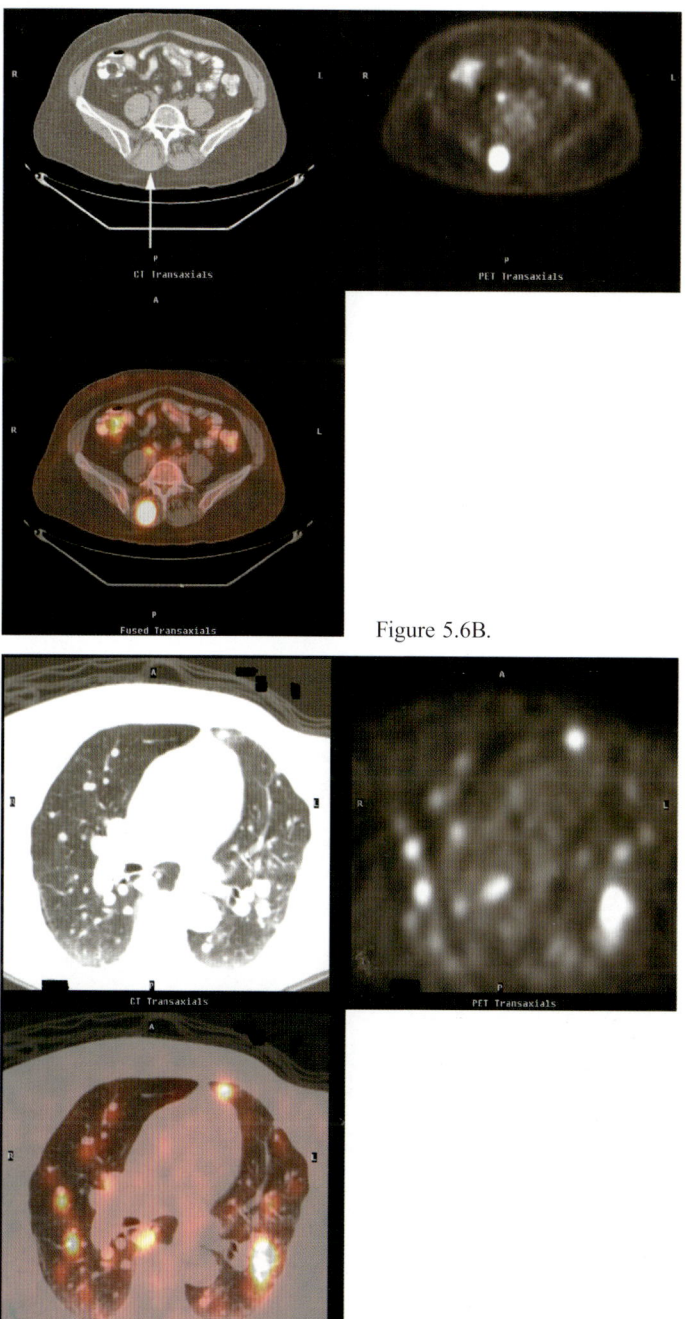

Figure 5.6B.

Figure 10.3C.

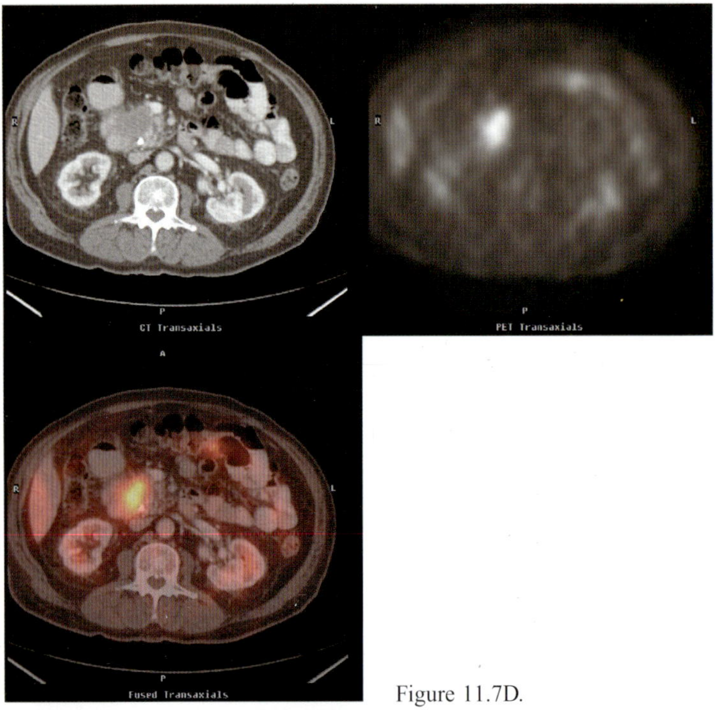

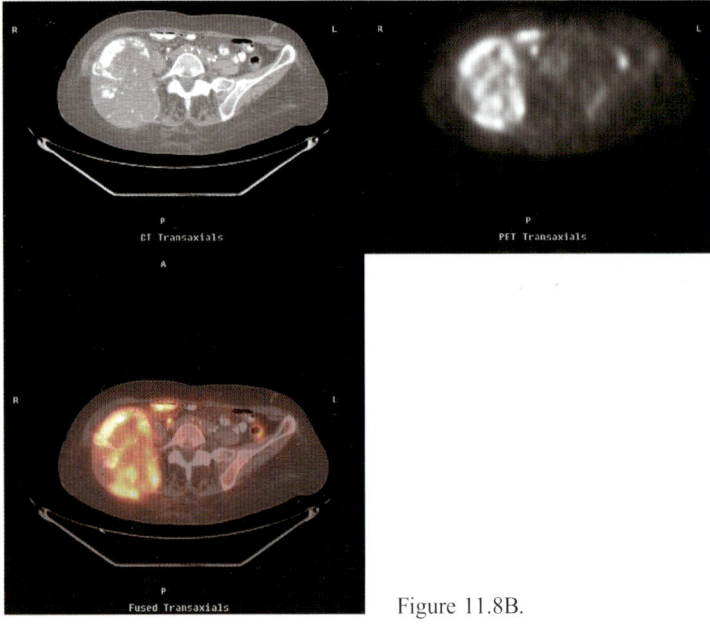

Figure 11.7D.

Figure 11.8B.

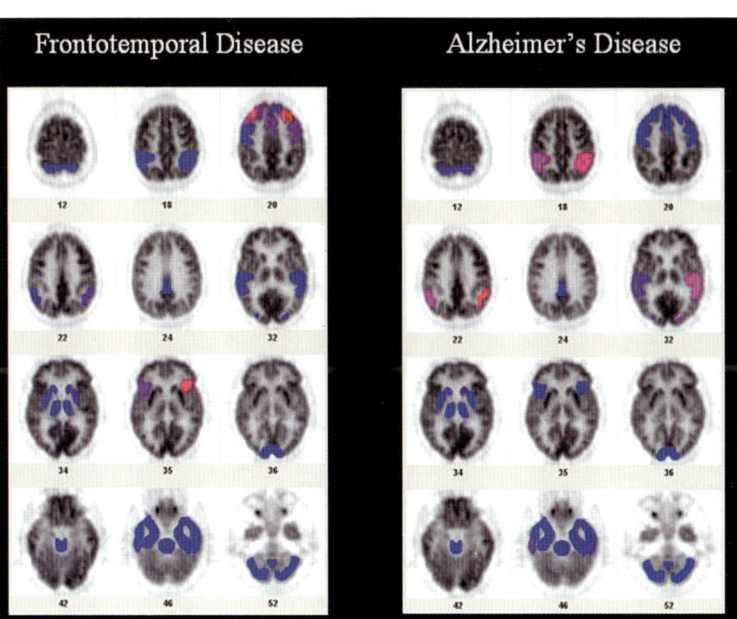

Figure 13.6.

Limitations of Fluorodeoxyglucose-Positron Emission Tomography Evaluation in Melanoma

The major limitation of FDG-PET imaging for melanoma is the reduced sensitivity for detecting small tumor foci. Wagner et al. [14] found that PET had a sensitivity of only 17% for regional lymph node metastases in patients with melanoma. This was likely related to the small tumor volumes (average 4.3 mm³) in these sentinel nodes, and the findings in this study and others with similar results served as the primary rationale for the denial of Medicare coverage for evaluating regional lymph node basins. In another study, Wagner et al. [15] correlated FDG-PET interpretations with the size of involved regional lymph node metastases from melanoma at pathology, and found that metastatic deposits with a minimum volume of 78 mm³ were detected with a sensitivity of 90%. On the other hand, PET was able to detect only 14% of involved lymph nodes with tumor volumes <78 mm³. Therefore, PET cannot substitute for sentinel lymph node pathology obtained during primary surgical resection, and provides an inadequate evaluation of the regional lymph node basin. The size-related sensitivity of FDG-PET also likely explains the decreased effectiveness of PET for evaluating stage I and II disease.

PET is less sensitive than CT for detecting pulmonary metastases. Gritters et al. [16] found that PET had a sensitivity of only 15% for detecting lung metastases, although 26 of the 27 pulmonary metastases in this study were less than 1 cm. In another study [13], CT was more sensitive (93%) than PET (57%) for detecting lung metastases, but PET was more specific (92% versus 70%). FDG-PET may also have reduced sensitivity for detecting liver metastases compared to MRI. Ghanem et al. [17] performed a study involving 39 MRI and PET scans in 35 patients; based on 34 lesions, the sensitivity of PET was 47% versus 100% for MRI. Size of the hepatic lesion was also significantly related to PET sensitivity in this study. Finally, FDG-PET is less sensitive than contrast-enhanced CT or MRI for detection of intracranial metastases. In a study of 38 metastatic lesions in 40 patients undergoing PET for extracranial malignancies, the sensitivity of FDG-PET was only 61% relative to MRI [18]. In addition to lesion size, sensitivity for intracranial metastases is also limited by the presence of high cerebral cortical activity, and contrast-enhanced MRI or CT is recommended if brain metastases are suspected.

An example of a patient with widespread metastatic melanoma is shown in Figure 5.3. Diffuse intensely hypermetabolic disease is present primarily in the mediastinum, lungs, liver, left inguinal region, and soft tissues of the lower extremities. An axial image in the thorax from the same PET/CT scan is presented in Figure 5.4, illustrating the benefit of combined PET and CT. In addition to providing accurate functional/anatomic correlation, the CT scan (Figure 5.4A) clearly detects smaller pulmonary metastases that are below the resolution of PET (Figure 5.4C). This patient also had multiple hemorrhagic intracranial metastases (Figure 5.5), which were not clearly apparent on the PET scan alone. Figure 5.6 presents examples of PET's benefit to CT. This patient not only has metastatic melanoma in the right hilar region, but also hematogenous

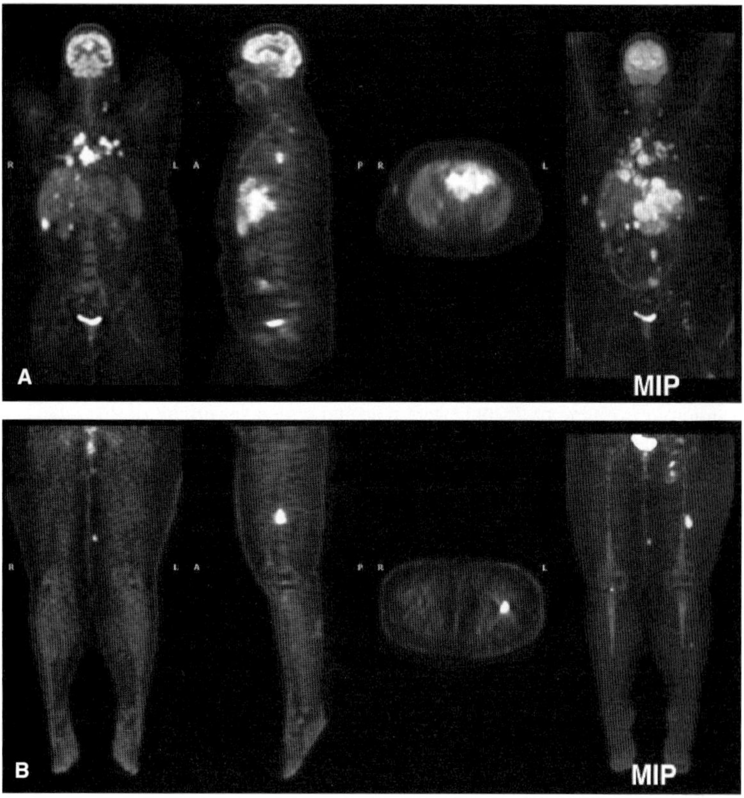

Figure 5.3. Coronal, sagittal, axial, and maximum intensity projection (MIP) FDG-PET images of a woman who presented with locally advanced melanoma in her left calf. Widespread metastases are identified throughout the chest and abdomen as well as both lower extremities.

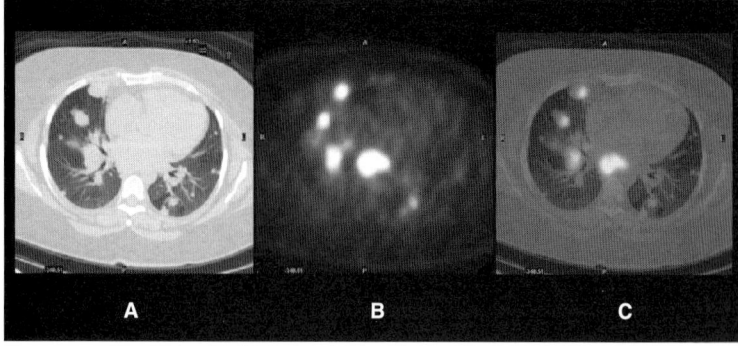

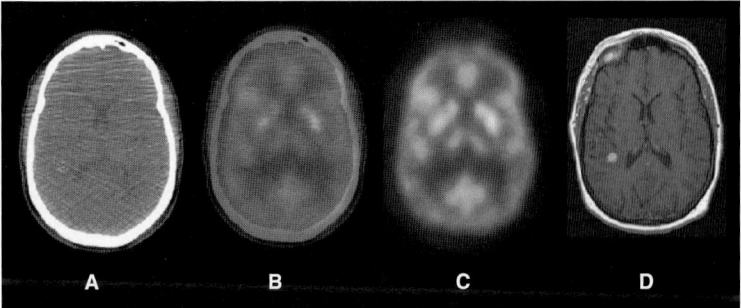

Figure 5.5. Same patient as in Figure 5.3. Limited sensitivity of FDG-PET for detecting intracranial metastases. CT from PET/CT **(A)** demonstrates subtle lesions having increased attenuation, compatible with hemorrhagic brain metastases. Attenuation-corrected PET **(C)**, and fused images **(B)** demonstrate no corresponding hypermetabolism in this region. MRI obtained 1 day later **(D)** confirmed the presence of multiple hemorrhagic metastases.

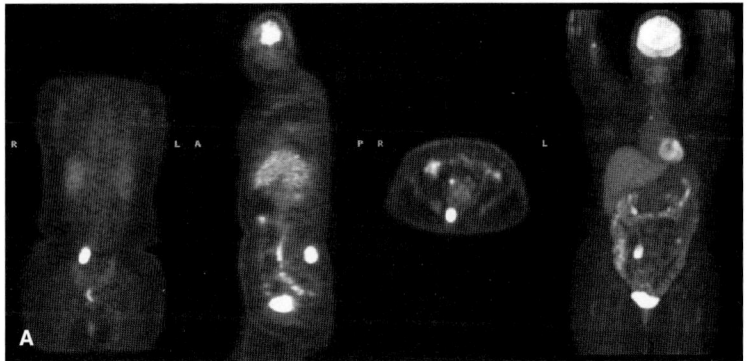

Figure 5.6. PET/CT images of a patient with metastatic melanoma. Whole-body FDG-PET images **(A)** demonstrate multiple abnormal foci of increased activity in the right hilar region as well as the right upper arm and right paraspinal region.

Continued.

◄ ─────────────────────────────────────

Figure 5.4. Same patient as in Figure 5.3. Axial **(A)** CT, **(B)** attenuation-corrected PET, and **(C)** fused PET/CT images demonstrate diffuse metastatic disease within the mediastinum along with innumerable pulmonary metastases. The larger pulmonary nodules demonstrate intense FDG accumulation, but the smaller pulmonary metastases can only be identified on CT.

84   T.Z. Wong et al.

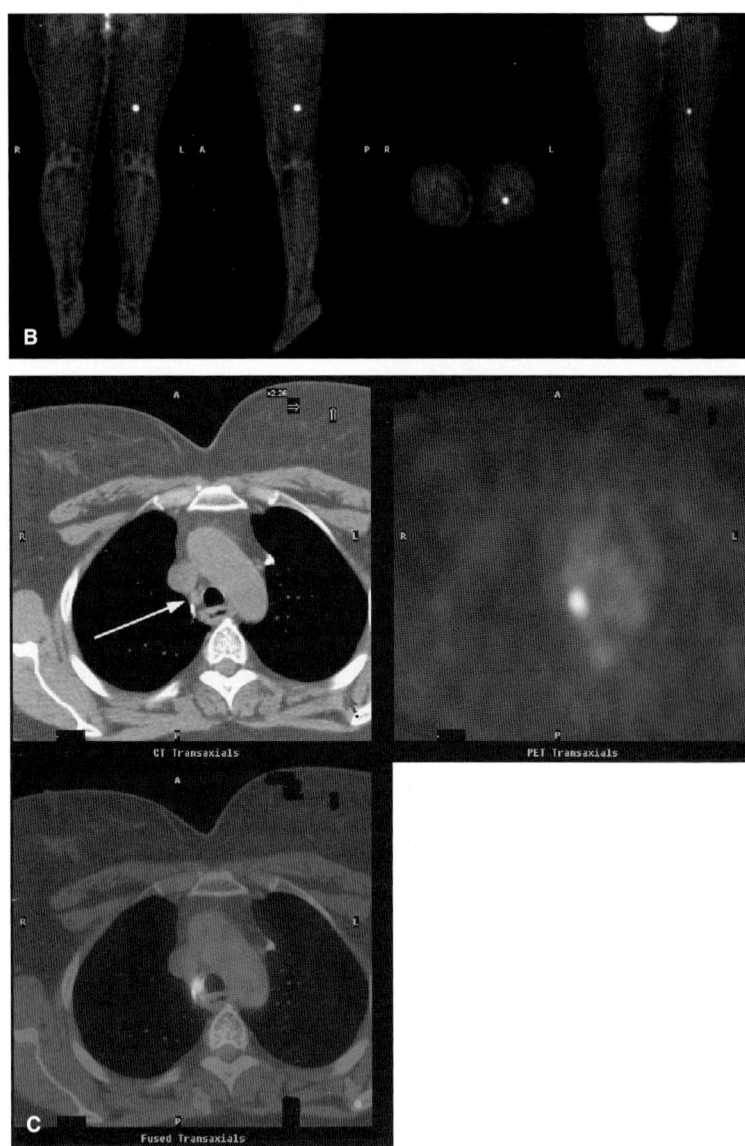

Figure 5.6. *Continued.* Lower extremity FDG-PET images **(B)** demonstrate a metastatic deposit in the left thigh. PET/CT images through the chest **(C)** localize the chest lesion to be a right paratracheal node (white arrow). PET/CT images through the pelvis and the lower extremities **(D** and **E)** reveal the metastatic melanoma deposits to be within right paraspinal and left thigh musculature (white arrows). (See part D only in the color insert.)

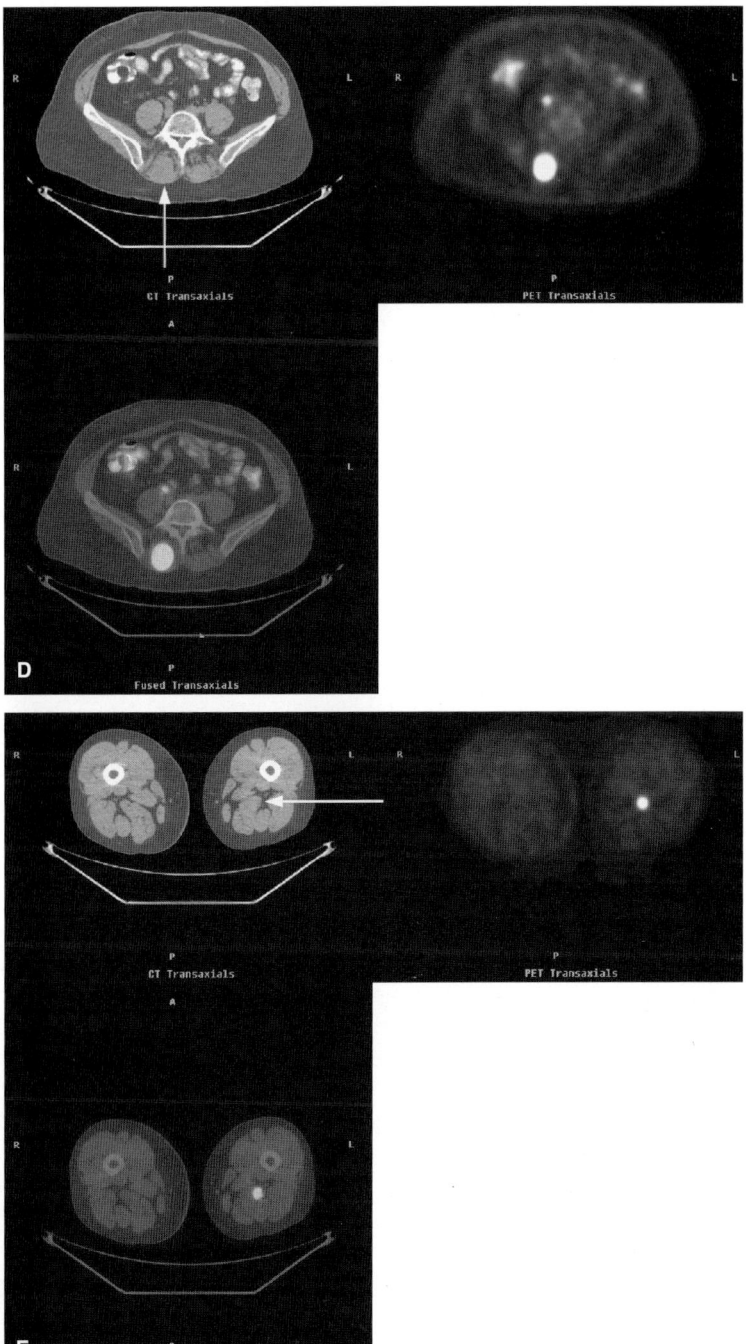

Figure 5.6. *Continued.*

deposits in the musculature of the right paraspinal, left thigh, and right upper arm regions (see also Plate 5.6D in the color insert).

Combined Positron Emission Tomography/Computed Tomography for Evaluation in Melanoma

Studies to date have been confined to FDG-PET alone for staging and restaging melanoma. The role of combined PET/CT remains to be studied. A reasonable hypothesis is that combined PET-DCT (PET with diagnostic-quality CT) will have improved sensitivity over PET alone, because of the ability to detect small pulmonary metastases that may be below the resolution of PET. Small liver metastases may also be apparent on CT. Based on our experience at Duke, oral contrast is essential for these DCT studies, particularly since melanoma can involve the bowel or mesentery (see Figure 5.2). Our experience and that of others is that low-density oral contrast does not cause significant attenuation-correction artifacts on the PET images. The routine use of intravenous contrast in these combined PET-DCT studies is a subject that requires further study.

Other potential benefits of PET-DCT are based on anecdotal experience. CT helps to confidently localize the abnormal FDG accumulation, an important consideration in diseases such as melanoma that can metastasize to any organ site. The sensitivity of combined PET-DCT is increased within the abdomen, where abnormalities on CT with associated hypermetabolism on PET confirm metastatic disease in the retroperitoneum, mesentery, or bowel wall that would otherwise be attributed to physiologic FDG accumulation if the PET study were performed alone. Small nodes that do not meet size criteria on CT for malignant disease can be intensely hypermetabolic on PET, indicating metastatic involvement. Conversely, large lymph nodes on CT may be hypometabolic on PET imaging, indicating benign nodes. Therefore, combined PET-DCT could potentially provide both higher sensitivity and specificity than either study alone, and may be the imaging technique of choice for evaluating patients with melanoma. However, further studies are needed to establish this, and to determine the cost-effectiveness of this approach.

Summary and Future Considerations

PET and PET/CT imaging can provide accurate staging for melanoma, and have most value in assessing stage III and stage IV disease. The improved accuracy in staging over other imaging methods provides important prognostic information and has a significant impact on management of patients with melanoma. The major limitation of PET imaging for evaluating melanoma is detection of small or microscopic disease. PET has limited utility in stage I or II melanoma. CT and MRI are more sensitive than PET for evaluating small pulmonary, hepatic, and intracranial metastases. In spite of these limitations, multiple studies have demonstrated that FDG-PET detects more metastatic lesions than CT imaging and is more accurate overall for evaluating metastatic disease in melanoma patients.

Further studies are needed to determine the potential additional value provided by PET/CT. The value of intravenous contrast in these combined studies has also yet to be determined. Both PET and CT studies are indicated in many patients with high-risk or advanced melanoma; combined PET/CT imaging provides a "one-stop" imaging approach for these patients, along with the additional mutual information delivered by these studies.

Advanced melanoma carries a poor prognosis, mandating development of new therapies. FDG-PET can provide an early indicator of response to therapy for a variety of malignancies [19], although little information is currently available regarding this application in melanoma therapy. This application of PET could significantly contribute to patient management by allowing treatment response to be predicted early during the treatment course. Therapy that shows no response could then be changed, saving the patient from ineffective therapy and associated toxicities.

At this time, there are few data regarding the effectiveness of combined PET/CT for evaluating melanoma, although anecdotal experience suggests that the combined studies may further improve accuracy. Additional studies are needed to support this contention, and research is needed to determine the most appropriate CT imaging protocols to use in these combined studies.

References

1. Jemal A, Murray T, Ward E, et al. Cancer statistics, 2005. CA Cancer J Clin 2005; 55:10–30.
2. Lens MB, Dawes M. Global perspectives of contemporary epidemiological trends of cutaneous malignant melanoma. Br J Dermatol 2004;150:179–185.
3. Gandini S, Sera F, Cattaruzza MS, et al. Meta-analysis of risk factors for cutaneous melanoma: II. Sun exposure. Eur J Cancer 2005;41:45–60.
4. Balch CM, Buzaid AC, Soong SJ, et al. Final version of the American Joint Committee on Cancer staging system for cutaneous melanoma. J Clin Oncol 2001;19: 3635–3648.
5. Yamada K, Brink I, Bisse E, Epting T, Engelhardt R. Factors influencing [F-18] 2-fluoro-2-deoxy-D-glucose (F-18 FDG) uptake in melanoma cells: the role of proliferation rate, viability, glucose transporter expression and hexokinase activity. J Dermatol 2005;32:316–334.
6. Holder WD, Jr., White RL, Jr., Zuger JH, Easton EJ, Jr., Greene FL. Effectiveness of positron emission tomography for the detection of melanoma metastases. Ann Surg 1998;227:764–769; discussion 769–771.
7. Eigtved A, Andersson AP, Dahlstrom K, et al. Use of fluorine-18 fluorodeoxyglucose positron emission tomography in the detection of silent metastases from malignant melanoma. Eur J Nucl Med 2000;27:70–75.

8. Tyler DS, Onaitis M, Kherani A, et al. Positron emission tomography scanning in malignant melanoma. Cancer 2000;89:1019–1025.

9. Harris MT, Berlangieri SU, Cebon JS, Davis ID, Scott AM. Impact of 2-deoxy-2[F-18]fluoro-D: -glucose positron emission tomography on the management of patients with advanced melanoma. Mol Imaging Biol 2005:1–5.

10. Gulec SA, Faries MB, Lee CC, et al. The role of fluorine-18 deoxyglucose positron emission tomography in the management of patients with metastatic melanoma: impact on surgical decision making. Clin Nucl Med 2003;28:961–965.

11. Friedman KP, Wahl RL. Clinical use of positron emission tomography in the management of cutaneous melanoma. Semin Nucl Med 2004;34:242–253.

12. Cormier JN, Xing Y, Ding M, et al. Population-based assessment of surgical treatment trends for patients with melanoma in the era of sentinel lymph node biopsy. J Clin Oncol 2005;23:6054–6062.

13. Fuster D, Chiang S, Johnson G, Schuchter LM, Zhuang H, Alavi A. Is 18F-FDG PET more accurate than standard diagnostic procedures in the detection of suspected recurrent melanoma? J Nucl Med 2004;45:1323–1327.

14. Wagner JD, Schauwecker D, Davidson D, et al. Prospective study of fluorodeoxyglucose-positron emission tomography imaging of lymph node basins in melanoma patients undergoing sentinel node biopsy. J Clin Oncol 1999;17:1508–1515.

15. Wagner JD, Schauwecker DS, Davidson D, Wenck S, Jung SH, Hutchins G. FDG-PET sensitivity for melanoma lymph node metastases is dependent on tumor volume. J Surg Oncol 2001;77:237–242.

16. Gritters LS, Francis IR, Zasadny KR, Wahl RL. Initial assessment of positron emission tomography using 2-fluorine-18-fluoro-2-deoxy-D-glucose in the imaging of malignant melanoma. J Nucl Med 1993;34:1420–1427.

17. Ghanem N, Altehoefer C, Hogerle S, et al. Detectability of liver metastases in malignant melanoma: prospective comparison of magnetic resonance imaging and positron emission tomography. Eur J Radiol 2005;54:264–270.

18. Rohren EM, Provenzale JM, Barboriak DP, Coleman RE. Screening for cerebral metastases with FDG PET in patients undergoing whole-body staging of non-central nervous system malignancy. Radiology 2003;226:181–187.

19. Weber WA. Use of PET for monitoring cancer therapy and for predicting outcome. J Nucl Med 2005;46:983–995.

6. Fluorodeoxyglucose-PET in Breast Cancer

Bennett B. Chin, Ronald B. Workman, Jr., and R. Edward Coleman

Similar to the previously discussed approved applications in oncology, FDG-PET in breast cancer has demonstrated superior diagnostic accuracy compared with conventional anatomic imaging for the detection of distant metastases. This increased accuracy in lesion detection has translated into improved staging, especially in cases with a high clinical suspicion or pre-test probability of distant metastases. In addition to staging and restaging, another application for FDG-PET covered by Medicare is in the evaluation of tumor response to therapy.

This chapter briefly reviews the basic classification and imaging aspects of breast cancer; describes the currently approved clinical indications, as defined by the Center for Medicare and Medicaid Services (CMS); and discusses the accuracy, strengths, and limitations of FDG-PET.

Epidemiology and Histopathology

Breast cancer is the most frequent tumor in women, with over 200,000 new cases each year in the US [1,2]. Women in the US have an approximately 1 in 7 lifetime risk of developing breast cancer. It is the second leading cause of cancer death in women with an approximately 15% mortality, or 40,000 deaths each year [1,2]. In men, only 1450 new cases occur each year in the US; however, mortality is approximately 450 each year [1,2].

Eighty percent of breast cancers are adenocarcinomas, 5–10% are lobular carcinomas, and 5% are medullary carcinomas. Other rare types of breast cancer include inflammatory breast carcinoma (1–3%), tubular carcinoma (2%), and Paget's disease of the breast (1%). Of the adenocarcinomas, approximately 20% are diagnosed at the early stage of intraductal carcinoma, also called ductal carcinoma in situ (DCIS).

Tumor Node Metastasis Staging

The tumor node metastasis (TNM) tumor staging of breast cancer is summarized in Table 6.1. Changes to the American Joint Committee on Cancer Staging (AJCC) in 2002 have been recently summarized [3]. New classifications

90   B.B. Chin et al.

Table 6.1. American Joint Committee on Cancer TNM staging for breast cancer

Stage	T	N	M
Stage 0	Tis	N0	M0
Stage I	T1	N0	M0
	T0	N1	M0
Stage IIA	T1	N1	M0
	T2	N0	M0
Stage IIB	T2	N1	M0
	T3	N0	M0
	T0	N2	M0
	T1	N2	M0
Stage IIIA	T2	N2	M0
	T3	N1	M0
	T3	N2	M0
	T4	N0	M0
Stage IIIB	T4	N1	M0
	T4	N2	M0
Stage IIIC	Any T	N3	M0
Stage IV	Any T	Any N	M1

Source: Used with permission of the American Joint Committee on Cancer (AJCC), Chicago, Illinois. The original source for this material is the AJCC Cancer Staging Manual, Sixth Edition (2002), published by Springer-Verlag, New York, www.springeronline.com.

have been added to incorporate lymph node metastases detected by sentinel lymph node biopsy and/or immunohistochemical staining or reverse transcriptase-polymerase chain reaction (RT-PCR). In addition, distinction is made between isolated tumor cells (≤ 0.2 mm) and micrometastatic disease (>0.2 mm and ≤ 2.0 mm). The number of positive lymph nodes is also incorporated into the nodal staging. Changes in staging criteria may influence the apparent survival data when comparing prognosis based on different staging criteria [4]. The more recent and more accurate pathologic staging may lead to an apparent increase in survival without true improvement [4].

Currently Approved Indications

In contrast to the other oncologic clinical indications, FDG-PET is currently not approved for the initial diagnosis of breast cancer. Mammography with ultrasound and biopsy is a highly sensitive approach for the majority of breast cancer initial diagnoses. Although the early reports of FDG-PET showed high sensitivity (>90%) for large lesions such as in locally advanced breast carcinoma [5,6], subsequent reports demonstrated significantly lower sensitivity in smaller primary lesions, predominantly related to the limited PET image resolution [7] (Figure 6.1). In a meta-analysis of the literature, FDG-PET on conventional whole-body scanners could not accurately classify a primary breast lesion as benign or malignant with sufficient sensitivity [8]. Promising devices currently under evaluation include novel PET instrumentation specifically designed for breast imaging which can improve sensitivity and accuracy for detection of smaller primary tumors [9–18]. See Figure 6.2 for a glimpse of a positron emission mammography (PEM) device and a representative FDG-PEM study.

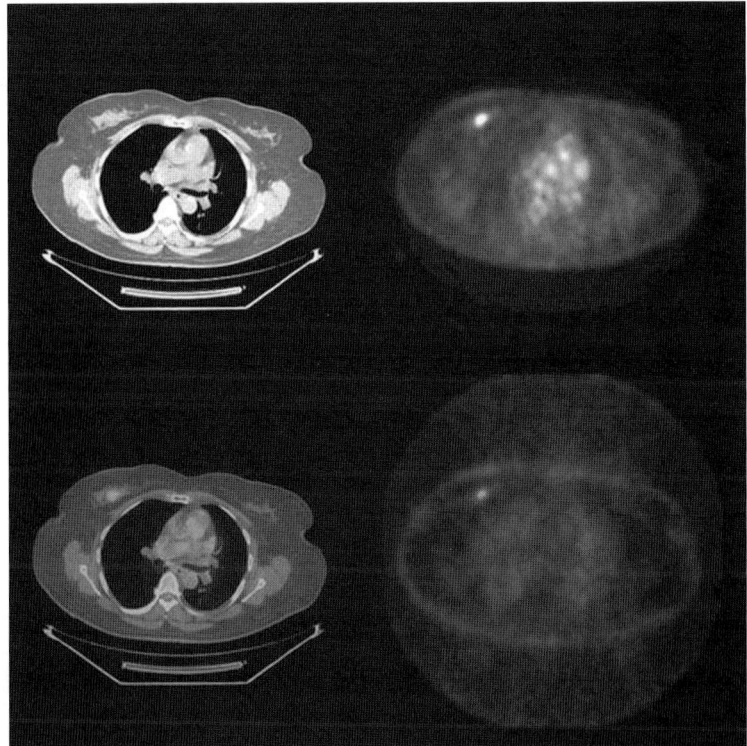

Figure 6.1. A 75-year-old woman who presented with a breast mass that was biopsied and demonstrated to be invasive ductal cancer. She was referred for a PET scan for initial staging, which was negative for disease other than the primary lesion in the right breast. The CT scan (upper left) reveals a right breast mass that is FDG avid on PET (upper right). The fused images (lower left) show the location of the cancer within the mass. The lower right image is the non-attenuation-corrected image.

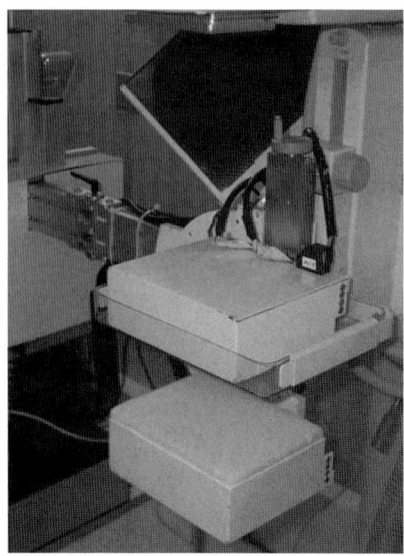 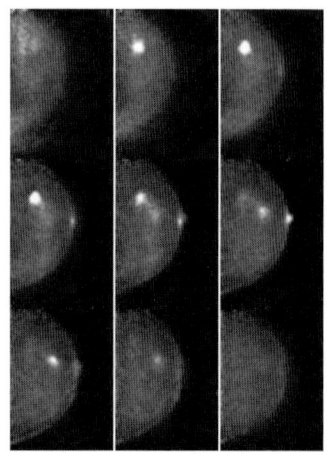

Figure 6.2. A positron emission mammography (PEM) device developed by Jefferson National Laboratory and being evaluated by Duke University Medical Center is shown on the left. The two detectors are placed on a mammography unit; the breast is positioned on the lower detector and the upper detector is lowered with the compression device for imaging. The tomographic images shown on the right reveal FDG accumulation in a large breast cancer.

Staging and Restaging of Breast Carcinoma

FDG-PET is currently approved for the staging and restaging of regional and distant metastatic disease. Advantages of FDG-PET include complete whole-body evaluation in a single study, and superior sensitivity and accuracy compared to conventional anatomic imaging modalities (Figure 6.3). Several review articles have summarized the higher accuracy of FDG-PET compared to conventional diagnostic modalities [19–22]. In a report of 60 patients with suspected breast cancer recurrence, FDG-PET sensitivity, specificity, and accuracy were 89%, 84%, and 87%, respectively, for the detection of local or regional recurrence [23]. For the detection of distant metastases, sensitivity, specificity, and accuracy were 100%, 97%, and 98%, respectively [23]. A meta-analysis of FDG-PET for detection of breast cancer recurrence or metastases in patients showed a pooled sensitivity of 90% (95% confidence interval = 86.8–93.2%), and a pooled false-positive rate of 11% (95% confidence interval = 7.8–14.6%) [24]. A number of other reports have shown significantly better sensitivity and accuracy of FDG-PET in detection of recurrence or distant metastases compared to conventional anatomic imaging modalities including CT [25–30]. Particular utility is demonstrated in the detection of mediastinal or internal mammary lymph node metastases [25,31–33]. Figures 6.3 and 6.4 demonstrates the ability of FDG-PET to identify sites of distant metastases.

Although FDG-PET has shown excellent sensitivity in the detection of distant recurrence or metastases, early micrometastatic disease to axillary lymph nodes may not be detected. In a blinded, prospective, multicenter study of FDG-PET in primary staging of the axillary lymph nodes, the sensitivity was 61% with a corresponding specificity of 80% [34]. Sentinel lymph node biopsy and

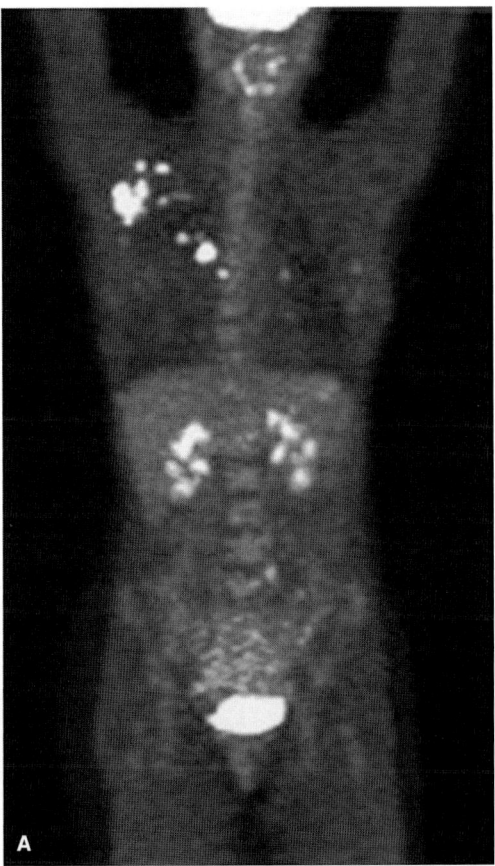

Figure 6.3. A 42-year-old woman with a history of breast cancer now with biopsy-proven axillary recurrence after mastectomy and radiation therapy. PET/CT scan was performed to determine extent of disease. Maximum intensity pixel projection image (A) demonstrates marked axillary nodal disease as well as disease in the right and left chest.

Continued.

focused histologic examination, which may include thin sectioning and immuno-histochemical staining [35], provide higher sensitivity compared to FDG-PET for axillary lymph node staging after initial diagnosis. Although intense foci were highly predictive of metastatic disease, this finding was relatively infrequent among those with axillary metastases, and routine staging of the axillary lymph nodes by FDG-PET is currently not recommended [34]. Other studies have confirmed a relatively low sensitivity compared to sentinel lymph node biopsy [35], and results from other studies have been recently summarized [36]. Thus, sentinel lymph node biopsy with dedicated histologic examination is recommended for initial axillary lymph node staging in the majority of cases clinically presenting with early stage disease.

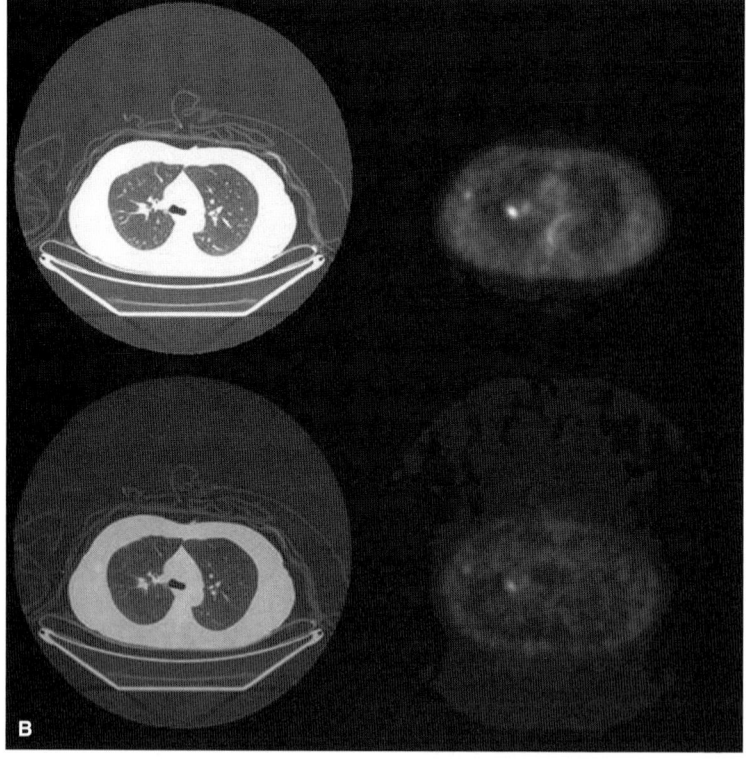

Figure 6.3. *Continued.* **(B)** Transaxial images of the chest demonstrate a lung metastasis (not obvious on CT) as well as hilar nodal metastases. The upper left image is the CT with lung windows, upper right is the attenuation-corrected PET image, the lower left is the fusion image, and the lower right is the non-attenuation-corrected PET image.

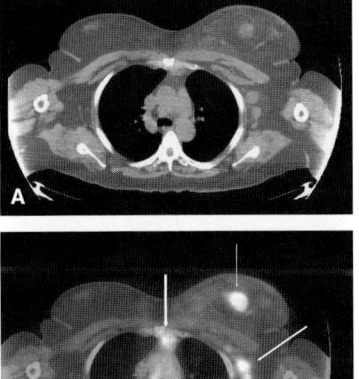
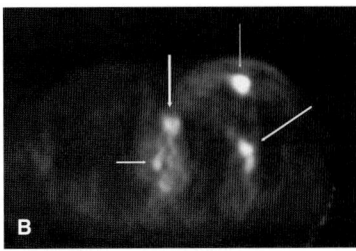

Figure 6.4. A 50-year-old woman presenting with inflammatory breast cancer. Left breast mass and palpable axillary lymph nodes. **(A)** Transaxial CT of the chest shows the left breast mass. **(B)** Transaxial PET at the same level shows intense FDG uptake in the breast mass (thin vertical arrow), in internal mammary lymph nodes (thick vertical arrow), in the left axillary lymph nodes (thick diagonal arrow), in the paratracheal lymph nodes (horizontal thick arrow), and in the soft tissues of the left breast. **(C)** Transaxial fusion of PET and CT co-localizes the same abnormalities described in **(B)**.

Evaluation of Response to Therapy

FDG-PET imaging is able to accurately predict response to therapy [26,33,37–40]. In a prospective study of patients with locally advanced breast cancer, FDG-PET was able to predict response to therapy after the first course of chemotherapy with a sensitivity of 100%, specificity of 91%, and overall accuracy of 88% [37]. A similarly designed study also showed a high sensitivity (90%) and a good specificity (74%) in prediction of response to chemotherapy after a single dose of chemotherapy [38]. Figure 6.5 demonstrates the ability of FDG-PET to predict response to chemotherapy.

FDG-PET after therapy has also demonstrated significantly higher accuracy in predicting disease relapse or death compared to conventional imaging [26,41,42]. Furthermore, preliminary results support the ability of FDG-PET to provide prognostic information in patients with bone-dominant metastatic disease [39,43].

FDG-PET can alter staging and patient management because of its high sensitivity and accuracy in detection of metastatic disease [33,44]. In a study of 125 patients with breast carcinoma, FDG-PET altered the therapeutic plan in 32% and directly supported the therapeutic plan in 27% of patients [33]. These

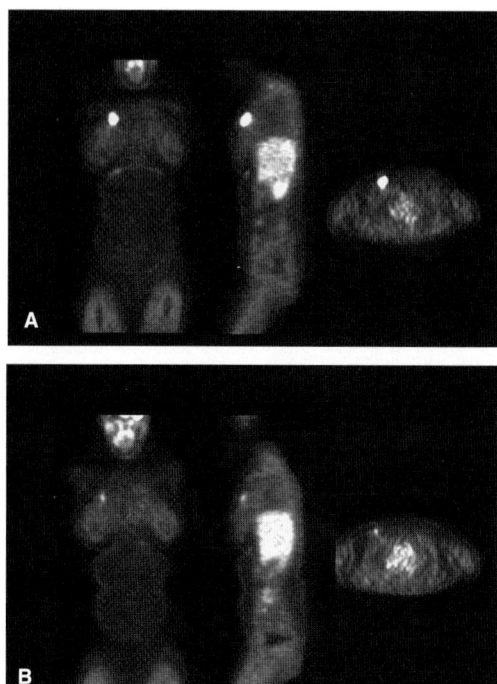

Figure 6.5. A 52-year-old woman with locally advanced, invasive intraductal breast carcinoma. **(A)** Prior to chemotherapy, FDG-PET (left) coronal, (middle) sagittal, and (right) transaxial images demonstrate intense uptake in the primary tumor. **(B)** After chemotherapy, FDG-PET (left) coronal, (middle) sagittal, and (right) transaxial images demonstrate marked reduction in tumor uptake compatible with tumor response to therapy.

results are very similar to an earlier study of FDG-PET that demonstrated a change in clinical stage (36%) and a greater than 30% change in patient management [44].

Potential Limitations

In patients with lobular breast carcinoma, FDG-PET has shown lower uptake and lower sensitivity in detection of the primary lesion [7,45]. Using a clinically relevant threshold for interpretation, 65% (15/23) of primary invasive lobular carcinomas were false negative [7]. A study of primary breast carcinoma also demonstrated a significantly lower FDG uptake in lobular compared to intraductal carcinoma [45]. A specific comparison of FDG uptake in metastatic lesions of lobular compared to intraductal histology has not been yet reported.

A potential limitation in detection of bone disease is in lesions that are osteoblastic. In a study of 23 patients comparing FDG-PET and ^{99m}Tc MDP, FDG-PET detection of bone metastases was reported to have a significantly lower sensitivity in osteoblastic compared to osteolytic bone metastases [46]. Several lesions did not show FDG-PET uptake in osteoblastic lesions that were positive on conventional bone scintigraphy with ^{99m}Tc MDP [46]. Although some patients had radiation therapy, these authors concluded that a significant number of osteoblastic metastases without prior radiotherapy were false negative on FDG-PET imaging. A larger series without segregation of type of bone metastases has demonstrated that the overall sensitivity and accuracy of FDG-PET was higher than that of ^{99m}Tc MDP scintigraphy [47]. Figure 6.6 is an example of

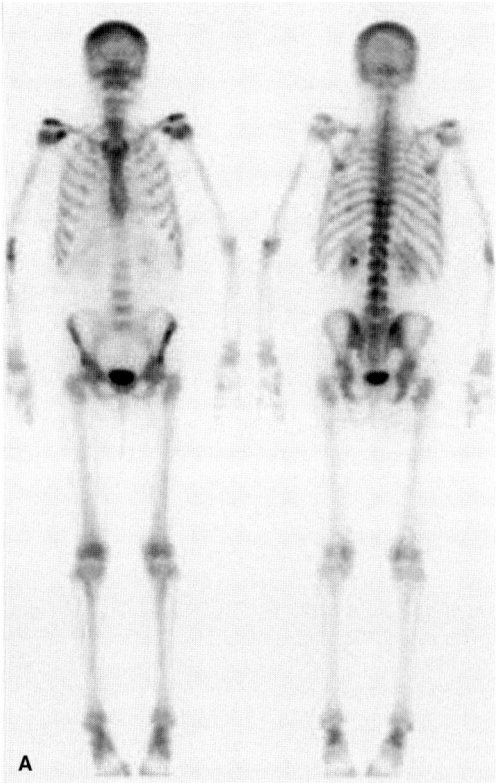

Figure 6.6. **(A)** Anterior and posterior whole-body planar images from a ^{99m}Tc methylene diphosphonate (MDP) bone scan in a patient with breast cancer demonstrates inhomogeneous uptake within the thoracolumbar spine. While this is suspicious for metastatic disease, it is not conclusive.

Continued.

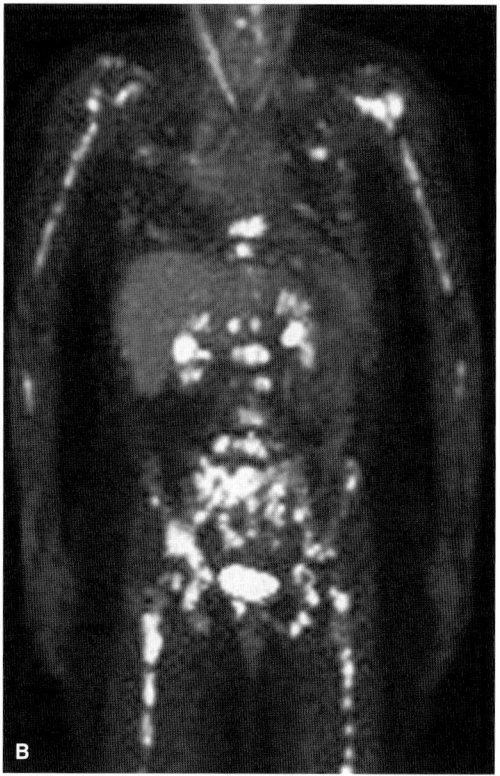

Figure 6.6. *Continued.* **(B)** Maximum intensity projection (MIP) image from an FDG-PET scan of the same patient obtained a few days following the bone scan demonstrates widespread osseous metastatic disease within the axial and proximal appendicular skeleton. Metastatic extent was significantly underestimated by the whole-body bone scan.

underestimation of osseous metastatic disease by bone scan compared to FDG-PET. Patients with osteoblastic bone metastases have better prognosis and survival, and thus, the clinical and biologic significance of reported decreased sensitivity in osteoblastic metastases requires further investigation [46].

As discussed previously, FDG-PET is unable to detect very small and micro-metastatic disease to lymph nodes because of limitations in spatial resolution. Sentinel lymph node biopsy and histologic evaluation is preferable in the staging for early axillary lymph node metastases. Sensitivity and accuracy in detection of primary breast cancer are similarly lower for detection of smaller tumors [7]. Multifocal breast cancer has also shown a relatively low FDG-PET sensitivity of 50–63% in recent studies [7,30]. Some of the new dedicated devices may improve the sensitivity for small lesions and multifocal disease.

The specificity of FDG-PET is relatively high. In a number of studies, specificities of greater than 90% have been reported. Studies are now being performed with co-registered CT which may further improve specificity [48,49]. Cases of false positives have included breast fibroadenoma, inflammation, dysplastic tissue [7], degenerative disease, infection [50], chronic infection, and non-specific lymph node uptake [27]. Physiologic FDG breast uptake is normally higher in patients with dense breasts [51], and in lactating women [52].

Future Directions

New PET radiotracers are currently being investigated to further characterize the biologic properties of breast cancer metabolism, receptor status, blood flow, hypoxia, proliferation [53], and response to hormonal therapy [54]. For example, ^{18}F fluoride may be more sensitive than conventional planar bone scintigraphy with ^{99m}Tc MDP in the detection of skeletal metastatic disease, and in addition, may be able to detect osteoblastic disease which may not have FDG uptake [46,55]. Advances in combined PET/CT are promising for improving accuracy in radiotherapy planning, and for improving accuracy in staging [20,48,49]. Research is currently being performed to determine the feasibility of using ^{18}F-FDG in high doses for radiotherapy [56].

References

1. Greenlee RT, Hill-Harmon MB, Murray T, Thun M. Cancer statistics, 2001. Ca-A Cancer Journal for Clinicians 2001;51:15–36.
2. American Cancer Society. Estimated new cancer cases and deaths by sex for all sites, US, 2004. American Cancer Society; 2004.
3. Singletary SE, Allred C, Ashley P, et al. Staging system for breast cancer: revisions for the sixth edition of the AJCC Cancer Staging Manual. Surg Clin North Am 2003; 83:803.
4. Woodward WA, Strom EA, Tucker SL, et al. Changes in the 2003 American Joint Committee on Cancer staging for breast cancer dramatically affect stage-specific survival. J Clin Oncol 2003;21:3244–3248.
5. Wahl RL, Cody RL, Hutchins GD, Mudgett EE. Primary and metastatic breast carcinoma: initial clinical evaluation with PET with the radiolabeled glucose analogue 2-[F-18]-fluoro-2-deoxy-D-glucose. Radiology 1991;179:765–770.
6. Nieweg OE, Kim EE, Wong WH, et al. Positron emission tomography with fluorine-18-deoxyglucose in the detection and staging of breast cancer. Cancer 1993;71: 3920–3925.
7. Avril N, Rose CA, Schelling M, et al. Breast imaging with positron emission tomography and fluorine-18 fluorodeoxyglucose: use and limitations. J Clin Oncol 2000; 18:3495–3502.

8. Samson DJ, Flamm CR, Pisano ED, Aronson N. Should FDG PET be used to decide whether a patient with an abnormal mammogram or breast finding at physical examination should undergo biopsy? Acad Radiol 2002;9:773–783.

9. Adler LP, Weinberg IN, Bradbury MS, et al. Method for combined FDG-PET and radiographic imaging of primary breast cancers. Breast J 2003;9:163–166.

10. Levine EA, Freimanis RI, Perrier ND, et al. Positron emission mammography: initial clinical results. Ann Surg Oncol 2003;10:86–91.

11. Raylman RR, Majewski S, Weisenberger AG, et al. Positron emission mammography-guided breast biopsy. J Nucl Med 2001;42:960–966.

12. Rosen EL, Turkington T, Soo MS, Baker JA, Coleman RE. Detection of primary breast carcinoma with a dedicated large field of view FDG-PET mammography device: initial experience. Radiology 2005;234:527–534.

13. Smith MF, Raylman RR, Majewski S, Weisenberger AG. Positron emission mammography with tomographic acquisition using dual planar detectors: initial evaluations. Phys Med Biol 2004;49:2437–2452.

14. Murthy K, Aznar M, Thompson CJ, Loutfi A, Lisbona R, Gagnon JH. Results of preliminary clinical trials of the positron emission mammography system PEM-I: a dedicated breast imaging system producing glucose metabolic images using FDG. J Nucl Med 2000;41:1851–1858.

15. Murthy K, Aznar M, Bergman AM, et al. Positron emission mammographic instrument: initial results. Radiology 2000;215:280–285.

16. Thompson CJ, Murthy K, Aznar M, Lisbona R, Loutfi A. Preliminary clinical evaluation of an instrument for "positron emission mammography" in the detection of breast cancer. Clin Positron Imaging 1998;1:265.

17. Doshi NK, Shao Y, Silverman RW, Cherry SR. Design and evaluation of an LSO PET detector for breast cancer imaging. Med Phys 2000;27:1535–1543.

18. Eubank WB, Mankoff DA. Current and future uses of positron emission tomography in breast cancer imaging. Semin Nucl Med 2004;34:224–240.

19. Zangheri B, Messa C, Picchio M, Gianolli L, Landoni C, Fazio F. PET/CT and breast cancer. Eur J Nucl Med Mol Imaging 2004;31(Suppl 1):S135–142.

20. Siggelkow W, Rath W, Buell U, Zimny M. FDG PET and tumour markers in the diagnosis of recurrent and metastatic breast cancer. Eur J Nucl Med Mol Imaging 2004; 31(Suppl 1):S118–124.

21. Lind P, Igerc I, Beyer T, Reinprecht P, Hausegger K. Advantages and limitations of FDG PET in the follow-up of breast cancer. Eur J Nucl Med Mol Imaging 2004; 31(Suppl 1):S125–134.

22. Kamel EM, Wyss MT, Fehr MK, von Schulthess GK, Goerres GW. [18F]-Fluorodeoxyglucose positron emission tomography in patients with suspected recurrence of breast cancer. J Cancer Res Clin Oncol 2003;129:147–153.

23. Eubank WB, Mankoff DA, Takasugi J, et al. (18)Fluorodeoxyglucose positron emission tomography to detect mediastinal or internal mammary metastases in breast cancer. J Clin Oncol 2001;19:3516–3523.

24. Isasi CR, Moadel RM, Blaufox MD. A meta-analysis of FDG-PET for the evaluation of breast cancer recurrence and metastases. Breast Cancer Res Treat 2005;90: 105–112.

25. Vranjesevic D, Filmont JE, Meta J, et al. Whole-body F-18-FDG PET and conventional imaging for predicting outcome in previously treated breast cancer patients. J Nucl Med 2002;43:325–329.

26. Dose J, Bleckmann C, Bachmann S, et al. Comparison of fluorodeoxyglucose positron emission tomography and "conventional diagnostic procedures" for the detection of distant metastases in breast cancer patients. Nucl Med Commun 2002; 23:857–864.

27. Goerres GW, Michel SCA, Fehr MK, et al. Follow-up of women with breast cancer: comparison between MRI and FDG PET. Eur Radiol 2003;13:1635–1644.

28. Gallowitsch HJ, Kresnik E, Gasser J, et al. F-18 fluorodeoxyglucose positron-emission tomography in the diagnosis of tumor recurrence and metastases in the follow-up of patients with breast carcinoma: a comparison to conventional imaging. Invest Radiol 2003;38:250–256.

29. van der Hoeven JJM, Krak NC, Hoekstra OS, et al. F-18-2-fluoro-2-deoxy-D-glucose positron emission tomography in staging of locally advanced breast cancer. J Clin Oncol 2004;22:1253–1259.

30. Schirrmeister H, Kuhn T, Guhlmann A, et al. Fluorine-18 2-deoxy-2-fluoro-D-glucose PET in the preoperative staging of breast cancer: comparison with the standard staging procedures. Eur J Nucl Med 2001;28:351–358.

31. Bellon JR, Livingston RB, Eubank WB, et al. Evaluation of the internal mammary lymph nodes by FDG-PET in locally advanced breast cancer (LABC). Am J Clin Oncol 2004;27:407–410.

32. Eubank WB, Mankoff DA, Shanley TJ, et al. Risk factors associated with metastasis to mediastinal or internal mammary (IM) nodes detected at FDG PET in breast cancer patients suspected of locoregional spread of disease. J Nucl Med 2000;41:28P.

33. Eubank WB, Mankoff D, Bhattacharya M, et al. Impact of FDG PET on defining the extent of disease and on the treatment of patients with recurrent or metastatic breast cancer. AJR Am J Roentgenol 2004;183:479–486.

34. Wahl RL, Siegel BA, Coleman RE, Gatsonis CG. Prospective multicenter study of axillary nodal staging by positron emission tomography in breast cancer: a report of the Staging Breast Cancer with PET Study Group. J Clin Oncol 2004;22:277–285.

35. van der Hoeven JJM, Hoekstra OS, Comans EFI, et al. Determinants of diagnostic performance of [F-18]fluorodeoxyglucose positron emission tomography for axillary staging in breast cancer. Ann Surg 2002;236:619–624.

36. Crippa F, Gerali A, Alessi A, Agresti R, Bombardieri E. FDG-PET for axillary lymph node staging in primary breast cancer. Eur J Nucl Med Mol Imaging 2004;31(Suppl 1):S97–102.

37. Schelling M, Avril N, Nahrig J, et al. Positron emission tomography using [F-18]fluorodeoxyglucose for monitoring primary chemotherapy in breast cancer. J Clin Oncol 2000;18:1689–1695.

38. Smith IC, Welch AE, Hutcheon AW, et al. Positron emission tomography using [F-18]-fluorodeoxy-D-glucose to predict the pathologic response of breast cancer to primary chemotherapy. J Clin Oncol 2000;18:1676–1688.

39. Stafford SE, Gralow JR, Schubert EK, et al. Use of serial FDG PET to measure the response of bone-dominant breast cancer to therapy. Acad Radiol 2002;9:913–921.

40. Kim SJ, Kim SK, Lee ES, Ro J, Kang S. Predictive value of [18F]FDG PET for pathological response of breast cancer to neo-adjuvant chemotherapy. Ann Oncol 2004;15:1352–1357.

41. Vranjesevic D, Filmont JE, Schiepers C, et al. Prognostic value of FDG-PET for predicting the outcome of re-staged breast cancer patients. J Nucl Med 2001;42: 81P.

42. Oshida M, Uno K, Suzuki M, et al. Predicting the prognoses of breast carcinoma patients with positron emission tomography using 2-deoxy-2-fluoro[F-18]-D-glucose. Cancer. 1998;82:2227–2234.

43. Biersack HJ, Bender H, Palmedo H. FDG-PET in monitoring therapy of breast cancer. Eur J Nucl Med Mol Imaging. 2004;31:S112–117.

44. Yap CS, Seltzer MA, Schiepers C, et al. Impact of whole-body F-18-FDG PET on staging and managing patients with breast cancer: the referring physician's perspective. J Nucl Med 2001;42:1334–1337.

45. Bos R, van der Hoeven JJM, van der Wall E, et al. Biologic correlates of (18)fluorodeoxyglucose uptake in human breast cancer measured by positron emission tomography. J Clin Oncol 2002;20:379–387.

46. Cook GJ, Houston S, Rubens R, Maisey MN, Fogelman I. Detection of bone metastases in breast cancer by (18)FDG PET: differing metabolic activity in osteoblastic and osteolytic lesions. J Clin Oncol 1998;16:3375–3379.

47. Yang SN, Liang JA, Lin FJ, Kao CH, Lin CC, Lee CC. Comparing whole body F-18–2-deoxyglucose positron emission tomography and technetium-99 m methylene diphosphonate bone scan to detect bone metastases in patients with breast cancer. J Cancer Res Clin Oncol 2002;128:325–328.

48. Tatsumi M, Cohade C, Mourtzikos K, Wahl RL. Initial experience with FDG PET/CT in the evaluation of breast cancer. J Nucl Med 2003;44:394p [abstract].

49. Buck A, Wahl A, Eischer U, et al. Combined morphological and functional imaging with FDG PET/CT for restaging breast cancer: impact on patient management. J Nucl Med 2003;44:78p [abstract].

50. Lonneux M, Borbath I, Berlière M, Kirkove C, Pauwels S. The place of whole-body PET FDG for the diagnosis of distant recurrence of breast cancer. Mol Imaging Biol 2000;3:45–49.

51. Vranjesevic D, Schiepers C, Silverman DH, et al. Relationship between F-18-FDG uptake and breast density in women with normal breast tissue. J Nucl Med 2003; 44:1238–1242.

52. Hicks RJ, Binns D, Stabin MG. Pattern of uptake and excretion of F-18-FDG in the lactating breast. J Nucl Med 2001;42:1238–1242.

53. Buck AK, Schirrmeister H, Mattfeldt T, Reske SN. Biological characterisation of breast cancer by means of PET. Eur J Nucl Med Mol Imaging 2004;31(Suppl 1): S80–87.

54. Mortimer JE, Dehdashti F, Siegel BA, Trinkaus K, Katzenellenbogen JA, Welch MJ. Metabolic flare: indicator of hormone responsiveness in advanced breast cancer. J Clin Oncol 2001;19:2797–2803.

55. Cook GJR, Fogelman I. Detection of bone metastases in cancer patients by F-18-fluoride and F-18-fluorodeoxyglucose positron emission tomography. Q J Nucl Med 2001;45:47–52.
56. Moadel RM, Nguyen AV, Lin EY, et al. Positron emission tomography agent 2-deoxy-2-[18F]fluoro-D-glucose has a therapeutic potential in breast cancer. Breast Cancer Res 2003;5:R199–205.

7. PET and PET/CT in Head and Neck Cancer

Nirav P. Shah, Ronald B. Workman, Jr., and R. Edward Coleman

Epidemiology

In 2005, head and neck cancer involving the nasopharynx, larynx, and hypopharynx collectively afflicted over 39,000 patients in the United States. These malignancies occur more often in men, especially over the age of 60, with higher prevalence in blacks than whites. Clinically, patients present with various signs and symptoms, including dysphagia, odynophagia, shortness of breath, palpable mass, hemoptysis, pain, bleeding, hoarseness, and hearing loss. According to the American Cancer Society, the most important risk factors related to the development of head and neck cancer are alcohol use, tobacco use, poor nutrition, chronic human papillomavirus infection, compromised immune function, and occupational exposure in industries such as metalworking, textiles, and petroleum [1].

Diagnosis of a head and neck cancer is usually made with a combination of history, physical examination, and either nasopharyngoscopy and/or laryngoscopy with directed biopsies or percutaneous fine-needle aspiration of clinically palpable masses and/or nodes. Panendoscopy (laryngoscopy, esophagoscopy, and possible bronchoscopy) may be necessary to reveal the true extent of tumor involvement. Anatomic imaging evaluation with head and neck computed tomography (CT) and/or magnetic resonance imaging (MRI) with intravenous contrast is often utilized either prior to panendoscopy to non-invasively assess the aerodigestive tract, or afterward to provide information about primary tumor size, penetration, involvement of surrounding structures, and regional nodal involvement. A chest radiograph or CT of the chest is also performed in the majority of patients to evaluate for lung or lower airway metastases or possible synchronous tumors.

Malignancies of the head and neck can be divided based upon their site of origin into several categories: lip and oral cavity, nasopharynx, larynx, hypopharynx, paranasal sinuses, and major salivary glands. Lymphoma and tumors involving the brain, thyroid, and skin are classified separately and are discussed elsewhere in this text. Accurate and complete staging is essential in order to most effectively categorize the primary tumor, provide prognostic **information**, and to plan appropriate therapy. Staging of head and neck cancers is most often performed using the *American Joint Committee on Cancer Staging Manual*, which utilizes a system based upon defining three components of malignancy: primary tumor size and extent (T), regional nodal involvement

(N), and distant metastases (M) [2]. The (T) staging is specific for the particular site of involvement of the primary tumor, but both the (N) and (M) staging for all head and neck sites are similar (except nodal staging for nasopharyngeal sites). See Tables 7.1 and 7.2 for the TNM staging of head and neck cancer.

Additional factors not included in determination of staging but important in therapy planning and prognosis are histologic type and grade of tumor, lymphatic and/or venous invasion, and patient performance status [2]. There are a wide variety of histologic tumor types, including large cell, giant cell, small cell, adenocarcinoma, adenoid cystic, mucoepidermoid, clear cell, oat cell, basal cell, squamous cell, and mixed variants. However, squamous cell carcinomas comprise the vast majority of head and neck cancers and will be the focus of this chapter because the use of PET and PET/CT is most documented with this tumor type.

Therapy for head and neck cancer is dependent upon staging and will generally include a combination of surgery, radiation therapy, and chemotherapy.

Table 7.1. TNM staging for head and neck cancer

Primary tumor (T): lip and oral cavity

TX	Primary tumor cannot be assessed
T0	No evidence of primary tumor
Tis	Carcinoma in situ
T1	Tumor 2 cm or less in greatest dimension
T2	Tumor more than 2 cm but not more than 4 cm in greatest dimension
T3	Tumor more than 4 cm in greatest dimension
T4	(Lip) Tumor invades through the cortical bone, inferior alveolar nerve, floor of mouth, or skin of face, i.e., chin or nose
T4a	(Oral cavity) Tumor invades through cortical bone, into deep (extrinsic) muscle of tongue (genioglossus, hyoglossus, palatoglossus, and styloglossus), maxillary sinus, or skin of face
T4b	Tumor invades masticator space, ptyergoid plates, or skull base, and/or encases internal carotid artery

Primary tumor (T): nasopharynx

TX	Primary tumor cannot be assessed
T0	No evidence of primary tumor
Tis	Carcinoma in situ
T1	Tumor confined to the nasopharynx
T2	Tumor extends to soft tissues
T2a	Tumor extends to the oropharynx and/or the nasal cavity without parapharyngeal extension*
T2b	Any tumor with parapharyngeal extension*
T3	Tumor involves bony structures and/or paranasal sinuses
T4	Tumor with intracranial extension and/or involvement of cranial nerves, infratemporal fossa, hypopharynx, orbit, or masticator space

Continued.

Table 7.1. *Continued.* TNM staging for head and neck cancer

Primary tumor (T): oropharynx

TX	Primary tumor cannot be assessed
T0	No evidence of primary tumor
Tis	Carcinoma in situ
T1	Tumor 2 cm or less in greatest dimension
T2	Tumor more than 2 cm but not more than 4 cm in greatest dimension
T3	Tumor more than 4 cm in greatest dimension
T4a	Tumor invades the larynx, deep/extrinsic muscle of tongue, medial ptyergoid, hard palate, or mandible
T4b	Tumor invades lateral ptyergoid muscle, ptyergoid plates, lateral nasopharynx, or skull base or encases carotid artery

Primary tumor (T): larynx – supraglottic

TX	Primary tumor cannot be assessed
T0	No evidence of primary tumor
Tis	Carcinoma in situ
T1	Tumor limited to one subsite of supraglottis with normal vocal cord mobility
T2	Tumor invades mucosa of more than one adjacent subsite of supraglottis or glottis or region outside the supraglottis without fixation of the larynx
T3	Tumor limited to larynx with vocal cord fixation and/or invades any of the following: post-cricoid area, pre-epiglottic tissues, paraglottic space, and/or minor thyroid cartilage erosion (e.g. inner cortex)
T4a	Tumor invades through the thyroid cartilage and/or invades tissue beyond the larynx
T4b	Tumor invades prevertebral space, encases carotid artery, or invades mediastinal structures

Primary tumor (T): larynx – glottic

TX	Primary tumor cannot be assessed
T0	No evidence of primary tumor
Tis	Carcinoma in situ
T1	Tumor limited to the vocal cord with normal mobility
T1a	Tumor limited to one vocal cord
T1b	Tumor involves both vocal cords
T2	Tumor extends to supraglottis and/or subglottis, or with impaired vocal cord mobility
T3	Tumor limited to larynx with vocal cord fixation, and/or invades paraglottic space, and/or minor thyroid cartilage erosion (e.g. inner cortex)
T4a	Tumor invades through the thyroid cartilage and/or invades tissues beyond the larynx
T4b	Tumor invades prevertebral space, encases carotid artery, or invades mediastinal structures

Continued.

Table 7.1. *Continued.*

Primary tumor (T): larynx – subglottic

TX	Primary tumor cannot be assessed
T0	No evidence of primary tumor
Tis	Carcinoma in situ
T1	Tumor limited to the subglottis
T2	Tumor extends to the vocal cord(s) with normal or impaired mobility
T3	Tumor limited to larynx with vocal cord fixation
T4a	Tumor invades cricoid or thyroid cartilage and/or invades tissues beyond the larynx
T4b	Tumor invades prevertebral space, encases carotid artery, or invades mediastinal structures

Primary tumor (T): hypopharynx

TX	Primary tumor cannot be assessed
T0	No evidence of primary tumor
Tis	Carcinoma in situ
T1	Tumor limited to one subsite of hypopharynx and 2 cm or less in greatest dimension
T2	Tumor invades more than one subsite of hypopharynx or an adjacent site, or measures more than 2 cm but not more than 4 cm in greatest dimension without fixation of hemilarynx
T3	Tumor measures more than 4 cm in greatest dimension or with fixation of hemilarynx
T4a	Tumor invades thyroid/cricoid cartilage, hyoid bone, thyroid gland, esophagus, or central compartment soft tissue
T4b	Tumor invades prevertebral fascia, encases carotid artery, or involves mediastinal structures

Primary tumor (T): major salivary glands

TX	Primary tumor cannot be assessed
T0	No evidence of primary tumor
T1	Tumor 2 cm or less in greatest dimension without extraparenchymal extension†
T2	Tumor more than 2 cm but not more than 4 cm in greatest dimension without extraparenchymal extension†
T3	Tumor more than 4 cm in greatest dimension and/or having extraparenchymal extension†
T4a	Tumor invades skin, mandible, ear canal and/or facial nerve
T4b	Tumor invades skull base and/or pterygoid plates and/or encases carotid artery

Primary tumor (T): paranasal sinuses – maxillary

TX	Primary tumor cannot be assessed
T0	No evidence of primary tumor
Tis	Carcinoma in situ
T1	Tumor limited to maxillary sinus mucosa with no erosion or destruction of bone

Continued.

Table 7.1. *Continued.* TNM staging for head and neck cancer

T2	Tumor causing bone erosion or destruction including extension into hard palate and/or middle nasal meatus, except extension to the posterior wall of maxillary sinus and pterygoid plates
T3	Tumor invades any of the following: bone of posterior wall of maxillary sinus, subcutaneous tissues, floor or medial wall of orbit, pterygoid fossa, ethmoid sinuses
T4a	Tumor invades anterior orbital contents, skin of cheek, pterygoid plates, infratemporal fossa, cribriform plate, sphenoid or frontal sinuses
T4b	Tumor invades any of the following: orbital apex, dura, brain, middle cranial fossa, cranial nerves other than maxillary division of trigeminal nerve V2, nasopharynx, or clivus

Primary tumor (T): paranasal sinuses: nasal cavity and ethmoid sinus

TX	Primary tumor cannot be assessed
T0	No evidence of primary tumor
Tis	Carcinoma in situ
T1	Tumor restricted to any one subsite, with or without bony invasion
T2	Tumor invading two subsites in a single region or extending to involve an adjacent region within the nasoethmoidal complex, with or without bony invasion
T3	Tumor extends to invade the medial wall or floor of the orbit, maxillary sinus, palate, or cribriform plate
T4a	Tumor invades any of the following: anterior orbital contents, skin of nose or cheek, minimal extension to anterior cranial fossa, pterygoid plates, sphenoid or frontal sinuses
T4b	Tumor invades any of the following: orbital apex, dura, brain, middle cranial fossa, cranial nerves other than maxillary division of trigeminal nerve V2, nasopharynx, or clivus

Regional lymph nodes (N): lip and oral cavity, oropharynx, larynx, hypopharynx, major salivary glands, and paranasal sinuses

NX	Regional lymph nodes cannot be assessed
N0	No regional lymph node metastasis
N1	Metastasis in a single ipsilateral lymph node, 3 cm or less in greatest dimension
N2	Metastasis in a single ipsilateral lymph node, more than 3 cm but not more than 6 cm in greatest dimension; or in multiple ipsilateral lymph nodes, none more than 6 cm in greatest dimension; or in bilateral or contralateral lymph nodes, none more than 6 cm in greatest dimension
N2a	Metastasis in a single ipsilateral lymph node more than 3 cm but not more than 6 cm in greatest dimension
N2b	Metastasis in multiple ipsilateral lymph nodes, none more than 6 cm in greatest dimension
N2c	Metastasis in bilateral or contralateral lymph nodes, none more than 6 cm in greatest dimension
N3	Metastasis in a lymph node more than 6 cm in greatest dimension

Table 7.1. *Continued.*

Regional lymph nodes (N): nasopharynx
NX   Regional lymph nodes cannot be assessed
N0   No regional lymph node metastasis
N1   Unilateral metastasis in lymph node(s), 6 cm or less in greatest
        dimension, above the supraclavicular fossa
N2   Bilateral metastasis in lymph node(s), 6 cm or less in greatest
        dimension, above the supraclavicular fossa
N3   Metastasis in a lymph node >6 cm, and/or to supraclavicular fossa
N3a   Greater than 6 cm in dimension
N3b   Extension to the supraclavicular fossa

Distant metastasis (M): ALL head and neck sites
MX   Distant metastasis cannot be assessed
M0   No distant metastasis
M1   Distant metastasis

---

* Parapharyngeal extension denotes posterolateral infiltration of tumor beyond the pharyngobasilar fascia.
† *Note*: Extraparenchymal extension is clinical or macroscopic evidence of invasion of soft tissues. Microscopic evidence alone does not constitute extraparenchymal extension for classification purposes.
Source: Used with permission of the American Joint Committee on Cancer (AJCC), Chicago, Illinois. The original source for this material is the *AJCC Cancer Staging Manual*, Sixth Edition (2002), published by Springer-Verlag, New York, www.springeronline.com.

Table 7.2. TNM stage grouping for head and neck cancer

Stage	**T**	**N**	**M**
Lip and oral cavity			
0	Tis	N0	M0
I	T1	N0	M0
II	T2	N0	M0
III	T3	N0	M0
	T1	N1	
	T2	N1	
	T3	N1	
IVA	T4a	N0	M0
	T4a	N1	
	T1	N2	
	T2	N2	
	T3	N2	
	T4a	N2	
IVB	Any T	N3	M0
	T4b	Any N	
IVC	Any T	Any N	M1

Continued.

Table 7.2. *Continued.* TNM stage grouping for head and neck cancer

Stage	T	N	M
Nasopharynx			
0	Tis	N0	M0
I	T1	N0	M0
IIA	T2a	N0	M0
IIB	T1	N1	M0
	T2	N1	
	T2a	N1	
	T2b	N0	
	T2b	N1	
III	T1	N2	M0
	T2a	N2	
	T2b	N2	
	T3	N0	
	T3	N1	
	T3	N2	
IVA	T4	N0	M0
	T4	N1	
	T4	N2	
IVB	Any T	N3	M0
IVC	Any T	Any N	M1
Oropharynx and hypopharynx			
0	Tis	N0	M0
I	T1	N0	M0
II	T2	N0	M0
III	T3	N0	M0
	T1	N1	
	T2	N1	
	T3	N1	
IVA	T4a	N0	M0
	T4a	N1	
	T1	N2	
	T2	N2	
	T3	N2	
	T4a	N2	
IVB	T4b	Any N	M0
	Any T	N3	
IVC	Any T	Any N	M1
Larynx (supraglottic, glottic, subglottic)			
0	Tis	N0	M0
I	T1	N0	M0
II	T2	N0	M0
III	T3	N0	M0
	T1	N1	
	T2	N1	
	T3	N1	

Table 7.2. *Continued.*

Stage	T	N	M
IVA	T4a	N0	M0
	T4a	N1	
	T1	N2	
	T2	N2	
	T3	N2	
	T4a	N2	
IVB	T4b	Any N	M0
	Any T	N3	
IVC	Any T	Any N	M1
Nasal cavity and paranasal sinuses			
0	Tis	N0	M0
I	T1	N0	M0
II	T2	N0	M0
III	T3	N0	M0
	T1	N1	
	T2	N1	
	T3	N1	
IVA	T4a	N0	M0
	T4a	N1	
	T1	N2	
	T2	N2	
	T3	N2	
	T4a	N2	
IVB	T4b	Any N	M0
	Any T	N3	
IVC	Any T	Any N	M1
Major salivary glands			
I	T1	N0	M0
II	T2	N0	M0
III	T3	N0	M0
	T1	N1	
	T2	N1	
	T3	N1	
IVA	T4a	N0	M0
	T4a	N1	
	T1	N2	
	T2	N2	
	T3	N2	
	T4a	N2	
IVB	T4b	Any N	M0
	Any T	N3	
IVC	Any T	Any N	M1

Source: Used with permission of the American Joint Committee on Cancer (AJCC), Chicago, Illinois. The original source for this material is the *AJCC Cancer Staging Manual*, Sixth Edition (2002), published by Springer-Verlag, New York, www.springeronline.com.

Neoadjuvant or adjuvant radiotherapy, and/or neoadjuvant chemotherapy can also be used to complement surgery, and it is generally now recognized that combination therapy is the best approach in the majority of patients, especially those with higher stage disease.

Positron Emission Tomography and Head and Neck Cancer

Positron emission tomography (PET) is a functional nuclear medicine imaging technique that is used to assess biochemical, metabolic, and physiologic parameters of disease. Many metabolic and cell biological processes are altered in neoplastic cells as compared to normal or non-neoplastic cells, including glucose consumption, DNA synthesis, amino acid synthesis, perfusion, oxygenation, and cell membrane synthesis among others. PET employs radioactive analogues of these biological substances and others and is able to provide images of their distribution and localization in the body, and how this is changed with disease involvement and therapy. The most common and studied PET radiotracer is ^{18}F-2-fluoro-2-deoxy-D-glucose (FDG), which is a Food and Drug Administration (FDA)-approved analogue of endogenous glucose and is used to detect areas of altered glucose utilization in the body. Many types of neoplastic cells take up glucose to a much greater degree than normal cells, because of the higher energy requirements and increased rates of cell growth and division. For more information on the fundamentals of PET and FDG, see Chapter 1. Head and neck squamous cell cancers (HNSCC) have been found to be very glucose-avid, and therefore FDG is an excellent tracer to study this malignancy [3].

The spatial resolution of PET is higher than that of SPECT or routine planar nuclear imaging studies, but less than either CT or MRI. The lower resolution of PET has been addressed with the development of combined PET/CT scanners, which house both a PET and CT mechanically integrated in one machine. The advent of the PET/CT now permits the evaluation of both metabolic and anatomic characteristics of disease, which has proven to be a major advance for diagnosis, initial staging, evaluation of therapy response, restaging, and evaluation of recurrence of head and neck cancer. The metabolic information provided by PET and PET/CT has been proven in many cases to be a more accurate predictor of malignant involvement, response to therapy, and presence of recurrent disease than anatomic imaging alone [4–6]. PET and PET/CT are also useful in guiding biopsy, predicting therapy response and prognosis, and characterizing indeterminate lesions found by other imaging. An important principle that underlies the utility of PET is that tumor involvement can occur in tissue that appears normal by anatomic imaging, and that resolution or eradication of disease with therapy is closely paralleled by changes in metabolism. Anatomic resolution of diseased tissues can many times lag behind the metabolic resolution. A whole-body PET can be completed in less than 1 hour, while a whole-body PET/CT can be obtained in less than 30 minutes, providing an effective means of evaluating total body involvement of malignancy and a very useful tool for staging.

PET imaging of head and neck cancer with ^{18}F FDG was approved by the Centers for Medicare and Medicaid Services (CMS) in 2001, and subsequently by most other private medical insurers, for reimbursement in the diagnosis, initial staging, and restaging of patients with suspected or confirmed head and neck cancer.

Diagnosis

PET and PET/CT are sensitive, specific, and accurate in the detection of primary squamous cell carcinomas of the head and neck. Minn et al. initially described increased uptake of FDG in primary tumors of the head and neck in 1988 [7]. Multiple subsequent studies have demonstrated high overall accuracy of PET in detection of primary lesions subsequently confirmed by histopathology [8–10] (Figure 7.1). PET has even been found to detect small tumors that may be missed by anatomic imaging [3]. The level of uptake within the primary tumor has been found to carry prognostic significance; Reisser et al. studied 50 patients with HNSCC and found that higher levels of FDG uptake carried a poorer prognosis [11]. However, the metabolic information from PET alone is not capable of providing the detailed anatomic information necessary for complete T staging of tumors, and small lesions or those with either low volume of tumor or very low histologic grade may fall below the spatial resolution limit of most PET scanners or have FDG uptake which is not clearly distinguishable from surrounding tissue. Therefore, in most centers, FDG-PET imaging is not used routinely for primary tumor detection and T staging. Visualization with nasopharyngoscopy, laryngoscopy, and/or panendoscopy with directed biopsy remains the standard for lesion detection and diagnosis. High resolution CT and/or MRI with intravenous contrast is also mandatory for accurate evaluation of tumor size, depth of invasion, and involvement of surrounding structures.

Recent advances with combined PET/CT imaging have improved the ability to detect primary lesions by accurately characterizing metabolically abnormal lesions with important complementary anatomic localization, and thus to differentiate pathology from normal biodistribution of FDG. Newer generation PET/CT scanners incorporating improved sensitivity detectors that provide better image resolution, along with multidetector CT technology able to image 0.5–1.0-mm slice thickness in multiple planes, provide improved lesion detection and characterization. The use of PET/CT provides opportunity to use intravenous contrast for the CT, and the combination of metabolic information provided by PET with the detailed anatomic information available with intravenous contrast-enhanced thin-slice CT will become an important non-invasive complement to endoscopy and biopsy for T staging in head and neck cancer.

PET and PET/CT imaging has been found particularly helpful at the time of diagnosis in two subsets of patients: those with carcinoma of unknown primary with evidence of neck nodal metastases, and those patients who have synchronous or second primary malignancies. Occasionally, patients present with confirmed neck nodal metastases in which the primary tumor site is uncertain. The conventional work-up usually includes anatomic imaging including CT/MRI of the neck along with whole-body CT imaging. In addition, panendoscopy is also

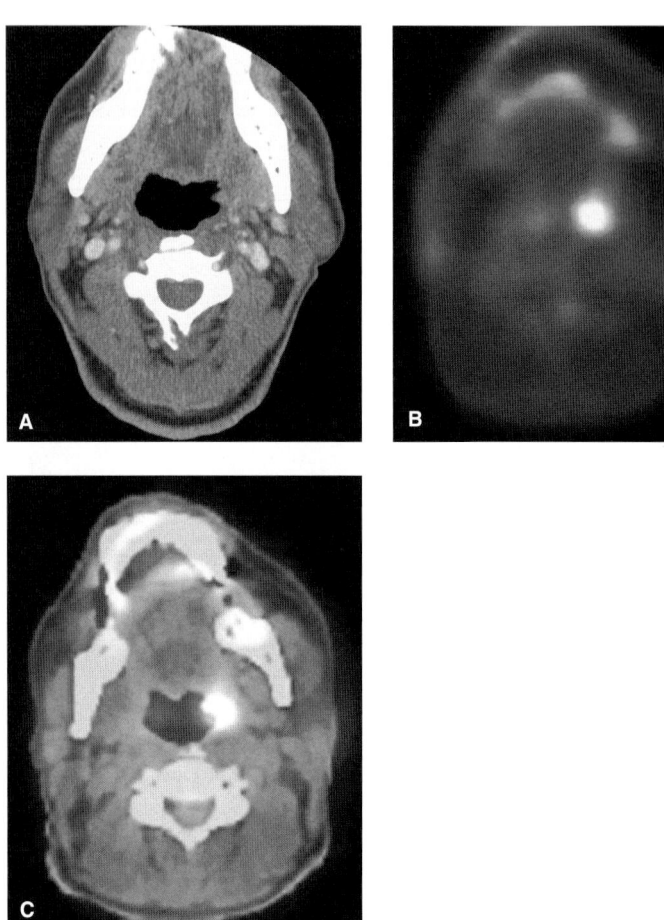

Figure 7.1. Left pharyngeal T1 squamous cell cancer (SCC). Axial CT with contrast **(A)**, PET **(B)**, and PET/CT fusion **(C)**. Both PET and PET/CT fusion reveal
focal hypermetabolic uptake localizing to left posterolateral pharynx near the
left palatine tonsil, corresponding to subtle soft tissue fullness on contrast-
enhanced CT.

performed with either directed biopsy of discovered lesions and/or random sampling of regions such as the tonsils and base of tongue. However, this work-up
fails to identify the primary site in a significant proportion of patients. PET and
PET/CT have been found to be very useful in these patients, discovering the
primary lesion in approximately 25% of cases [12,13] (Figure 7.2).

Patients with head and neck cancers are also at significant risk of developing second primaries, either in the head and neck or elsewhere in the body. Patients with head and neck cancer have a 4% incidence per year of developing second primary neoplasms, with approximately 30% of these lesions outside the head and neck, including the lungs, esophagus, and colon [14] (Figure 7.3). The incorporation of whole-body PET and PET/CT imaging into the staging and

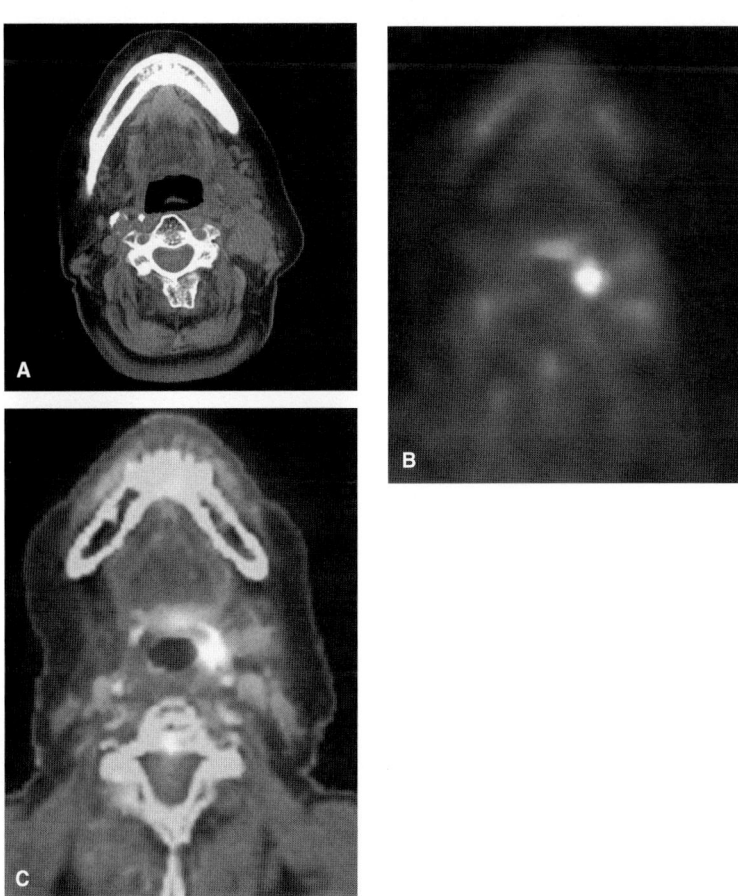

Figure 7.2. Carcinoma of unknown primary. Axial CT with contrast **(A)**, PET **(B)**, and PET/CT fusion **(C)**. Initial CT reveals conglomerate left level 2 lymph nodes, biopsied as squamous cell carcinoma. Initial endoscopic evaluation was negative. Subsequent PET and PET/CT fusion reveal focal hypermetabolic uptake within the left lateral hypopharyngeal wall near aryepiglottic fold. Follow-up biopsies revealed primary SCC.

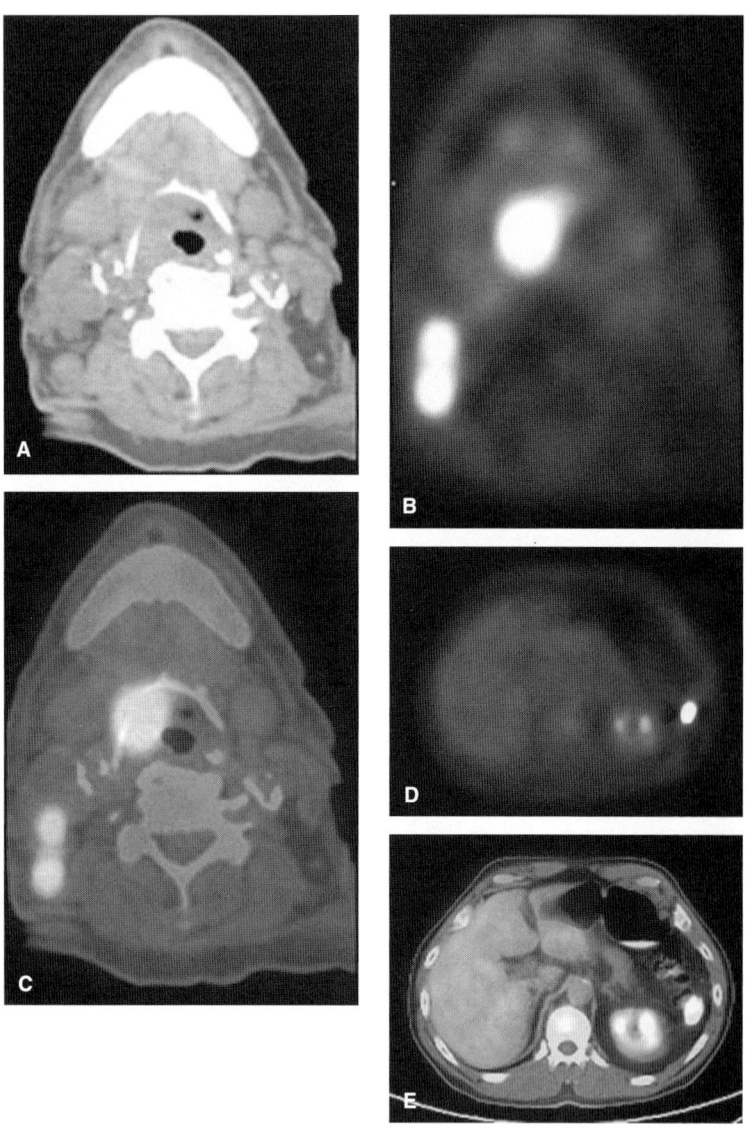

Figure 7.3. Unsuspected second primary. Axial CT **(A)**, PET **(B)**, and PET/CT fusion **(C)** reveal known right supraglottic T2 SCC with ipsilateral level 3 nodes during initial staging work-up. However, incidental finding of focal hypermetabolic uptake within left colon on other PET **(D)**, and PET/CT fusion **(E)** images from same study. Colonoscopy revealed colorectal adenocarcinoma.

restaging algorithms of head and neck cancer patients can be very effective in discovering these lesions.

Staging

Accurate staging of head and neck cancer involvement is essential for effective therapy planning and prognosis. Usually, a combination of primary site biopsy (tumor type and grade) along with anatomic imaging with either contrast-enhanced CT or MRI of the neck is performed to fully assess T and N staging. About 10–15% of patients with head and neck cancer have distant metastatic disease, usually involving the lungs or bone. Accordingly, many patients also undergo either a chest radiograph or CT of the chest to assess for both metastatic disease and synchronous primaries. Depending on symptoms and other findings, initial staging studies may also include whole-body bone scanning and CT scanning of the abdomen and pelvis.

The use of PET and PET/CT as an adjunctive tool for T staging has been discussed above (see Diagnosis section). After determination of accurate T stage, the assessment of regional nodal involvement is of paramount importance. The most critical factors that need to be elucidated regarding regional nodal involvement include total number of nodes, size of nodes, location (unilateral or bilateral), morphology (central necrosis, conglomerate appearance, loss of normal nodal contour), specific levels of involvement, and extracapsular spread. All of these factors directly influence stage, therapy decision-making, and prognosis. Traditionally, either CT or MRI has been utilized to provide non-invasive characterization of regional nodal disease. However, purely anatomic assessment of nodal regions does not provide for a high overall accuracy. CT and MRI use size criteria for determination of nodal disease, with a 1.0-cm long axis being considered pathologic except for jugulodigastric nodes where 1.5 cm is considered abnormal. The main confounding factor with this system is that neck nodes can be infiltrated with tumor and still measure less than 1 cm in size (false negative), or reactive and/or inflammatory nodes may be present that are greater than 1.0 cm (false positive). In addition, involved nodes may contain only micrometastatic disease, which again will result in normal appearing nodes on CT and/or MRI. Because of these factors, conventional imaging may not identify clinically silent (non-palpable) but diseased nodes, resulting in under-staging of disease.

The incorporation of metabolic data from FDG-PET and PET/CT has been shown to significantly improve sensitivity, specificity, and overall accuracy of non-invasive regional nodal staging. PET has the ability to detect diseased nodes that appear normal on anatomic imaging but have altered metabolism present secondary to tumor infiltration (Figure 7.4). Although PET imaging cannot detect microscopic disease involvement, it can accurately characterize nodes with smaller volume disease than either contrast-enhanced CT or MRI. An additional benefit of PET/CT is that its results can provide biopsy and surgical guidance, which may result in fewer false-negative findings and more accurate surgical staging.

Several studies have compared PET to CT and MRI for the non-invasive staging of regional nodes, with surgical neck dissection as the gold standard.

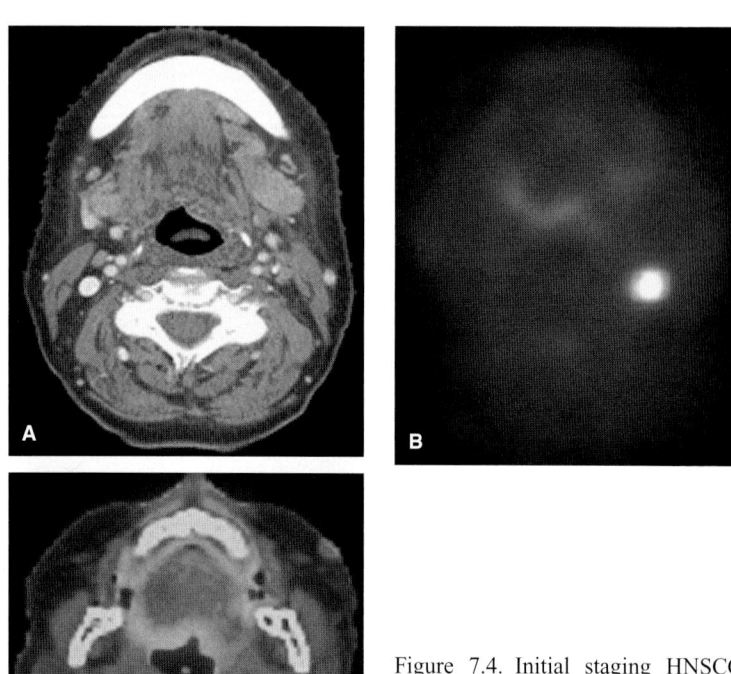

Figure 7.4. Initial staging HNSCC. Axial CT with contrast **(A)**, PET **(B)**, and PET/CT fusion **(C)**. Both PET and PET/CT fusion reveal hypermetabolic 7–9-mm left level 2 lymph nodes, which appeared equivocal and normal in size on diagnostic CT. Subsequent dissection confirmed metastatic involvement.

Kau et al. compared PET, CT, and MRI with surgical results in 70 patients with various stage HNSCC and found both higher overall sensitivity (87%) and specificity (94%) with PET, compared with sensitivities of 65–88% and specificities of 41–47% for CT/MRI [15]. Hannah et al. looked at 40 patients with various stage HNSCC and found significantly higher specificity with PET (95%) than with CT (81%) when both were compared to surgical neck dissection [16]. Multiple other studies have found higher overall sensitivity, specificity, and accuracy for PET when compared to CT/MRI for detection of regional nodal disease [17–20].

The advent of PET/CT has been a major advance in the assessment of regional nodal disease. Because PET alone is limited in detecting extracapsular spread and in evaluating morphology (central necrosis, conglomerate nodes), the combined metabolic and anatomic information obtained with PET/CT will allow

Table 7.3. Assessment of regional nodal disease

Number of nodes	PET
Distribution (unilateral, bilateral, contralateral)	PET
Size	PET and CT
Level	PET and CT
Morphology (central necrosis, conglomerate)	CT
Extracapsular spread	CT

the most accurate estimation of all crucial aspects of nodal involvement. The specific strength of PET in looking at metabolism complements the anatomic detail afforded by CT and provides a very comprehensive evaluation of disease involvement (Table 7.3).

The inclusion of PET for the detection of distant metastatic disease has been found to improve both initial staging and restaging. The discovery of distant metastases upgrades patients to stage IV disease, and almost always warrants the inclusion of systemic therapy such as chemotherapy. PET can more fully characterize equivocal abnormalities found on anatomic imaging and can detect metastatic disease in otherwise normal appearing tissue on CT and MRI (Figure 7.5). As mentioned previously, the whole-body nature of PET allows for the

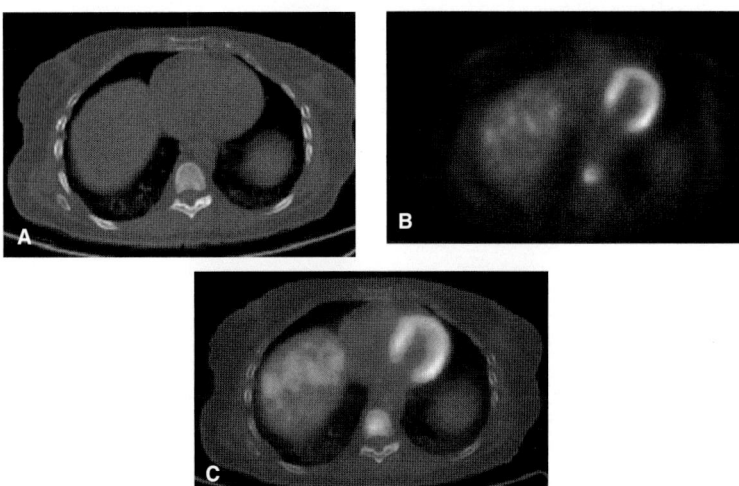

Figure 7.5. Unsuspected osseous metastasis. Axial CT **(A)**, axial PET **(B)**, axial PET/CT fusion **(C)**, sagittal PET **(D)**, and sagittal PET/CT fusion **(E)** reveal focal increased uptake within T9 vertebral body. CT images appear normal, but subsequent T1 **(F)** and T2 **(G)** MRI images confirm metastasis. Biopsy revealed metastatic disease.

Continued.

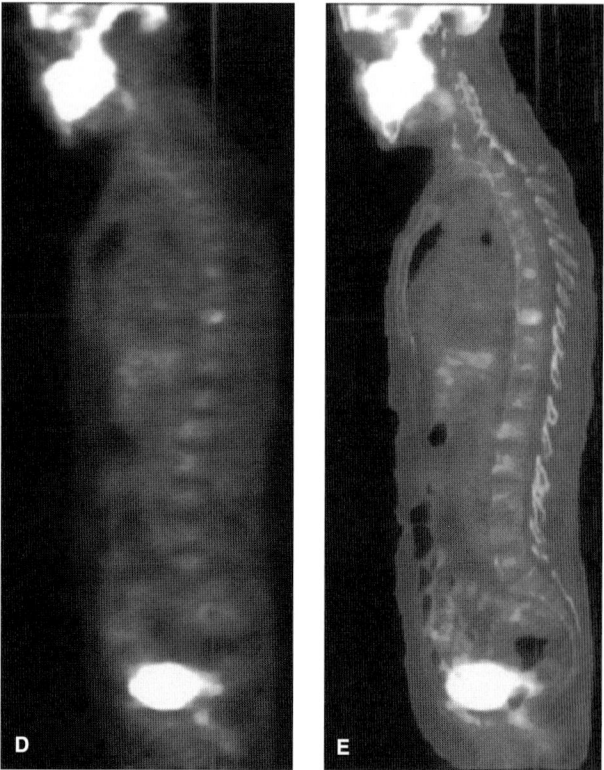

Figure 7.5. *Continued.*

detection of second primary malignancies, as over 30% of these lesions are outside the head and neck [14]. Schmid et al. studied patients with advanced HNSCC and found that the addition of PET to initial staging evaluation resulted in a change in management in approximately 10% of patients, either by upstaging or downstaging regional nodal disease or by detecting unsuspected distant metastases [21]. Their conclusion was that "PET is superior to CT for detection of metastatic disease." Multiple other studies have also confirmed the added value of PET in the initial and restaging evaluation of distant metastatic disease, with PET detecting unsuspected metastatic disease that was confirmed in 6–16% of patients [22–24].

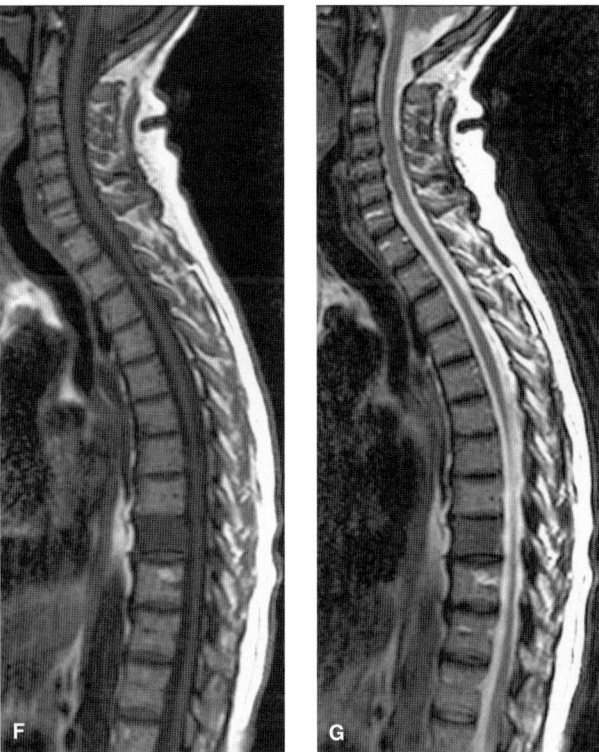

Figure 7.5. *Continued.*

Restaging and Therapy Response

Therapy for head and neck cancer involves some combination of surgery, radiation, and chemotherapy. Surgery and radiation therapy, either for treatment of the primary tumor and/or for regional nodal disease, often result in significant alteration of normal anatomy. In addition, local therapy result in inflammation with or without edema and/or hemorrhage, production of granulation tissue and fibrosis, and soft tissue vasculitis. The post-surgical/post-therapy head and neck is a notoriously difficult region to evaluate with imaging, and assessing for recurrent malignancy and gauging efficacy of therapy under these conditions can be very difficult. Enlarged reactive and inflammatory nodes may be present, normal anatomic landmarks may be absent, contrast-enhancing granulation tissue may form, and post-therapy fibrotic changes may mimic residual or recurrent tumor. Anatomic resolution of disease may lag behind the metabolic resolution, resulting in residual masses and nodes that do not have malignancy and an inability to fully evaluate therapy response with anatomic imaging alone.

Although decreased size of lymph nodes and primary tumor sites after therapy suggests a satisfactory response, it is often difficult to estimate residual tumor based on anatomic factors in isolation.

PET imaging is an excellent imaging tool to assess for residual malignancy after completion of therapy and when clinical signs and symptoms occur which suggest recurrence. Metabolic characterization with glucose utilization is a very sensitive, specific, and accurate method to determine the presence of viable tumor and can provide a very effective adjunct to anatomic imaging for biopsy guidance, radiation therapy, and surgery (Figure 7.6). However, it is important

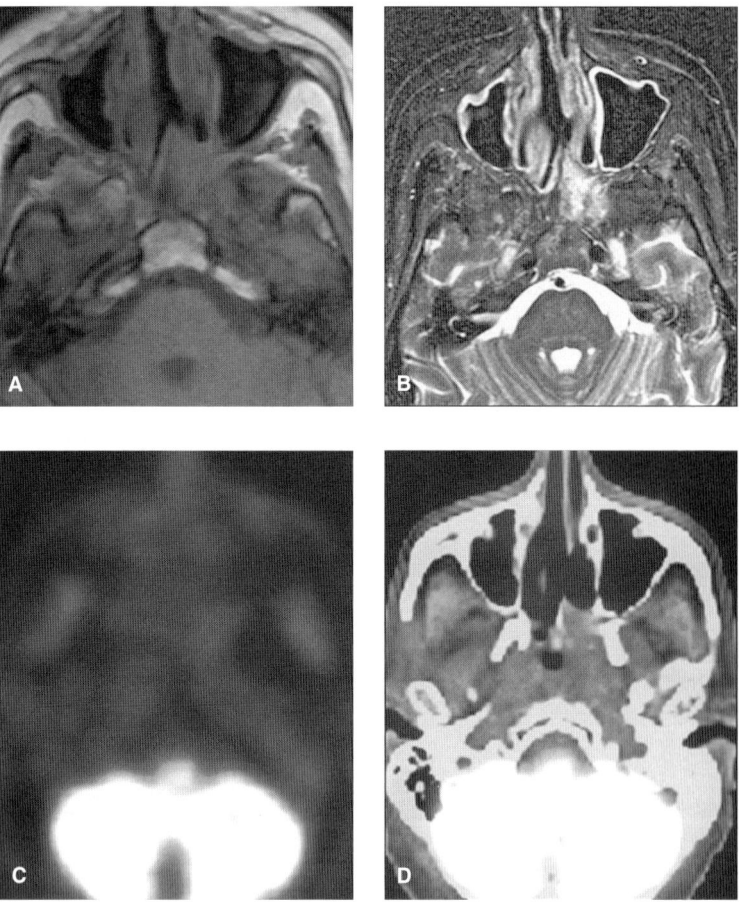

Figure 7.6. Nasopharyngeal SCC after radiation therapy: Axial T1 **(A)** and T2 **(B)** MRI images reveal persistent posterior nasopharyngeal soft tissue mass; subsequent PET **(C)** and PET/CT fusion **(D)** reveal no abnormal FDG uptake within the mass, consistent with treated disease and no viable tumor.

to delay evaluation with PET at least 6–8 weeks after completion of therapy to minimize false-positive uptake due to resultant inflammatory tissue. Given this fact, PET has a very high negative predictive value after therapy; a negative PET after completion of therapy has very strong positive prognostic value. Porceddu et al. evaluated 39 patients with HNSCC 3 months after completion of either radiation and/or chemotherapy with PET imaging. All patients had evidence of residual masses and nodes and were followed for 3 years. The negative predictive value of PET was found to be 97% [25]. Lonneux et al. studied 44 patients with HNSCC after completion of primary therapy with clinically suspected recurrence and found higher accuracy for PET in confirming recurrent disease. The sensitivity, specificity, and accuracy of PET were 96%, 61%, and 81%, respectively; corresponding values for CT/MRI were 73%, 50%, and 64% [26]. In any event, it is imperative to closely follow patients for at least 2 years after therapy, as local recurrence is most likely to occur within this time interval.

Velazquez et al. found poor correlation between CT findings and subsequent surgical dissection in 43 patients with stage III/IV HNSCC who had completed chemotherapy [27]. All patients had clinically positive necks and were scheduled for either unilateral or bilateral neck dissections. CT had a sensitivity, specificity, and positive predictive value of 85%, 24%, and 40%, respectively, when compared to surgical results. Goerres et al. evaluated 26 patients with stage III/IV HNSCC after completion of chemotherapy and found very good correlation between PET and subsequent surgical dissection and clinical follow-up results [28]. PET had a sensitivity and specificity of 91% and 94%, respectively. Multiple other studies have found higher overall sensitivity and specificity for PET in detection of local recurrence or residual disease when compared to CT/MRI [29–31] (Figure 7.7).

Horizons

The incorporation of PET imaging in the diagnosis, staging, and restaging of patients with head and neck cancer has been clearly documented to have a significant impact on accuracy of staging, prognosis, and assessment of therapy. The advent of combined PET/CT scanners has been a major advance in imaging evaluation of these patients. Image fusion of anatomic information provided by state-of-the-art multidetector contrast-enhanced CT with metabolic information provided by PET, all during the course of one patient visit and scan, increases the accuracy of both PET and CT by minimizing false positives and false negatives (Figure 7.8), provides more precise biopsy guidance, and leads to more accurate patient staging. Image guidance with PET detecting probes and developing software has the possibility to provide surgeons with very meticulous intraoperative direction and targeting of nodal disease and recurrent lesions. The use of PET/CT has already had a tremendous impact on radiation therapy planning. The incorporation of metabolic data provided by PET has already been shown to decrease tumor volume delineation and more accurately guide radiation therapy dose planning [32]. The increasing use of intensity-modulated radiation therapy (IMRT) is complemented nicely by PET/CT, as maximal radiation dose can now be directed toward areas of metabolically active disease with

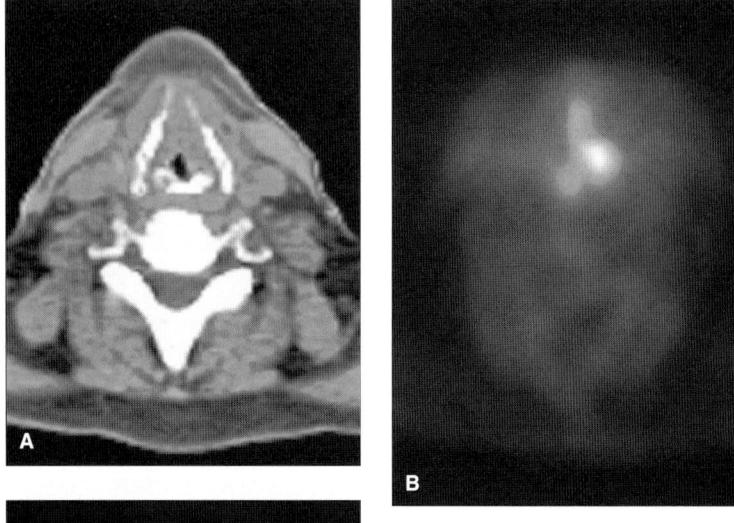

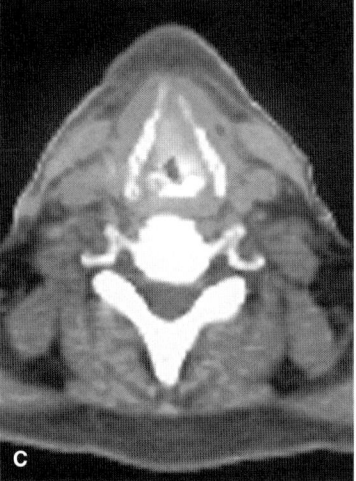

Figure 7.7. Laryngeal SCC after chemoradiation, presenting with persistent laryngeal edema and multiple negative random endoscopic biopsies. Axial CT (A), PET (B), and PET/CT fusion (C) reveal focal hypermetabolic uptake within left posterior larynx, guiding endoscopy and confirming recurrent malignancy.

sparing of other tissues. In addition, the continual development of other PET tracers will increase the use of PET imaging. There are now over 100 different PET tracers currently being investigated around the world, studying a myriad of biologic and therapeutic processes, from DNA synthesis to enzyme kinetics to hormonal and antibody function. It is now possible to "target" imaging to

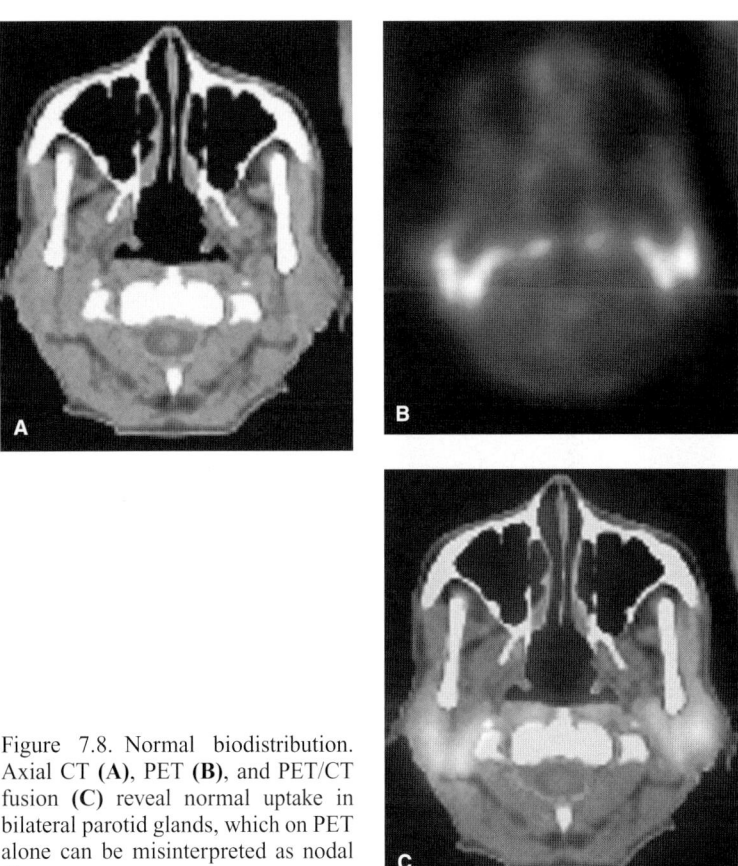

Figure 7.8. Normal biodistribution. Axial CT **(A)**, PET **(B)**, and PET/CT fusion **(C)** reveal normal uptake in bilateral parotid glands, which on PET alone can be misinterpreted as nodal disease.

different diseases and malignancies, taking advantage of biochemical differences by employing disease-specific PET ligands for their detection.

Limitations

PET is primarily a metabolic imaging modality, and therefore the anatomic resolution of PET scanners is limited. Even with combined PET/CT, the spatial resolution of PET limits the accurate characterization of lesions to those over approximately 6–8 mm in diameter. Uptake in lesions less than 1 cm is underestimated unless corrections for resolution effects are made. And, as in any imaging modality, PET cannot detect microscopic disease.

In addition, there is tremendous variation in normal physiologic activity in the head and neck. Normal FDG uptake can be seen in the major and minor salivary glands, lymphoid tissue such as the tonsils, optic nerves, vocalis muscles, muscles of mastication, secreted saliva, and base of tongue (genioglossus) (Figure 7.9). This normal variation can at times be difficult to distinguish from abnormal uptake, especially if it is asymmetric. There can also be FDG uptake in metabolically active fat (brown fat), which on PET imaging can be challenging to separate from malignant nodal uptake. The increasing use of PET/CT imaging helps diagnostic accuracy by correctly localizing most physiologic uptake to normal appearing structures.

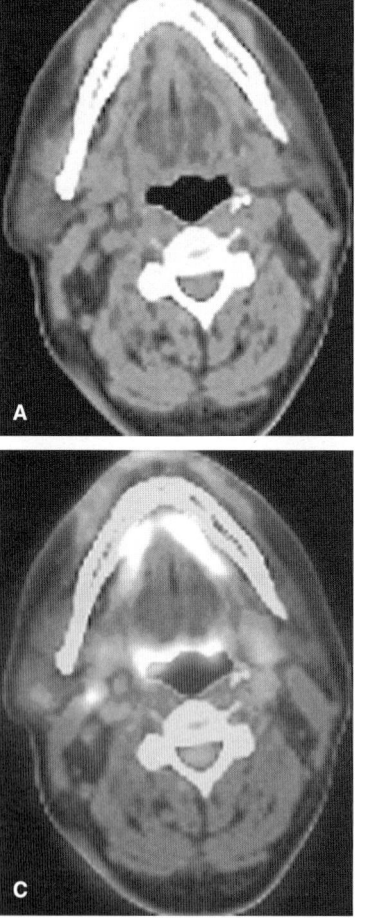
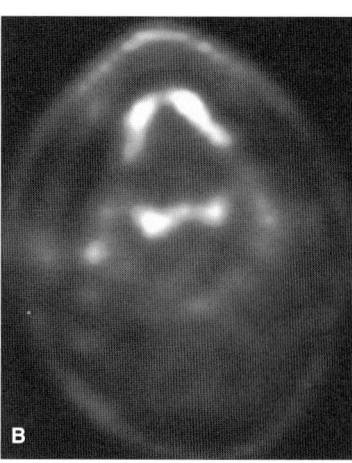

Figure 7.9. Nodal disease coexistent with normal biodistribution: Axial CT (A), PET (B), and PET/CT fusion (C) reveal right level 2A nodal disease, along with normal uptake in the genioglossus, parotid glands, palatine tonsils, and submandibular glands. The fusion of metabolic PET with anatomic CT images allows correct identification of normal uptake versus pathology.

There are causes of false-positive FDG uptake which must be recognized, including therapy-induced inflammatory and active granulation tissue, muscle uptake due to tension or hyperglycemia, nodal uptake due to infection or active inflammatory disease, benign tumors (pleomorphic adenoma and Warthin's tumors), chemotherapy-induced bone marrow hyperplasia, radiation-induced osteoradionecrosis, and variable laryngeal uptake (vocal cord paralysis, talking after FDG injection, and Teflon implants).

References

1. American Cancer Society (www.cancer.org); 2005 Accessed March 2005.
2. Greene FL, Page DL, Fleming ID, et al. AJCC Cancer Staging Manual, sixth edition. New York: Springer-Verlag; 2002.
3. Bailet JW, Abemayor E, Jabour BA, et al. Positron emission tomography: a new, precise imaging modality for detection of primary head and neck tumors and assessment of cervical adenopathy. Laryngoscope 1992;102(3):281–288.
4. von Schulthess GK. Positron emission tomography versus positron emission tomography/computed tomography: from "unclear" to "new-clear" medicine. Mol Imaging Biol 2004;6(4):183–187.
5. Cerfolio RJ, Ojha B, Bryant AS, et al. The accuracy of integrated PET-CT compared with dedicated PET alone for the staging of patients with nonsmall cell lung cancer. Ann Thorac Surg 2004;78(3):1017–1023.
6. Rusthoven KE, Koshy M, Paulino AC. The role of PET-CT fusion in head and neck cancer. Oncology (Huntingt) 2005;19(2):241–246.
7. Minn H, Paul R, Ahonen A. Evaluation of treatment response to radiotherapy in head and neck cancer with fluorine-18 fluorodeoxyglucose. J Nucl Med 1988;29(9):1521–1525.
8. Laubenbacher C, Saumweber D, Wagner-Manslau C, et al. Comparison of fluorine-18-fluorodeoxyglucose PET, MRI and endoscopy for staging head and neck squamous-cell carcinomas. J Nucl Med 1995;36(10):1747–1757.
9. Wong WL, Chevretton EB, McGurk M, et al. A prospective study of PET-FDG imaging for the assessment of head and neck squamous cell carcinoma. Clin Otolaryngol 1997;22(3):209–214.
10. Paulus P, Sambon A, Vivegnis D, et al. 18FDG-PET for the assessment of primary head and neck tumors: clinical, computed tomography, and histopathological correlation in 38 patients. Laryngoscope 1998;108(10):1578–1583.
11. Reisser C, Haberkorn U, Dimitrakopoulou-Strauss A, et al. Chemotherapeutic management of head and neck malignancies with positron emission tomography. Arch Otolaryngol Head Neck Surg 1995;121:272–276.
12. Johansen J, Eigtved A, Buchwald C, et al. Implication of 18F-fluoro-2-deoxy-D-glucose positron emission tomography on management of carcinoma of unknown primary in the head and neck: a Danish cohort study. Laryngoscope 2002;112(11):2009–2014.

13. Jungehulsing M, Scheidhauer K, Damm M, et al. 2[F]-fluoro-2-deoxy-D-glucose positron emission tomography is a sensitive tool for the detection of occult primary cancer (carcinoma of unknown primary syndrome) with head and neck lymph node manifestation. Otolaryngol Head Neck Surg 2000;123(3):294–301.

14. Leon X, Quer M, Diez S, et al. Second neoplasm in patients with head and neck cancer. Head Neck 1999;21(3):204–210.

15. Kau RJ, Alexiou C, Laubenbacher C, et al. Lymph node detection of head and neck squamous cell carcinomas by positron emission tomography with fluorodeoxyglucose F 18 in a routine clinical setting. Arch Otolaryngol Head Neck Surg 1999; 125(12):1322–1328.

16. Hannah A, Scott AM, Tochon-Danguy H, et al. Evaluation of 18 F-fluorodeoxyglucose positron emission tomography and computed tomography with histopathologic correlation in the initial staging of head and neck cancer. Ann Surg 2002;236(2): 208–217.

17. Laubenbacher C, Saumweber D, Wagner-Manslau C, et al. Comparison of fluorine-18-fluorodeoxyglucose PET, MRI and endoscopy for staging head and neck squamous-cell carcinomas. J Nucl Med 1995;36(10):1747–1757.

18. Adams S, Baum RP, Stuckensen T, et al. Prospective comparison of 18F-FDG PET with conventional imaging modalities (CT, MRI, US) in lymph node staging of head and neck cancer. Eur J Nucl Med 1998;25(9):1255–1260.

19. Di Martino E, Nowak B, Hassan HA, et al. Diagnosis and staging of head and neck cancer: a comparison of modern imaging modalities (positron emission tomography, computed tomography, color-coded duplex sonography) with panendoscopic and histopathologic findings. Arch Otolaryngol Head Neck Surg 2000;126(12):1457–1461.

20. Nowak B, Di Martino E, Janicke S, et al. Diagnostic evaluation of malignant head and neck cancer by F-18-FDG PET compared to CT/MRI. Nuklearmedizin 1999;38(8): 312–318.

21. Schmid DT, Stoeckli SJ, Bandhauer F, et al. Impact of positron emission tomography on the initial staging and therapy in locoregional advanced squamous cell carcinoma of the head and neck. Laryngoscope 2003;113(5):888–891.

22. Keyes JW, Jr., Chen MY, Watson NE Jr., et al. FDG PET evaluation of head and neck cancer: value of imaging the thorax. Head Neck 2000;22(2):105–110.

23. Wax MK, Myers LL, Gabalski EC, et al. Positron emission tomography in the evaluation of synchronous lung lesions in patients with untreated head and neck cancer. Arch Otolaryngol Head Neck Surg 2002;128(6):703–707.

24. Kitagawa Y, Nishizawa S, Sano K, et al. Whole-body (18)F-fluorodeoxyglucose positron emission tomography in patients with head and neck cancer. Oral Surg Oral Med Oral Pathol Oral Radiol Endod 2002;93(2):202–207.

25. Porceddu SV, Jarmolowski E, Hicks RJ, et al. Utility of positron emission tomography for the detection of disease in residual neck nodes after (chemo)radiotherapy in head and neck cancer. Head Neck 2005;27(3):175–181.

26. Lonneux M, Lawson G, Ide C, et al. Positron emission tomography with fluorodeoxyglucose for suspected head and neck tumor recurrence in the symptomatic patient. Laryngoscope 2000;110(9):1493–1497.

27. Velazquez RA, McGuff HS, Sycamore D, et al. The role of computed tomographic scans in the management of the N-positive neck in head and neck squamous cell carcinoma after chemoradiotherapy. Arch Otolaryngol Head Neck Surg 2004;130(1): 74–77.

28. Goerres GW, Schmid DT, Bandhauer F, et al. Positron emission tomography in the early follow-up of advanced head and neck cancer. Arch Otolaryngol Head Neck Surg 2004;130(1):105–109.

29. Lapela M, Grenman R, Kurki T, et al. Head and neck cancer: detection of recurrence with PET and 2-[F-18] fluoro-2-deoxy-D-glucose. Radiology 2002;197:205–211.

30. Farber LA, Benard F, Machtay M, et al. Detection of recurrent head and neck squamous cell carcinomas after radiation therapy with 2–18F-fluoro-2-deoxy-D-glucose positron emission tomography. Laryngoscope 1999;109(6):970–975.

31. Fischbein NJ, AAssar OS, Caputo GR, et al. Clinical utility of positron emission tomography with 18F-fluorodeoxyglucose in detecting residual/recurrent squamous cell carcinoma of the head and neck. AJNR Am J Neuroradiol 1998;19(7):1189–1196.

32. Daisne JF, Duprez T, Weynand B, et al. Tumor volume in pharyngolaryngeal squamous cell carcinoma: comparison at CT, MR imaging, and FDG PET and validation with surgical specimen. Radiology 2004;233(1):93–100.

8. PET in Colorectal Carcinoma

Martin J. O'Connell, Ronald B. Workman, Jr., and R. Edward Coleman

Colorectal cancer is the third most common malignancy in the United States, excluding skin carcinoma, and is the second leading cause of cancer-related death. The American Cancer Society estimated that approximately 145,000 new cases of colorectal cancer would be diagnosed in 2005 and approximately 56,000 people would die of the disease [1]. Colorectal cancer death rates have been steadily declining over the past 15 years due to increased public awareness, emphasis on early detection, and improvements in therapy.

Risk factors for developing colorectal cancer include age greater than 50, a positive family history, known genetic factors such as familial adenomatous polyposis and hereditary non-polyposis colorectal cancer, a history of colon polyps or inflammatory bowel disease, smoking, diabetes, and a diet which is high in fat, especially animal fat.

The obligatory precursor of colorectal cancer is the adenomatous polyp. While some patients may have occult bleeding and present with weakness related to anemia, the majority of patients with neoplastic colon polyps are asymptomatic and have hematologic indices that are within normal limits. If left undiagnosed, potentially curable disease can progress to an advanced stage. This is why colorectal cancer screening is so important. See Table 8.1 for the current American Cancer Society colorectal cancer screening guidelines [2]. Screening with stool guaiac testing, air contrast barium enema examination, and conventional optical colonoscopy have enabled physicians to detect the disease at an earlier and more successfully treatable stage. Computed tomography virtual colonoscopy is a relatively new and accurate screening technique which compares favorably with conventional colonoscopy. Its precise role in screening for colorectal neoplasm is continuing to grow and evolve. The 5-year survival rate for those with colorectal cancer detected early, before metastasis, can be better than 90%. See Table 8.2 for a breakdown of 5-year survival based on cancer stage [3].

Once cancer is detected, surgical options are available, and neoadjuvant and adjuvant chemoradiation therapy may be used to improve prognosis [4]. When metastasis occurs, surgical treatment may include local tumor resection, hepatic resection or pulmonary wedge resection. For liver or pulmonary metastasis radiofrequency ablation is used in selected patients. Despite advances, colon carcinoma remains a major cause of cancer-related deaths. Colon carcinoma recurrence is typically distant from the original tumor site, whereas locoregional recurrence is more common in rectal carcinoma. Colorectal cancer recurs in 37–45% of patients within 2 years of curative resection with early recurrence typically occurring at an average of 14 months after resection [5]. When cancer recurs locally, radical resection is the treatment of choice; however, few

Table 8.1. American Cancer Society colorectal cancer screening guidelines*

1. Fecal occult blood test (FOBT)† or fecal immunochemical test (FIT)
   every year, or
2. flexible sigmoidoscopy every 5 years, or
3. an FOBT† or FIT every year plus flexible sigmoidoscopy every 5 years
   (of these first three options, the combination of FOBT or FIT every year
   plus flexible sigmoidoscopy every 5 years is preferable), or
4. double-contrast barium enema every 5 years, or
5. colonoscopy every 10 years.

* Beginning at age 50, men and women who are at average risk for developing colorectal cancer should have one of the five screening options listed. Those at increased risk for colorectal cancer should undergo screening earlier and at more frequent intervals.
† For FOBT or FIT, the take-home multiple sample method should be used.
Source: From, "Can colorectal polyps and cancer be found early?" American Cancer Society (www.cancer.org); 2005 Accessed August 2005.

candidates are suitable for surgery. Surgery for palliation may include relief of obstruction by enteroenterostomy or stoma, adhesion lysis or removal of tumor causing hemorrhage. Research has shown the importance of good surgical technique, particularly in removing rectal cancers. Modifications of the surgical technique aimed at reducing local recurrence include wide and anatomic resection of the primary lesion with high vascular ligation and total mesorectal excision. The rectal stump is also subsequently washed with cytotoxic agents.

The locoregional recurrence rate of colorectal carcinoma has previously been described as high as 50% [6]. However, with modern surgical techniques recurrence rates are likely to be lower, typically in the range of 5–15% [7]. Only 4% of patients with locoregional recurrence who do not have re-resection are alive at 5 years [6]. Retroperitoneal recurrence is seen in 18% of patients, with 33%

Table 8.2. Five-year colorectal cancer survival rates by American Joint Committee on Cancer Stage

Stage	Five-year survival
I	93%
IIA	85%
IIB	72%
IIIA	83%
IIIB	64%
IIIC	44%
IV	8%

Source: From O'Connell, Maggard, Ko [3], by permission of the *Journal of the National Cancer Institute*.

of recurrence occurring in the liver; 25% of these patients with recurrence in the liver are suitable for curative resection. The 5-year survival post partial liver resection is 25–44% [8]. Liver resection itself has an operative mortality of 2–7% [9]. Lung metastasis occurs in 22% of patients for which resection potentially offers a cure. Pulmonary wedge resection, video-assisted pulmonary nodule resection or lobectomy have low perioperative mortality [10]. In patients with prior resection of hepatic metastasis, pulmonary metastasectomy also offers survival benefit [10].

The major role of ^{18}F fluorodeoxyglucose (FDG) PET imaging in colorectal carcinoma is in restaging and in the determination of the extent of metastatic disease prior to liver resection or pulmonary resection. For initial staging, CT, and in the case of rectal carcinoma, MRI, combined with operative lymph node resection of mesenteric lymph nodes remain the gold standard.

Technical Considerations

Oral contrast improves image interpretation on the CT scan, and, in many centers, is used routinely. Assessment of bowel wall lesions is improved by distension of the small or large bowel, which helps to eliminate the possibility of an erroneous CT correlate for focal physiologic bowel activity on the PET scan. Oral contrast was reported in early studies to cause artifacts on PET imaging in the bowel within areas of dense barium concentration because it causes overestimation of tissue FDG concentration. This appearance is readily recognizable on direct comparison with co-registered CT images. With the use of less dense oral contrast agents and improved reconstruction algorithms, oral contrast does not cause artifacts in the PET imaging from a PET/CT scanner. Many centers recommend the routine use of endorectal contrast in CT staging of rectal cancer, but this use has not gained acceptance in PET/CT. Intravenous contrast is used in CT to assess liver lesions and to distinguish retroperitoneal lesions from adjacent vascular structures. In PET/CT, intravenous contrast is used to improve accuracy of interpretation. The importance of using intravenous contrast with PET/CT is under evaluation.

Mucinous Adenocarcinoma

Mucinous colorectal carcinoma has been reported as demonstrating less uptake than non-mucinous carcinoma on FDG-PET imaging. The reduced uptake may reflect reduced cells per unit volume (tumor cells are surrounded by secreted mucin) or alterations in the intracellular metabolism of FDG. Sensitivity of PET for detection of primary and recurrent mucinous carcinomas has been reported to be as low as 58% [11]. Co-registered CT as part of PET/CT imaging is likely to increase sensitivity for mucinous tumor detection, especially if intravenous contrast is used.

Diagnosis

PET imaging is rarely used for colon cancer diagnosis, but may be used in the identification of a primary lesion in the colon in a patient presenting with metastatic carcinoma of unknown primary. Incidental gastrointestinal tract lesions are detected in 3% of all patients undergoing FDG-PET imaging for a variety of indications [2]. Of these lesions, 60% turn out to be cancers or pre-cancerous lesions [12]. In colorectal carcinoma, the primary lesion is detected in 95% of patients (Figure 8.1); however, specificity is limited to 43%. Lesions of 11–14 mm may be detected [13]. However, the relatively low specificity makes screening with PET imaging impractical. The low specificity also reflects detection of colonic adenomas that, despite being associated with a risk of progression to colon carcinoma, are regarded as false positives. The degree of uptake in adenomas does not correlate with the degree of dysplasia. Low-grade radio-tracer uptake can rarely be seen in hyperplastic polyps or thrombosed hemorrhoids. However, hyperplastic polyps typically demonstrate no FDG uptake. One study demonstrated adenomas having lower FDG uptake (SUV 3.56 ± 0.68) than colonic carcinomas (SUV 5.74 ± 2.26); however, this difference is not likely to be a useful discriminator [14]. The sensitivity for detecting adenomas is low for small lesions, with 24% of polyps measuring 5 mm or smaller identified [12], which is close to the lower limit of PET image resolution. Ninety percent of lesions measuring greater than 13 mm are identified. PET demonstrates a higher sensitivity for detecting adenomas in the cecum, ascending colon, and descending colon [13], which may relate to the relative lack of movement with respiration of these regions of the colon that are predominantly retroperitoneal. The lifetime risk of an adenoma progressing to cancer is up to 10%, and endoscopic or surgical resection is indicated [15].

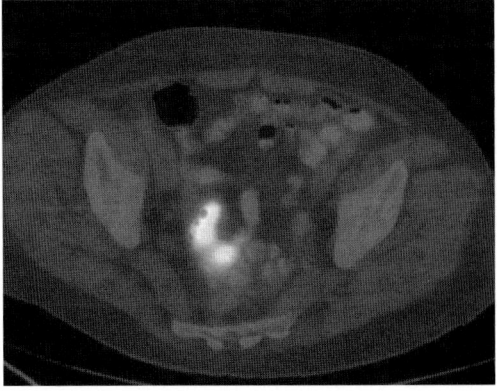

Figure 8.1. Axial fusion PET/CT image demonstrates intense focal radiotracer uptake in a primary sigmoid colon mass.

Initial Staging

PET imaging is reimbursed by the Centers for Medicare and Medicaid Services (CMS) for primary staging of colorectal carcinoma, but in many centers it is not used for this purpose, with operative staging of lymph node involvement by the TNM (Table 8.3) or Dukes' staging system being used instead. PET/CT is superior to CT in the detection of lymph node metastasis at initial staging, with the gold standard being surgical resection. When PET imaging is used in initial staging, it influences management mainly in the identification of liver or distal metastasis. Despite the presence of metastasis, surgery may still be performed to prevent colonic obstruction. In the presence of metastasis, con-

Table 8.3. TNM staging of colorectal carcinoma

Primary tumor (T)	
TX	Primary tumor cannot be assessed
T0	No evidence of primary tumor
Tis	Carcinoma in situ: intraepithelial or invasion of lamina propria*
T1	Tumor invades submucosa
T2	Tumor invades through muscularis propria
T3	Tumor invades through muscularis propria into subserosa or into non-peritonealized pericolic or perirectal tissues
T4	Tumor directly invades other organs or structures, and/or perforates visceral peritoneum (direct invasion in T4 includes invasion of other sections of the colon or rectum through the serosa)†,‡
Regional lymph nodes (N)	
NX	Regional lymph nodes cannot be assessed
N0	No regional lymph node metastasis
N1	Regional lymph node metastasis in 1 to 3 lymph nodes
N2	Regional lymph node metastasis in 4 or more lymph nodes
Distant metastasis (M)	
MX	Distant metastasis cannot be assessed
M0	No distant metastasis
M1	Distant metastasis

* Includes cancers confined within the glandular basement membrane (intraepithelial) or lamina propria (intramucosal) with no extension through the muscularis mucosae into the submucosa.
† Direct invasion in T4 includes invasion of other segments of the colorectum by way of the serosa; for example, invasion of the sigmoid colon by a carcinoma of the cecum.
‡ Tumor that is adherent to other organs or structures, macroscopically, is classified T4. However, if no tumor is present in the adhesion, microscopically, the classification should be pT3. The V and L substaging should be used to identify the presence or absence of vascular or lymphatic invasion.
Source: Used with permission of the American Joint Committee on Cancer (AJCC), Chicago, Illinois. The original source for this material is the *AJCC Cancer Staging Manual*, Sixth Edition (2002), published by Springer-Verlag, New York, www.springeronline.com.

servative treatment options are available and include metallic colonic stent placement. Because metastatic disease only occurs if the submucosa is involved, PET is not likely to be useful in initial staging of carcinoma in situ or post polypectomy with no evidence of residual tumor, and therefore PET imaging as part of initial staging is not recommended in most patients presenting with colorectal cancer [16].

PET imaging cannot exclude microscopic metastatic disease, and lymph node excision at initial surgery remains the gold standard for N staging. CT for colonic tumors and MRI for rectal tumors are used for nodal staging prior to surgery. MRI performed with an endorectal coil has an accuracy of 80% in local nodal staging [17], with similar results for external array MRI coils. In addition, local extension of rectal tumors into the mesorectal fascia can be identified. CT is used primarily to assess for retroperitoneal, hepatic, and pulmonary metastasis. PET may be used in selected patients where distal metastases are suspected at diagnosis. For CT and MRI, size criteria are used in the evaluation of perirectal nodes and 5 mm is used as the upper limit of normal lymph node size, rather than 6–10 mm as at other sites in the retroperitoneum or mediastinum [17]. In addition, the architecture of local lymph nodes on T2-weighted MRI is also useful. In locoregional lymph node staging, similar to PET imaging in esophageal cancer, peri-tumoral hypermetabolic lymph nodes can be missed because of "blooming" of intense radiotracer activity in an adjacent colonic primary lesion.

Restaging

The major role of PET in colorectal carcinoma is in restaging. Indications for restaging of colorectal carcinoma are potential curative surgery for isolated metastatic disease, differentiation of scar from recurrent tumor, particularly in the pre-sacral space, and evaluation of increased carcinoembryonic antigen level (CEA). Although restaging PET was initially used only in patients with abnormal CEA levels, currently PET is indicated in restaging colorectal carcinoma in patients with normal or elevated CEA levels. Colon carcinoma and rectal carcinoma behave differently in terms of recurrence site, with colon carcinoma typically recurring distant from the original site, either within the abdomen, retroperitoneum or the liver, whereas locoregional recurrence is more common in rectal carcinoma, typically in the pre-sacral region.

Neoadjuvant chemotherapy is used in colorectal carcinoma; however, the role of restaging in this context has had very limited evaluation. PET was superior to CT and MRI in detecting treatment response in rectal carcinoma in one study that demonstrated PET as having positive and negative predictive values of 77% and 100%, respectively. In comparison CT had positive and negative predictive values of 78% and 57%, respectively, with MRI at 83% and 50%, respectively [18]. Local radiotherapy has the potential to give false-positive findings relating to inflammation or inflammation with fibrosis. Restaging should be performed 6 months after radiation treatment to reduce false-positive results. This interval is often not practical, with earlier follow-up more frequently employed. Rarely, post-radiation changes may persist after 6 months.

PET, in common with imaging modalities including CT and MRI, may not detect very low-volume disease and microscopic disease cannot be excluded. In addition, PET has been reported as having lower sensitivity for detection of peritoneal carcinomatosis, likely related to the relatively small volume of peritoneal deposits. The lesion resolution of most standard PET imaging systems is 8–10 mm and small peritoneal deposits may be below this range in size. However, PET/CT helps to overcome this limitation, where the superior spatial resolution of CT avoids a misdiagnosis (Figure 8.2).

In evaluation of local or pelvic recurrence and distant metastasis, PET has higher sensitivity and accuracy than CT, with sensitivity of 79–100%, specificity of 58–100%, and accuracy of 83–100% [4] (Figure 8.3). CT has a reported sensitivity of 47–86%, specificity of 36–100%, and accuracy of 56–83% [4].

In rectal carcinoma PET is commonly used to differentiate post-surgical changes on CT from recurrent tumor in the pre-sacral space. Using CT alone, the only option for evaluation of soft tissue at this site is short interval follow-up CT at 2–3 months or image-guided biopsy. These approaches lead to a delay in the diagnosis of recurrence and unnecessary biopsy procedures. Increased FDG uptake may be identified in postoperative soft tissue in the pre-sacral space for up to 4 months after surgery [19]. When evaluation is made for recurrence at the anastomosis site, false-positive results have been described to result from postoperative inflammation or healing. PET is useful in the evaluation of small lymph nodes in the retroperitoneum or mesentery that may be considered within normal limits for size or indeterminate by CT criteria. In unusual cases where suspicious lymph nodes identified at CT are negative at PET, biopsy should nonetheless be performed. False-positive results on PET are rarely seen in reactive lymphadenopathy. PET/CT can be useful to identify small focal areas of pericolic tumor that may otherwise be difficult to identify on CT. Oral contrast is likely to improve sensitivity in this context.

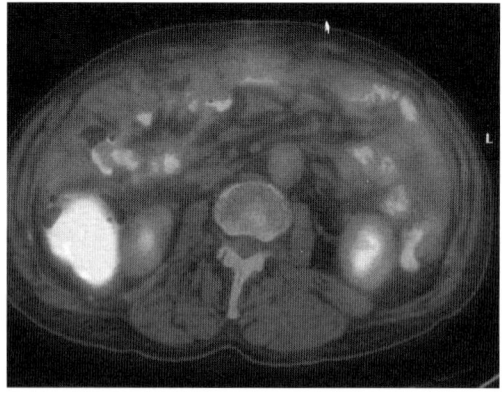

Figure 8.2. Intense hypermetabolic activity in a cecal carcinoma primary lesion with multiple adjacent foci of uptake identified consistent with diffuse peritoneal metastasis.

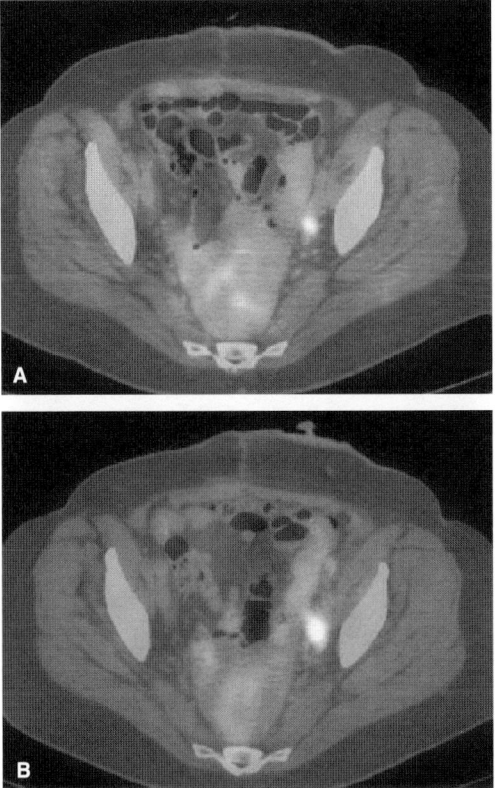

Figure 8.3. (A) Focal intense radiotracer uptake in a subcentimeter left pelvic side wall lymph node is consistent with metastasis. (B) Axial fusion PET/CT image in the same patient 3 months later demonstrates enlargement of the same pelvic side wall lymph node.

Partial hepatic resection is associated with a high rate of recurrence in patients with colorectal carcinoma, which suggests that current pre-surgical evaluation is suboptimal. PET may be used to reduce morbidity and mortality associated with inappropriate liver resection surgery. Five-year survival increases from 30% to 58% when PET imaging is negative for *extra hepatic disease* prior to resection [20]. In evaluation of recurrent liver metastasis, PET has higher specificity and accuracy than CT. In a lesion-by-lesion analysis, PET demonstrates 70% of liver masses identified histologically at liver resection, but with small lesions less apparent, where contrast MRI is superior in the detection of sub centimeter metastases [21]. The main added benefit of PET, however, is in the improved detection of extrahepatic metastatic disease. Other imaging modalities such as MRI and CT arterial-portography are limited in the detection of

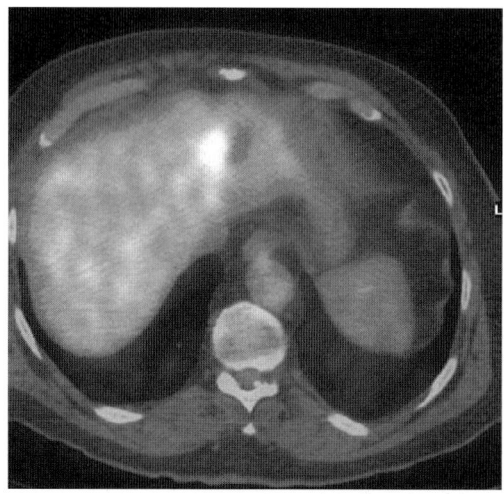

Figure 8.4. Axial fusion PET/CT demonstrates intense focal radiotracer uptake on the lateral margin of a radiofrequency ablation site in the liver. Recurrent disease was not apparent on conventional imaging.

extrahepatic disease. In potential partial resection candidates, PET changes management in 18–29% of patients [22]. In liver metastases, uptake in lesion margins with central photopenia (low uptake) indicates central necrosis, and confirmatory biopsy should be from the lesion margin. PET has been demonstrated to improve sensitivity in restaging liver metastasis following radiofrequency ablation (Figure 8.4). This improved sensitivity is likely to have an impact in the earlier detection of recurrence at the margin of the ablation site, in one study detecting tumor 3 months earlier by PET than on CT [23].

Interpretation Considerations

Bowel accumulation of FDG is identified in the colonic mucosa and is rarely in the bowel lumen. Bowel wall activity can be distinguished from recurrent tumor by lack of a CT soft tissue mass correlate or by demonstration of a typical pattern of bowel uptake. A "string of beads" appearance is used to describe the appearance of physiologic radiotracer uptake in bowel on PET imaging. Diffuse, intermediate level uptake is commonly identified in colon and small bowel. Although several methods of decreasing bowel accumulation of FDG have been tried, no technique has been demonstrated to consistently decrease bowel uptake of radiotracer. More focal uptake may be seen in diverticulitis, focal colitis, or following polypectomy. Focal physiologic activity may occasionally be very intense and close correlation is needed with associated CT images to assess for focal wall thickening to rule out an associated lesion. Crohn's disease is a cause of potential false-positive colonic uptake that may be distinguished from tumor by the presence of diffuse bowel wall thickening, multifocal involvement, associated mesenteric changes, and characteristic or prior history. More diffuse colitis is clearly identified corresponding to longer segments of colonic involvement and is not likely to be mistaken for tumor. PET has the potential to identify synchronous bowel lesions, but colonoscopy, or in the case of narrow strictures, virtual colonoscopy, is more commonly used for this purpose.

PET/CT reduces false-positive results and leads to more definitive reports, improving accuracy from 78% to 89% in patients with colorectal cancer [24]. Accumulation of FDG may be seen in radiation proctitis, postoperative granulomas, peristomal colon, and laparoscopy ports. To reduce false-positive results, correlation with the patient's clinical history is needed. A patient questionnaire can confirm dates of surgery, radiotherapy, and current symptoms. On PET images focal accumulation of radiotracer in the ureter may have very intense activity similar to renal or bladder activity and should not be mistaken for metastasis. PET/CT allows direct correlation of this activity with a normal retroperitoneal ureter.

Pulmonary nodules less than 5–10 mm in size may have false-negative uptake because of relative motion in the lungs during normal respiration and the limited resolution of PET. Evaluation of non-attenuation-corrected PET images is recommended routinely in the assessment of radiotracer activity in small pulmonary nodules, especially in patients with significant misregistration of PET and CT images resulting from motion. Pulmonary nodules only partially consist of tumor, and the CT or radiographic opacity reflects tumor surrounded by inflammation, hemorrhage, necrosis or atelectasis within the adjacent lung, which results in relatively lower or a smaller focus of uptake on PET. In addition, respiratory motion artifactually lowers apparent radiotracer uptake particularly in lower lobe pulmonary lesions. This motion can be overcome by respiratory gating at the cost of extra scanning time, with the PET image acquisition time for the thorax typically being increased by a factor of 4. Respiratory gating is currently not widely available or utilized. If small pulmonary nodules are not identified on PET imaging, they may be identified on the CT portion of PET/CT imaging. So-called "cold" nodules require standard CT follow-up at 3 and 6 month intervals for stability, whereas wedge resection or chemotherapy may be indicated for "hot" or hypermetabolic lesions. The CT portion of PET/CT is commonly performed in either the end-tidal volume phase or during quiet respiration, which provide the closest match to PET for image co-registration. However, these phases of respiration lower CT sensitivity for detection of very small pulmonary nodules. Alternatively, a separate dedicated inspiratory CT may be performed as part of the imaging protocol solely for pulmonary nodule evaluation.

The accuracy and effectiveness of PET imaging in colorectal cancer has been well studied. In the assessment of data in the literature from the previous 10 years studying PET sensitivity for nodal involvement and distal metastatic disease, there are multiple confounding factors including the use of PET versus PET/CT, the use of emission only versus attenuation-corrected PET images, and the use of single versus multidetector CT scanning (MDCT). In addition, surgical gold standard staging varies in terms of number of lymph nodes resected,

Table 8.4. Limitations of PET in colorectal cancer

(a) False positives:
Physiologic colonic radiotracer uptake
Colonic adenoma (premalignant lesion)
Thrombosed hemorrhoid
Acute diverticulitis
Colonic fistula
Liver abscess
Post-radiation colitis/proctitis
Postoperative uptake – scar, stoma, laparoscopy ports, pre-sacral soft tissue
   (for up to 4 months postoperatively)
Crohn's disease

(b) False negatives:
Mucinous colorectal carcinoma (uncommon)
Peritoneal carcinomatosis (PET/CT may help to overcome this limitation)
Low volume nodal or metastatic disease (in common with all current imaging
   modalities)
Pulmonary nodules <1 cm on PET (PET/CT will identify small pulmonary
   nodules)
Liver metastases less than 1 cm in size detected by contrast MRI, but may be
   detected by contrast enhanced PET/CT

---

limited sampling of local lymph nodes, and whether total mesocolon resection is routinely performed. Histologic techniques also vary, with conventional histology demonstrating less nodal involvement in comparison to molecular biology techniques. Only limited data on the accuracy of PET/CT in terms of long-term follow-up or prognosis are available as yet. The ability of the radiologist or nuclear medicine physician to interpret both modalities of PET/CT is likely to increase the added benefit of the combination modality, with a recent study demonstrating 18% increased accuracy when dedicated reporting of the CT portion of a PET/CT examination was performed [25].

Postneoadjuvant chemotherapy, liver lesions with residual abnormality detected by CT, or MRI may no longer demonstrate increased FDG uptake at PET/CT consistent with treatment response by PET criteria. As a result these lesions are no longer identified on the PET component of the PET/CT study but are identified on the contrast CT component of PET/CT. Microscopic residual disease should be considered in such lesions prior to liver resection.

Conclusion

The limitations of PET in colorectal cancer are presented in Table 8.4. The strongest indications for PET or PET/CT imaging in colorectal carcinoma are in the diagnosis of recurrent disease, exclusion of extrahepatic metastasis prior to liver resection, exclusion of extrapulmonary metastasis prior to lung resection, or in the evaluation of a rising CEA level. Optimal imaging assessment prior to liver resection is with a combination of PET/CT and contrast MRI. Despite the relatively increased cost of FDG-PET imaging in comparison to other modalities, it is cost-effective because of increased diagnostic accuracy in comparison to CT. The information provided by PET/CT is likely to combine the best imaging features of both modalities and become the gold standard for staging in colorectal carcinoma.

References

1. What are the key statistics for colorectal cancer? American Cancer Society (www.cancer.org); 2005 Accessed August 2005.
2. Can colorectal polyps and cancer be found early? American Cancer Society (www.cancer.org); 2005 Accessed August 2005.
3. O'Connell JB, Maggard MA, Ko CY. Colon cancer survival rates with the new American Joint Committee on Cancer sixth edition staging. J Natl Cancer Inst 2004;96(19):1420–1425.
4. Kitapci MT, Coleman RE. Colorectal cancer. In: Oehr P, Biersack HJ, Coleman E, editors. PET and PET/CT in Oncology. Berlin: Springer; 2003;20:213–226.
5. American Cancer Society 2003. Facts and figures. Atlanta, GA: ACS.
6. Nyam DC, Ho YH, Leong AF, Seow-Choen F. Palliative surgery for locally recurrent colorectal cancer. Singapore Med J 1999;40:333–335.
7. Heald RJ, Karanjia ND. Results of radical surgery for rectal cancer. World J Surg 1992;16:848–857.
8. Fuhrman GM, Curley SA, Hohn DC, Roh MS. Improved survival after resection of colorectal liver metastasis. Ann Surg Oncol 1995;2:537–541.
9. Holm A, Bradley E, Aldrete JS. Hepatic resection of metastasis for colorectal carcinoma: mortality, morbidity and pattern of recurrence. Ann Surg 1989;209:428–434.
10. Labow DM, Buell JE, Yoshida A, Rosen S, Posner MC. Isolated pulmonary recurrence after resection of colorectal hepatic metastasis – is resection indicated? Cancer J 2002;8:342–347.
11. Whiteford MH, Whiteford HM, Yee LF, et al. Usefulness of FDG PET scan in the assessment of suspected metastatic or recurrent adenocarcinoma of the colon and rectum. Dis Colon Rectum 2000;34:759–770.
12. Kamel EM, Thumshirn M, Truninger K, et al. Significance of incidental FDG accumulation in the gastrointestinal tract on PET/CT. Correlation with endoscopic and histologic results. J Nucl Med 2004;45:1804–1810.
13. Yasuda S, Hirofumi F, Nakahara T, et al. 18F-FDG PET in detection of colonic adenomas. J Nucl Med 2001;42:989–992.
14. Chen YK, Kao CH, Liao AC, Shenn YY, Su CT. Colorectal cancer screening in asymptomatic adults. The role of FDG PET scan. Anticancer Res 2003;23:4357–4361.
15. McArdle CS, Kerr DJ, Boyle P, editors. Colorectal Cancer. Oxford: Isis Medical Media; 2000.

16. Iyer RB, Silverman PM, DuBrow RA, Charnsangavej C. Imaging in the diagnosis, staging and follow-up of colorectal cancer. AJR Am J Roentgenol 2002;179:3–13.

17. Detry RJ, Kartheusen AH, Lagneaux G, Rahier J. Preoperative lymph node staging in rectal cancer: a difficult challenge. Int J Colorectal Dis 1996;11:217–221.

18. Denecke T, Rau B, Hoffmann KT, et al. Comparison of CT, MRI and FDG-PET in response predication of patients with locally advanced rectal cancer after multimodal preoperative therapy. Eur Radiol 2005;15:1658–1666.

19. Gordon BA, Flanagan FL, Dehdashti F. Wholebody PET: Normal variations, pitfalls and technical considerations. AJR Am J Roentgenol 1997;169:1675–1680.

20. Fernandez FG, Drebin JA, Linehan DC, et al. Five year survival after resection of hepatic metastasis from colorectal cancer in patients screened by PET with F18-FDG. Ann Surg 2004;240:438–447.

21. Fong Y, Saldinger PF, Akhurst T, et al. Utility of 18F-FDG PET scanning in selection of patients for resection of hepatic colorectal metastases. Am J Surg 1999; 178:282–287.

22. Flamen P, Strobaarts S, Van Cutsem E, et al. Additional value of wholebody PET with F18 FDG in recurrent colorectal cancer. J Clin Oncol 1999;17:894–901.

23. Blokhuis TJ, van der Schaaf MC, van den Tol MP, Comans EF, Manoliu RA, van der Sijp JR. Results of radiofrequency ablation of primary and secondary liver tumours: long term follow-up with CT and F18 PET scanning. Scand J Gastroenterol Suppl 2004;241:93–97.

24. Cohade C, Osman M, Leal J, Wahl RL. Direct comparison of 18F-FDG PET and PET/CT in patients with colorectal carcinoma. J Nucl Med 2003;44:1804–1805.

25. Kamel IR, Cohade C, Neyman E, Fishman EK, Wahl RL. Incremental value of CT in PET/CT of patients with colorectal carcinoma. Abdom Imaging 2004;29:663–668.

9. PET in Esophageal Cancer

Martin J. O'Connell, Ronald B. Workman, Jr., and R. Edward Coleman

Epidemiology

The American Cancer Society estimates that 14,250 people will be diagnosed with esophageal cancer in 2005, and 13,570 will die of the disease. Because it is usually advanced at diagnosis, most people eventually die of esophageal cancer. In the 1960s, overall 5-year survival rates were less than 5%, and today overall 5-year survival is 9–16% [1]. While improvements in diagnosis and treatment have taken place, without an effective screening tool most cases remain advanced at diagnosis unless detected incidentally.

There are several known risk factors associated with esophageal cancer. Esophageal cancer is three to four times as common in men as in women, and 50% more common in African Americans than in white Americans. African Americans are more likely to have squamous cell esophageal cancer, whereas white Americans are more likely to develop adenocarcinoma. Chronic gastroesophageal reflux disease (GERD) can lead to metaplasia of the epithelial lining of the lower esophagus from normal squamous cells to columnar cells. This condition, known as Barrett's esophagus, carries a high risk of cellular dysplasia. Dysplastic cells are premalignant, and patients with Barrett's esophagus are strongly encouraged to undergo frequent upper endoscopy. Additional risk factors for esophageal cancer, particularly squamous cell, include tobacco and alcohol use, especially when combined. Obesity and a diet low in fruits and vegetables have been linked to an increased risk of esophageal adenocarcinoma. Chemical exposure, especially lye ingestion, tylosis (a rare autosomal dominant genetic abnormality characterized by hyperkeratosis of volar surfaces), and esophageal web formation are also strongly associated with esophageal cancer.

Esophageal carcinoma typically occurs in the distal esophagus, with surgery being potentially curative. Palliative options include surgery, radiotherapy/brachytherapy, or metallic stent placement. Combination therapy consisting of surgery, chemotherapy, and radiation therapy can increase survival [2]. Combination modality therapy is associated with morbidity and expense; it could delay potentially curative surgery in some patients with early stage disease, risking progression of disease to an incurable stage if treatment is unsuccessful. Nodal status is extremely important in determining prognosis. Five-year survival for N0 disease is rated at 42–72%, and with N1 disease is 10–12% [3]. Reduced survival reflects the likelihood of distal metastatic disease. Most esophageal carcinomas present at an advanced stage at diagnosis, with 30–50% of cases being stage IV at presentation [4].

Patients with esophageal carcinoma frequently present with symptoms related to obstruction (dysphagia), with dysphagia for solid foods preceding dysphagia

Table 9.1. PET imaging versus conventional imaging in esophageal cancer

	Sensitivity	**Specificity**
Metastatic disease:		
PET	47–78%	89–93%
CT	33–46%	74–96%
Stage IV disease:		
PET	74%	90%
CT	41%	83%
EUS	42%	94%
Locoregional lymph nodes (within 3 cm of primary tumor):		
PET	22–89%*	78–100%
CT	15–87%*	73–100%
EUS	85–95%	54–80%

* In comparison to extensive lymph node dissection PET had sensitivity of 52% versus CT sensitivity of 15% [16].

for liquids. Initial staging modalities include barium swallow followed by endoscopy and biopsy. Because of the relative insensitivity for detecting local lymphadenopathy by all imaging modalities, local lymph nodes are resected at the time of surgery. Unlike breast or colon carcinoma, node positivity on surgically resected esophageal specimens does not affect future treatment. Thirty-month survival with local disease is 60% and with distant metastatic disease is 20% [5].

Investigative options in staging locoregional nodal disease (i.e., nodal disease within 3 cm of the primary lesion) include CT, endoscopic ultrasound (EUS), and endoscopic ultrasound with fine-needle aspiration biopsy (FNA). Initial staging can also include thoracoscopic sampling of mediastinal lymph nodes and abdominal laparoscopy and sampling of upper abdominal lymph nodes. CT and EUS-guided biopsy are only able to evaluate certain lymph node groups. Surgical lymph node sampling is associated with some morbidity and is limited to sampling certain lymph node groups. MRI has been used in selected patients, but in general it does not provide additional information over CT. ^{18}F fluorodeoxyglucose (FDG) positron emission tomography (PET) imaging has been used as a non-invasive method of staging local and distal disease in esophageal carcinoma. PET or PET/CT imaging, when used in selected patients, has a significant role in improving staging and leads to more effective treatment (Table 9.1).

Technical Considerations for Positron Emission Tomography Imaging

Imaging is performed 60–90 minutes after FDG injection. Imaging from the skull base to mid-thigh is usually adequate unless disease is suspected outside of those limits. In general the target to background uptake of radiotracer, representing metabolic activity in the tumor in comparison to surrounding tissues, increases over time to a peak level (typically at 2 hours) and then declines. Visual analysis of the images is usually adequate for interpretation, but semi-quantitation of lesions can be performed using region-of-interest analysis with or without determining the standardized uptake value (SUV). Uptake in a lesion can be compared to a region of interest placed in the mediastinal blood pool activity or the liver. In the assessment of SUV, the timing of PET imaging after FDG injection must be standardized as SUV values vary for an individual tumor depending on the time after injection at which imaging is performed. SUV measurement is subject to many potential causes of variability and many PET physicians do not use SUV measurement in routine clinical practice, but only as a research tool. In this case visual assessment of the intensity of FDG uptake is made.

Diagnosis

PET is highly sensitive at identifying the primary tumor, with reported sensitivity for lesion detection of 83–96% [6]. However, PET is rarely used to identify the primary tumor. The SUV, which is a measure of the intensity of metabolic activity in a lesion, can be used to predict survival. An SUV >7.0 is associated with a significantly lower survival rate in comparison to patients with lower values [7]. Although the SUV may correlate with the depth of invasion, it cannot define T stage.

There is no difference in uptake values between squamous carcinomas and adenocarcinomas [6]. PET scanning has been reported as having false-negative results in esophageal cancer in patients with small volume disease (T1 or T in situ) and in 10–15% of undifferentiated esophageal adenocarcinomas [3]. Some tumors located at the gastroesophageal junction, particularly with signet ring conformation or mucin-containing tumors, may have reduced or very low uptake of FDG. Therefore, FDG-PET accuracy for lesions in the esophagus may not necessarily apply to tumors at the gastroesophageal junction.

There are numerous potential mechanisms for low FDG uptake including differences in GLUT-1 or GLUT-3 receptor expression, reduced intracellular hexokinase activity, or a low volume of tumor cells per unit volume of tumor mass. In uncommon cases in which a tumor of T2 stage or greater demonstrates no FDG uptake, then PET should not be relied upon to accurately stage disease, as metastases from such lesions are also non-FDG avid. If a T1 primary lesion is not identified because of small volume, it is not clear whether the tumor can be followed accurately with PET.

Low-grade physiologic uptake in the esophagus may be a normal variant (Figure 9.1). Focal radiotracer may be identified in Barrett's esophagus or severe reflux esophagitis but it is usually more linear-appearing and not to the amount and extent as seen with cancer. However, correlation with endoscopic and biopsy findings may be necessary to differentiate esophagitis from distal esophageal cancer. Because of potential false positives and the inability to detect certain types of early stage disease, including tumor in situ (TIS) and T1a stage tumors, PET imaging is not useful in screening for esophageal primary lesions.

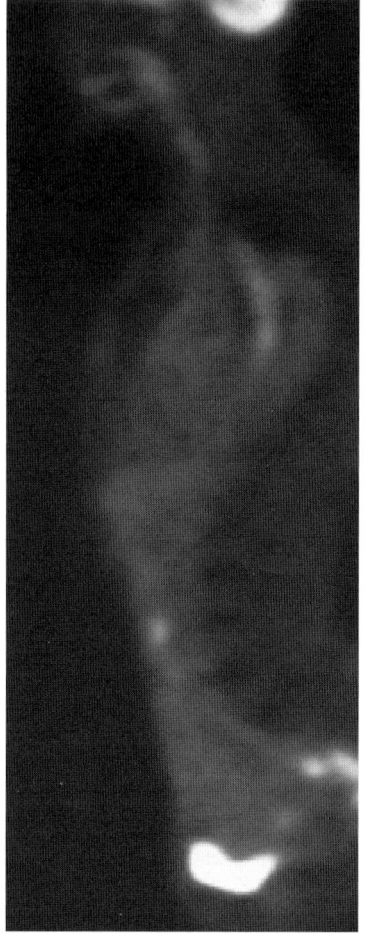

Figure 9.1. Sagittal PET image demonstrates diffuse, moderately increased radiotracer uptake throughout the esophagus, which is a normal variant. Uptake of this intensity can also be identified in reflux esophagitis. Rarely, benign physiologic uptake can be focal and intense, simulating a primary tumor.

Staging

TNM staging is determined by the depth of wall invasion of the primary lesion (T stage), the presence of local lymphadenopathy (N stage), and the presence of distal metastasis (Table 9.2). Esophageal carcinoma has an unpredictable pattern of lymph node spread, with both distal and proximal esophageal lesions potentially spreading to abdominal (celiac), retroperitoneal, mediastinal, and cervical lymph nodes. For example, the probability of both mid and distal esophageal tumors spreading to cervical lymph nodes is relatively similar at 27–29% [8]. The extent of lymph node involvement strongly correlates with patient prognosis and response to neoadjuvant chemotherapy.

Standard imaging in CT covers from the lower neck to the lower abdomen. In some patients, this limited coverage can mean that metastatic lesions in the neck or pelvis are not identified. CT uses various criteria for predicting lymph node involvement with tumor, with 10 mm being regarded as the maximum size in short axis for reactive or benign lymph nodes in the mediastinal region and 6–10 mm used as a cutoff in the cervical region, retroperitoneum, and upper abdomen. However, in a study of lung carcinoma staging, up to 40% of enlarged

Table 9.2. TNM staging of esophageal cancer

Primary tumor	
TX	Primary tumor cannot be assessed
T0	No evidence of primary tumor
Tis	Carcinoma in situ
T1	Tumor invades lamina propria or submucosa
T2	Tumor invades muscularis propria
T3	Tumor invades adventitia
T4	Tumor invades adjacent structures
Regional lymph nodes	
NX	Regional lymph nodes cannot be assessed
N0	No regional lymph node metastasis
N1	Regional lymph node metastasis
Distant metastasis	
MX	Distant metastasis cannot be assessed
M	No distant metastasis
M1	Distant metastasis
Tumors of the lower thoracic esophagus	
M1a	Metastasis in celiac lymph nodes
M1b	Other distant metastasis
Tumors of mid-thoracic esophagus	
M1a	Not applicable
M1b	Non regional lymph nodes and/or other distant metastasis
Tumors of the upper thoracic esophagus	
M1a	Metastasis in cervical nodes
M1b	Other distant metastasis

Source: Used with permission of the American Joint Committee on Cancer (AJCC), Chicago, Illinois. The original source for this material is the *AJCC Cancer Staging Manual*, Sixth Edition (2002), published by Springer-Verlag, New York, www.springeronline.com.

mediastinal lymph nodes by CT criteria did not contain tumor cells [9]. The presence of a fatty hilum in a lymph node has previously been used to suggest a benign etiology. Both surgery and PET imaging have demonstrated that lymph nodes measuring less than 10 mm in size and with a fatty hilum may contain tumor deposits.

EUS uses both size criteria and lesion echogenicity to assess whether a lymph node is involved with tumor; however, although having a high sensitivity, it is associated with reduced specificity [10]. The accuracy of EUS is increased when combined with endoscopic fine-needle aspiration biopsy (FNA). EUS is limited in local staging because of the small field of view and the ultrasound device being in the gastroesophageal lumen. It is limited to examining structures adjacent to the esophagus, stomach, or duodenum. In addition, esophageal narrowing cannot be passed in approximately 30% of cases, causing an inability to complete local staging [11]. Air-containing structures may be obscured or may reduce the field of view of EUS, because air blocks ultrasound transmission. The technique has high accuracy for assessment of both T stage and N stage, with a sensitivity of 62–95% and specificity of 54–80% for nodal disease [10–13]. EUS is limited in distinguishing T1 tumors from T2 tumors and also in distinguishing T3 from T4 tumors [11]. CT is less sensitive for T staging in comparison to EUS and has reduced sensitivity for detection of local lymphadenopathy (N stage). CT has better sensitivity and specificity in evaluating for T4 and stage IV disease in comparison to EUS.

CT assesses mediastinal fat invasion and invasion of structures adjacent to the esophagus, often using the lack of an intervening fat plane as an important sign in the assessment of invasion. To assess direct invasion of mediastinal vessels, intravenous contrast is used. The extent to which a vascular structure is surrounded by tumor predicts vascular invasion, with structures surrounded by greater than 180 degrees likely to have invasion, with a very high probability of invasion if 270 degrees or more is surrounded by tumor [14]. Stage IV disease is missed by CT in 18–29% of patients staged by surgery [13]. CT is not accurate in evaluating the pericardium in patients with esophageal cancer who may lose a fat plane between the esophagus and the pericardium secondary to cachexia, causing a misdiagnosis of local invasion. In addition, endoscopic ultrasound and CT cannot distinguish carcinoma from inflammation. PET is not an anatomic imaging modality and is limited in the assessment of local invasion. However, the combination of contrast-enhanced CT and co-registered PET images at PET/CT can overcome this problem.

Surgery is the gold standard in evaluating the accuracy of staging. EUS is the most accurate imaging modality in the evaluation of metastatic mediastinal lymph nodes with an accuracy of 64–80%, with CT having an accuracy of 45–74%. The combination of the two modalities has 70–90% accuracy [15]. In the assessment of diagnostic accuracy for distal lymphadenopathy, results are influenced by the extent of surgical resection. Gold standard evaluation is further limited by non-standard surgical technique with inter-institutional variations. In comparison to two- or three-field lymph node dissection, PET has sensitivity, specificity, and accuracy of 52%, 94%, and 84%, respectively, with CT having sensitivity, specificity, and accuracy of 15%, 97%, and 77%, respectively [16].

There is still limited information on the added value of PET/CT, but it is expected to combine the best features of both PET and CT, reducing false positives on PET and false negatives on CT. PET/CT is recommended in patients in whom the standard staging algorithm of CT followed by EUS suggests resectable disease. In these patients PET particularly improves the detection of metastatic disease (stage IV) and improves the specificity of local lymph node staging, having a greater positive predictive value than CT or EUS (Figure 9.2). If conventional imaging is negative for metastasis, PET imaging has been demonstrated to identify metastatic disease in 3–37% of patients [17]. Conversely, PET imaging can also be used to downstage patients by demonstrating no FDG accumulation in lesions suspected to be metastatic disease on other imaging examinations.

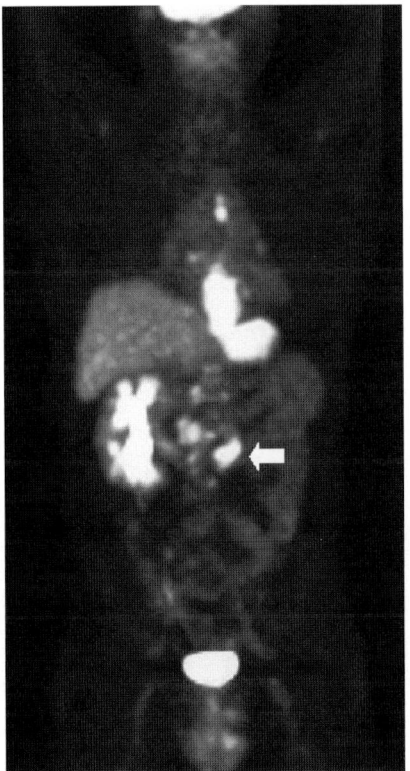

Figure 9.2. Initial staging coronal PET scan demonstrates a long segment tumor of the distal esophagus extending into gastric cardia. Metastatic hypermetabolic lesions are identified in the mediastinum and the retroperitoneum.

Considerations in Positron Emission Tomography and Positron Emission Tomography/Computed Tomography Interpretations in Staging

Results suggest that PET/CT fusion improves detection and characterization of metastatic sites. PET imaging may not be as sensitive as CT and EUS in detecting some peri-esophageal and left gastric lymph nodes because of reduced spatial resolution and proximity to the primary lesion (Figure 9.3).

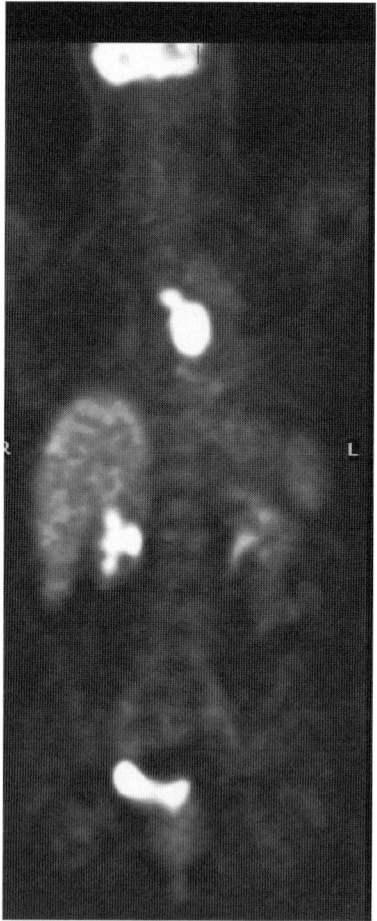

Figure 9.3. Coronal PET image demonstrates intense radiotracer up-take in a mid-esophageal squamous cell carcinoma. Adjacent intense activity is identified in a subcarinal lymph node. The intensity of uptake in the primary lesion almost masks the activity in the adjacent node. This is one of the proposed mechanisms that reduces sensitivity for detection of local lymph nodes in PET imaging.

Areas of tumor necrosis can cause heterogeneous uptake in the primary lesion, simulating lymphadenopathy adjacent to the primary lesion. In addition, small liver and lung lesions may not appear to be metabolically active because their small size is below the resolution of PET. Histologic confirmation of lesions that would prevent a patient from being selected for curative therapy is recommended. Failure to prove metastatic disease on image-guided or excisional biopsy can lead to uncertainty as to the stage of disease. A biopsy may be avoided if a typical pattern of metastatic disease is present. In one study PET incorrectly increased the N stage of T1 and T2 lesions (reflecting false-positive radiotracer uptake), but correctly staged T3 and T4 tumors [6]. Therefore, the accuracy and incremental value of PET is greatest in patients with a higher probability of metastasis. The diagnostic yield for metastatic disease in T1 tumors and carcinoma in situ lesions is very low, and PET is not routinely recommended in these patients. As with breast carcinoma and melanoma, PET cannot exclude locoregional microscopic disease diagnosed at surgery or laparoscopic staging, although it is superior to conventional modalities in detecting this disease.

Evaluating Response to Treatment and Restaging

The diagnostic accuracy of metabolism-based PET in response assessment appears more precise than anatomic based methods such as CT or EUS because of increased specificity in distinguishing post-surgical or post-treatment-related changes from residual disease [17]. PET is becoming more commonly used for restaging after surgery or assessment of treatment response to neoadjuvant or induction chemoradiation. Early response assessment evaluates tumor sensitivity to treatment and late response assessment evaluates for residual viable tumor. The Centers for Medicare and Medicaid Services (CMS) provide reimbursement of restaging in esophageal carcinoma, but do not cover early response evaluation at present, but this will be covered under the Registry (see Chapter 2). Up to 50% of patients with esophageal cancer will not respond to neoadjuvant chemoradiation, and these patients are at risk for disease progression during the period prior to surgery, which is delayed to facilitate neoadjuvant treatment [17]. The absence of an early PET-based restaging response can identify non-responders to chemoradiation even before treatment is completed. Early response to chemoradiation therapy can be measured up to 2 weeks after initiation of treatment. Response is more typically measured immediately following completion of a full chemoradiation therapy protocol. After 2 weeks of neoadjuvant treatment, an SUV reduction of 35% or greater predicts an ultimate histopathologic response to therapy with a sensitivity of 93% and specificity of 95% [18]. Fifty-three percent of patients with a metabolic response demonstrate subtotal or complete histopathologic response, with only 5% of patients without a metabolic response demonstrating the same findings [18].

Typical or late response assessment occurs after a complete course of chemoradiation therapy. Major responders at the primary tumor site can be defined by a >80% reduction of the tumor to liver uptake ratio, this response correlating with survival [17]. After induction therapy, in one study, an SUV reduction less than 52% in the primary lesion indicated a poor response [19]. A

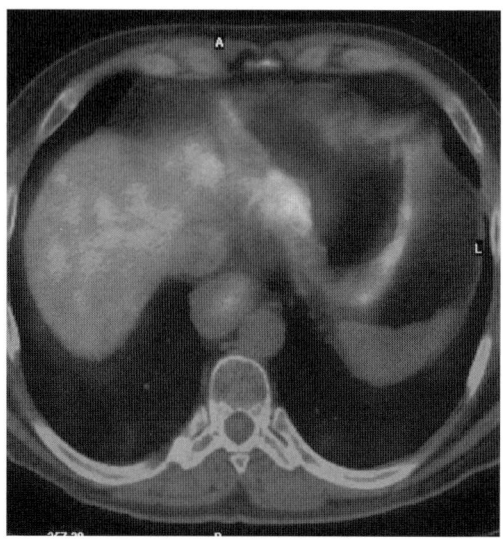

Figure 9.4. Axial restaging PET/CT fusion image at the level of the gastroe-sophageal junction demonstrates diffuse abnormal radiotracer uptake in the wall of the stomach and distal esophagus post-radiation therapy. The distal esophagus is dilated.

diagnosis of treatment response based on an SUV reduction of 52% or greater had sensitivity of 100% and specificity of 55%. The reduced specificity reflects treatment-related inflammation that may be related to chemotherapy or radiation therapy. Metabolically active radiation esophagitis proven histologically can be identified in up to 60% of patients after therapy (Figure 9.4). However, in general, a strong correlation is seen between response assessment at PET and histopathologic changes at surgery, and the response assessment is superior to that identified by CT. In the evaluation of therapeutic response, the negative predictive value of PET is particularly useful. Analyzing the primary tumor and metastatic lymphadenopathy, PET has a sensitivity of 71% and specificity of 82% in identifying major responders [19]. Sensitivity and specificity for pathologic complete response are 67% and 50%, respectively [19]. Therefore, a pathologic complete response cannot be predicted by a negative PET scan, because of the possibility of microscopic residual disease. Discordant response, with primary tumor SUV reduction but increased uptake in lymphadenopathy, can be identified, mainly in non-responders. The least responding PET-positive lesion determines prognosis. Flamen et al. demonstrated that response to neoadjuvant treatment could be predicted by nodal status on the basis of initial staging PET imaging with 33% response in N1 patients in comparison to 82% response in N0 patients [20]. Reduction in post-treatment SUV can also predict disease-free survival after neoadjuvant radiotherapy, with a 60% reduction in SUV representing a significantly longer 2-year disease-free period. However, the overall survival was not significantly altered. PET can also provide prognostic information for T3–T4 tumors with survival of 20–31% at 5 years in responders versus 0% in patients with no response [3]. CT, EUS, and MRI have significantly lower accuracy in assessing response to neoadjuvant therapy.

Assessment of response to treatment evaluation is an evolving area of PET imaging currently. It is likely that patients who are not benefiting from induction treatment will be imaged earlier than they are now and have treatment altered at an earlier stage with lower cumulative treatment toxicity. FDG-PET can also play a role in patient selection for continued treatment in non-responders.

Despite aggressive therapy, esophageal carcinoma recurrence is common. The survival benefit of early detection of recurrent disease is uncertain [17]. In the evaluation of recurrent tumors there are few data on the added benefit of PET, especially if CT demonstrates macroscopic metastasis. PET of esophageal cancer has not been studied as extensively as other cancers and the restaging indication is the least studied subgroup of esophageal cancer with relatively few studies in the literature. In the evaluation of tumor recurrence, one study demonstrated that PET provides up to 27% additional information (Figure 9.5) [21].

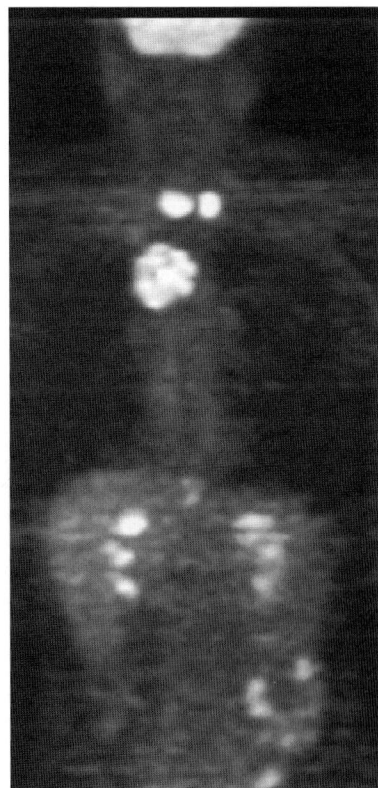

Figure 9.5. Coronal restaging PET scan demonstrates multiple foci of intense uptake at the gastroesophageal anastomosis site following esophagectomy and gastric pull-up. Recurrent adenocarcinoma was confirmed at biopsy.

This additional information may be relevant in an individual patient in determining prognosis and future treatment options. In comparison to conventional imaging, PET has increased sensitivity and accuracy for detection of recurrent local lymphadenopathy and distal metastatic disease.

Considerations in Positron Emission Tomography and Positron Emission Tomography/Computed Tomography Interpretations in Monitoring Response and Restaging

False-positive PET results in evaluation of response to treatment or restaging can be caused by radiation esophagitis. Longer segment involvement may help in some cases. In cases where the original tumor involved a long segment of the esophagus, this distinction may be difficult to make. PET may also underestimate response to treatment by failing to distinguish residual disease from the inflammatory and immune system responses to the primary lesion that can be hypermetabolic. PET is less susceptible to misdiagnosis of post-treatment changes as residual tumor in comparison to CT or EUS. False positives have also been described in patients with a history of recent dilatation of the esophagus or at the gastroesophageal anastomosis following resection secondary to inflammation. The specificity of a positive PET study at the gastroesophageal anastomosis has been found to be 57% in comparison to 93% on conventional imaging [17]. Conventional imaging requires a more significant volume of recurrent tumor in order to confirm disease recurrence in comparison to PET. Most recurrences after surgery are distal metastases that may be less affected by local treatment. Non-responders by PET criteria may demonstrate a histopathologic response at surgery [17].

Sarcoidosis is a potential cause of false-positive hypermetabolic lymphadenopathy in the neck, mediastinum, or retroperitoneum. Such patients may be asymptomatic. Correlation with any prior history of respiratory disease, examination for lung parenchymal abnormalities on co-registered CT, or a characteristic distribution of lymph nodes may help suggest false-positive uptake. Discussion of individual patients at a multidisciplinary team conference may help identify potential causes of false-positive nodal uptake. There is no definitive way at present to exclude sarcoidosis as a cause of hypermetabolic lymphadenopathy apart from image-guided biopsy, mediastinoscopy, or surgical resection. Abnormal hypermetabolic activity in thyroid or parathyroid adenomas or carcinoma can be identified by confirming co-registration to the thyroid gland or immediately posterior to the thyroid. Ultrasound-guided fine-needle aspirate biopsy is recommended to confirm or exclude a primary or secondary thyroid tumor.

Conclusion

Table 9.3 presents the limitations of PET in esophageal cancer. PET/CT scanning has a major role in the algorithm of initial staging and assessment of response to neoadjuvant treatment in cancer of the esophagus. In a large study with a heterogeneous population for staging, evaluation of response to treatment and restaging of esophageal cancer, conventional PET altered management in 14% of patients [22]. The majority of postoperative tumor recurrences of esophageal cancer are distant metastases. PET is superior to CT in detecting distant metastases at diagnosis and should be routinely employed in patients who have potentially resectable disease on the basis of CT and EUS evaluation, to exclude spread of tumor beyond the operative field. In the assessment of locoregional lymph nodes (within 3 cm of the primary tumor) PET is used as an adjunct to CT and EUS to improve the specificity of lymph node involvement. Therefore a combination of EUS with FNA biopsy with FDG-PET/CT is the most accurate initial staging method for esophageal cancer. Despite potential false-positive findings, especially from radiation esophagitis, FDG-PET is superior to conventional imaging in the evaluation of response to treatment. Patients with a less than 52% reduction in SUV following neoadjuvant treatment are non-responders. More data are needed to ascertain the optimum time to assess response to neoadjuvant treatment. PET is useful in restaging esophageal cancer but the impact of added benefit of the modality for this indication has been studied less well than in other cancers. A proportion of esophageal and gastroesophageal junction tumors do not take up FDG and therefore cannot be followed using PET imaging. The number of studies in the literature on the role of PET/CT in esophageal cancer is increasing, and it is anticipated that PET/CT will

Table 9.3. Limitations of PET in esophageal cancer

(a) False positives:
Barrett's esophagus
Hiatus hernia
Esophagitis – reflux, infective or radiation-induced
Inflammation at postoperative anastomosis
Severe bacterial infections, for example lobar pneumonia, possibly secondary to aspiration
Thyroid adenoma or carcinoma uptake simulating cervical metastasis
Sarcoid lymphadenopathy
Anthracosilicosis lymphadenopathy
(b) False negatives:
Early T stage lesions (Tis, T1)
Signet ring adenocarcinomas and some poorly differentiated adenocarcinomas of the gastroesophageal junction
Locoregional lymph nodes immediately adjacent to the primary lesion
Cannot predict complete histopathologic tumor response

significantly improve the evaluation of patients with esophageal cancer by combining the best features of both PET and CT, significantly lowering false-positive and false-negative results.

References

1. What are the key statistics about cancer of the esophagus? American Cancer Society (www.cancer.org); 2005 Accessed August 2005.
2. Vermund H, Pories WJ, Hillard J, Wiley AL, Youngblood R. Neoadjuvant chemoradiation therapy in patients with surgically treated esophageal cancer. Acta Oncol 2001;40:558–565.
3. Flamen P, Mortelmans L. Gastro-esophageal cancer. In: Oehr P, Biersack HJ, Coleman E, editors. PET and PET-CT in Oncology. Berlin: Springer; 2003;18:187–202.
4. Flanagan FL, Dehdashti F, Siegel BA, et al. Staging of esophageal cancer with FDG PET. AJR Am J Roentgenol 1997;168:417–424.
5. Luketich JD, Friedman DM, Weigel TL, et al. Evaluation of distant metastasis in esophageal cancer. 100 consecutive PET scans. Ann Thorac Surg 1999;68:1135–1137.
6. Heeren PA, Jager PL, Bongaerts F, van Dullemen H, Sluiter W, Plukker JT. Detection of distant metastasis in esophageal cancer with F-18 FDG PET. J Nucl Med 2004; 45:980–987.
7. Fukunaga T, Okazumi S, Koide Y, et al. Evaluation of esophageal cancers using F18-FDG PET. J Nucl Med 1998;39:1002–1007.
8. Akiyama H, Tsurumaru M, Udagawa H, Kajiyama Y. Radical lymph node dissection for carcinoma of the thoracic esophagus. Ann Surg 1994;220:364–373.
9. McLoud TC, Bourjoin PM, Greenberg RW, et al. Bronchogenic carcinoma: analysis of staging in the mediastinum with CT by comparison with lymph node mapping and sampling. Radiology 1992;182:319–323.
10. Flamen P, Lerut A, Van Cutsem E, et al. Utility of positron emission tomography for staging of patients with potentially operable esophageal carcinoma. J Clin Oncol 2000;18:3202–3210.
11. Fickling WE, Wallace MB. Endoscopic ultrasound and upper gastrointestinal disorders. J Clin Gastroenterol 2003;36:103–110.
12. Rasanen JV, Sihvo EI, Knuuti MJ, et al. Prospective analysis of the accuracy of positron emission tomography, computed tomography and endoscopic ultrasonography in staging of adenocarcinoma of the esophagus and the gastroesophageal junction. Ann Surg Oncol 2003;10:954–960.
13. Wren SM, Stijins P, Srinivas S. Positron emission tomography in the initial staging of esophageal cancer. Arch Surg 2002;137:1001–1006.
14. Megibow AJ, Zhou XH, Rotterdam H, et al. Pancreatic adenocarcinoma: CT versus MR imaging in the evaluation of respectability. Radiology 1995;195:327–332.
15. Lerut T, Flamen P, Ectors N, et al. Histopathologic validation of lymph node staging with FDG-PET scan in cancer of the esophagus and gastroesophageal junction. A

prospective study based on primary surgery with extensive lymphadenectomy. Ann Surg 2000;232:743–752.

16. Kim K, Park SJ, Kim BT, Lee KS, Shim YM. Evaluation of lymph node metastases in squamous cell carcinoma of the esophagus with positron emission tomography. Ann Thorac Surg 2001;71:290–294.

17. Dehdashti F, Siegel BA. Neoplasms of the esophagus and stomach. Semin Nucl Med 2004;34(3):198–208.

18. Weber WA, Ott K, Becker K, et al. Predication of response to preoperative chemotherapy in adenocarcinomas of esophagogastric junction by metabolic imaging. J Clin Oncol 2001;19:3058–3065.

19. Brucher BL, Weber W, Bauer M, et al. Neoadjuvant therapy of esophageal squamous cell carcinoma: response evaluation by positron emission tomography. Ann Surg 2001; 233:300–309.

20. Flamen P, Van Cutsem E, Lerut A, et al. Positron emission tomography for assessment of response to induction radiochemotherapy in locally advanced esophageal carcinoma. Ann Oncol 2002;13:361–368.

21. Flamen P, Lerut A, Van Cutsem E, et al. The utility of positron emission tomography for the diagnosis and staging of recurrent esophageal cancer. J Thorac Cardiovasc Surg 2000;120:1085–1092.

22. Yeung HW, Macapinlac HA, Mazumdar M, Bains M, Finn RD, Larson SM. FDG-PET in esophageal cancer – incremental value over computed tomography. Clin Positron Imaging 1999;2(5):255–260.

10. PET in Thyroid Cancer

Ronald B. Workman, Jr. and R. Edward Coleman

Epidemiology

In 2005 it was estimated that 25,690 new cases of thyroid cancer would be diagnosed and approximately 1490 people would die of thyroid cancer that year in the United States. Furthermore, the number of new cases of thyroid cancer continues to rise due to a 3% per year increase in the incidence per 100,000 people [1]. The majority of thyroid cancer cases arise from follicular cell origin and have well-differentiated histopathology. Papillary and follicular carcinomas are the most common cell types. Hürthle cell (a subtype of follicular) and anaplastic (or undifferentiated) thyroid cancers are less common yet more aggressive variants, with anaplastic among the most lethal of all malignancies. Medullary thyroid cancer is of distinct histopathology, arising from parafollicular, calcitonin-producing cells (also called C cells).

Papillary cancer is the most common thyroid malignancy, comprising 80–85% of cases. These tumors are usually unifocal, but can be multifocal, involving both lobes in 10–20% of cases. Although slow growing, they often metastasize early to regional lymph nodes. Follicular cancers tend to arise in countries with iodine-deficient diets, and they comprise about 5–10% of thyroid cancer cases. These tumors usually do not metastasize early, but when they do, it is usually to distant sites (e.g. lungs and bone). Lymph nodes are less often involved than in papillary thyroid cancer. The well-differentiated thyroid cancers are treated both surgically by thyroidectomy and with radioiodine therapy. Because these tumors arise from the cells responsible for thyroid hormone synthesis, they are amenable to radioiodide treatment with iodine-131 (^{131}I) sodium iodide administered orally, either in liquid or capsule form. The normal thyroid gland and well-differentiated thyroid tumors do not distinguish between radioactive and non-radioactive iodide. Because they are well-differentiated, papillary and follicular tumors retain their iodide-concentrating characteristics and are therefore exquisitely sensitive to the tissue-damaging effects of the beta particle emitting ^{131}I.

Because medullary thyroid cancer and anaplastic carcinoma do not concentrate iodide, they are not candidates for radioiodide ablation. If resectable, these cancers are treated surgically with neoadjuvant and/or adjuvant chemoradiation. Medullary thyroid cancer can be treated with ^{131}I metaiodobenzylguanidine (MIBG).

Thyroid malignancy is staged according to the Tumor, Node, Metastasis (TNM) framework created by the American Joint Committee on Cancer [2]. Table 10.1 provides the TNM staging of thyroid cancer.

Medicare has coverage policies for several indications in many malignancies (see Chapter 2). The following is the policy for thyroid cancer coverage:

Table 10.1. TNM staging for thyroid cancer

Primary tumor (T)
TX   Primary tumor cannot be assessed
T0   No evidence of primary tumor
T1   Tumor 2 cm or less in greatest dimension limited to the thyroid
T2   Tumor more than 2 cm but not more than 4 cm in greatest dimension
       limited to the thyroid
T3   Tumor more than 4 cm in greatest dimension limited to the thyroid or
       any tumor with minimal extrathyroidal extension (e.g. extension to
       sternothyroid muscle or perithyroid soft tissues)
T4a   Tumor of any size extending beyond the thyroid capsule to invade
       subcutaneous soft tissues, larynx, trachea, esophagus, or recurrent
       laryngeal nerve
T4b   Tumor invades prevertebral fascia or encases carotid artery or
       mediastinal vessels

       All anaplastic carcinomas are considered T4 tumors
T4a   Intrathyroidal anaplastic carcinoma – surgically resectable
T4b   Extrathyroidal anaplastic carcinoma – surgically unresectable

Regional lymph nodes (N)
NX   Regional lymph nodes cannot be assessed
N0   No regional lymph node metastasis
N1   Regional lymph node metastasis
N1a   Metastasis to level VI (pretracheal, paratracheal, and
       prelaryngeal/Delphian lymph nodes)
N1b   Metastasis to unilateral, bilateral, or contralateral cervical or superior
       mediastinal lymph nodes

Distant metastasis (M)
MX   Distant metastasis cannot be assessed
M0   No distant metastasis
M1   Distant metastasis

Stage grouping

Papillary or follicular (under 45 years):

| Stage I | Any T | Any N | M0 |
| Stage II | Any T | Any N | M1 |

Papillary or follicular (45 years and older):

Stage I	T1	N0	M0
Stage II	T2	N0	M0
Stage III	T3	N0	M0
	T1	N1a	M0
	T2	N1a	M0
	T3	N1a	M0
Stage IVA	T4a	N0	M0
	T4a	N1a	M0
	T1	N1b	M0
	T2	N1b	M0

Continued.

Table 10.1. *Continued.* TNM staging for thyroid cancer

	T3	N1b	M0
	T4a	N1b	M0
Stage IVB	T4b	Any N	M0
Stage IVC	Any T	Any N	M1
Medullary carcinoma:			
Stage I	T1	N0	M0
Stage II	T2	N0	M0
Stage III	T3	N0	M0
	T1	N1a	M0
	T2	N1a	M0
	T3	N1a	M0
Stage IVA	T4a	N0	M0
	T4a	N1a	M0
	T1	N1b	M0
	T2	N1b	M0
	T3	N1b	M0
	T4a	N1b	M0
Stage IVB	T4b	Any N	M0
Stage IVC	Any T	Any N	M1
Anaplastic carcinoma (all anaplastic carcinomas are considered stage IV):			
Stage IVA	T4a	Any N	M0
Stage IVB	T4b	Any N	M0
Stage IVC	Any T	Any N	M1

Source: Used with permission of the American Joint Committee on Cancer (AJCC), Chicago, Illinois. The original source for this material is the *AJCC Cancer Staging Manual*, Sixth Edition (2002), published by Springer-Verlag, New York, www.springeronline.com.

Only thyroid cancers of follicular cell origin that have been previously treated by thyroidectomy and radioiodine ablation and have a rising serum thyroglobulin level (greater than 10 ng/ml) but a negative iodine-131 whole-body scan are covered by the Centers for Medicare and Medicaid Services (CMS) at this time.

Positron Emission Tomography and Positron Emission Tomography/Computed Tomography versus Conventional Imaging in Thyroid Cancer

Thyroid nodules are quite prevalent (roughly 5%), and most are benign [3]. However, to appropriately and quickly identify the approximately 15% that are malignant, clinicians, radiologists, and nuclear medicine physicians should work together from a common understanding of the natural history of thyroid pathology. The management of patients with thyroid nodules can be both complex and controversial. As such, the initial management of these patients is outside the scope of this book. Suffice it to say, a systematic approach includes obtaining a full history, physical examination, thyroid function testing, and possibly thyroid ultrasound and radionuclide thyroid scintigram (usually with ^{99m}Tc pertechnetate or ^{123}I sodium iodide). Each of these steps may have a role in evaluating and characterizing thyroid abnormalities. Furthermore, in most patients who have a palpable thyroid nodule and particularly in those who are high risk, who have lesions which exhibit suspicious behavior, or who have lesions that exhibit worrisome imaging characteristics, cytologic correlation via fine-needle aspiration (FNA) is very important. FNA has proven to be sensitive, specific, and well-accepted because of its minimal discomfort and low risk of complications and is the procedure of choice in the initial evaluation of most solitary nodules [4]. Now, FDG-PET is finding a useful clinical niche in management as well.

The role of FDG-PET in cases of known thyroid cancer is well documented; yet, although there are several cases of incidental thyroid cancer detection with FDG-PET, its precise role in the diagnosis of thyroid malignancy has not been well defined [5]. Kresnik and colleagues evaluated FDG-PET in the preoperative assessment of suspicious thyroid nodules and found it helpful in selecting patients for surgery, especially if cytology is inconclusive. They found that using an SUV cutoff of 2.0 led to 100% sensitivity, 63% specificity, and 100% negative predictive value in diagnosing thyroid carcinoma [6].

FDG-PET can also incidentally detect thyroid cancer. In cases where whole-body FDG-PET scanning for a non-thyroidal malignancy incidentally detects a focal area of hypermetabolism within the thyroid gland, the literature strongly supports investigation to rule out a second primary [7]. Diffuse thyroid gland uptake raises the question of thyroiditis, but focal FDG uptake carries an approximately 25–50% chance of thyroid cancer and should be worked up [8] (Figures 10.1 and 10.2). In one small series, Van den Bruel and colleagues reported on

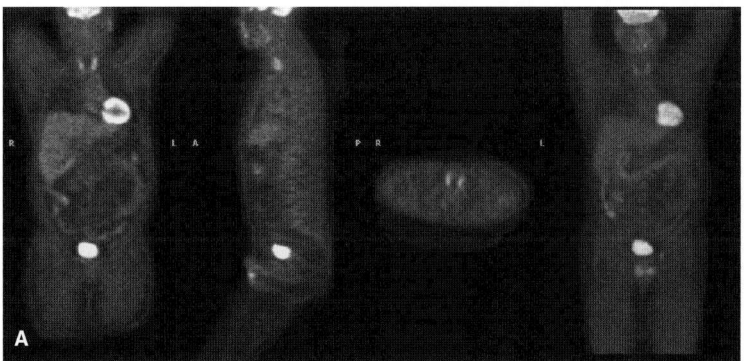

Figure 10.1. Diffuse thyroid uptake consistent with thyroiditis (**A** and **B**). Whole-body FDG-PET/CT images demonstrate moderate diffuse uptake within the thyroid gland. This activity has frequently been described in association with thyroiditis, but it can also be seen in patients without known thyroid disease.

Continued.

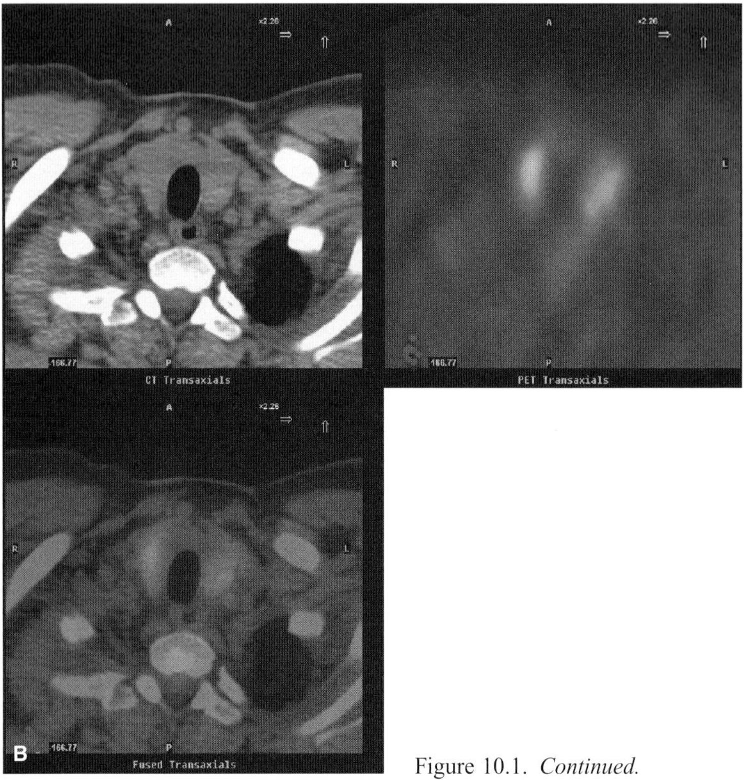

Figure 10.1. *Continued.*

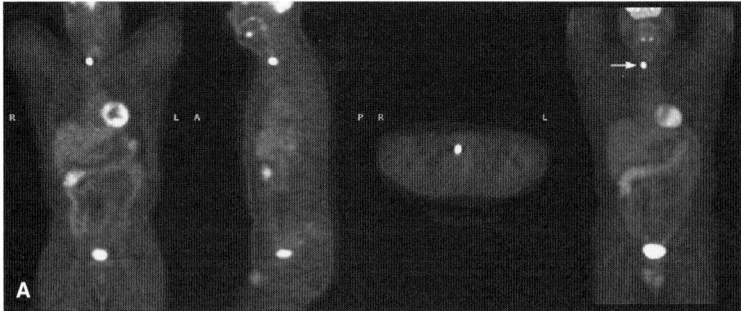

Figure 10.2. Incidental detection of thyroid malignancy. **(A)** Whole-body FDG-PET/CT scan of a patient who is status post chemotherapy for B-cell lymphoma. No evidence of active lymphoma is seen. However, there is an intense focus of increased FDG uptake in the right neck region (white arrow).

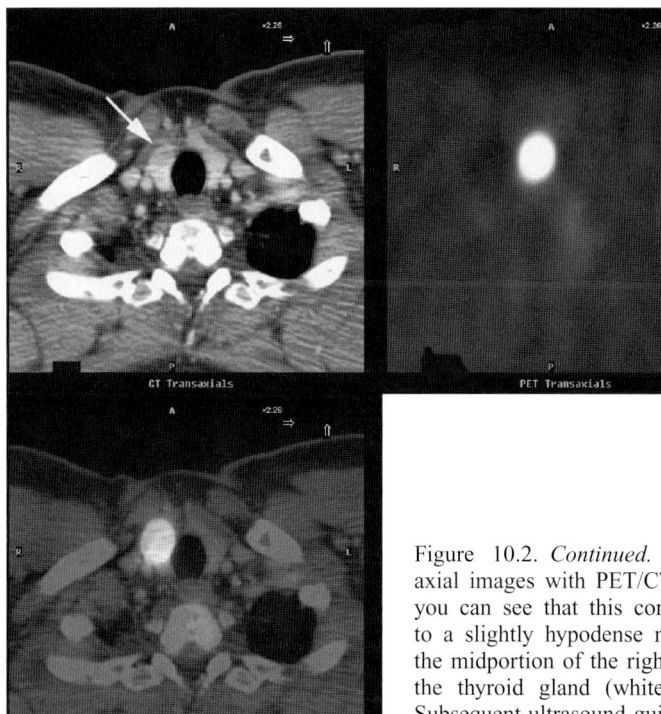

Figure 10.2. *Continued.* **(B)** On axial images with PET/CT fusion, you can see that this corresponds to a slightly hypodense nodule in the midportion of the right lobe of the thyroid gland (white arrow). Subsequent ultrasound-guided fine-needle aspiration revealed papillary carcinoma.

eight patients who demonstrated focal thyroid "hot spots" on FDG-PET scanning for non-thyroidal malignancy. Each patient underwent fine-needle aspiration cytology of these "incidentalomas." At surgery, five patients had thyroid cancer (three papillary and two medullary), and two patients had benign follicular adenomas (one patient had not undergone surgery at the time of publication) [9].

Positron Emission Tomography and Well-Differentiated Thyroid Cancer

Thyroid tumors are usually first detected when either the patient or the physician detects a painless nodule in the thyroid gland. After establishing a diagnosis, depending on lesion size and other risk factors, the initial management of well-differentiated thyroid cancer (WDTC) includes near total or total

thyroidectomy with or without node dissection. Postoperative radioiodine ablation is often performed, especially in cases in which there is increased potential
for recurrence (e.g. large tumors, aggressive subtypes, nodal spread, etc.).
Follow-up with physical examination is recommended every 3 to 6 months for
2 years, and then annually thereafter. Serum thyroglobulin levels are also recommended at 6 and 12 months, and then annually. Total body iodine (TBI) scans
with ^{131}I are also done annually [10]. Because WDTC is responsive to thyroid-
stimulating hormone (TSH), high levels of TSH increase the sensitivity of the
TBI scan. Following thyroidectomy, TBI scanning is done after thyroid hormone
withdrawal for 3–4 weeks when endogenous TSH levels should ideally be elevated in the 30–50 mU/ml range [11]. In patients who cannot tolerate hormone
withdrawal, recombinant human TSH can be administered to achieve comparable results. A low iodine diet is also recommended for 1–2 weeks prior to TBI
scanning.

In WDTC, FDG-PET does not typically enter the clinical picture until
patients show biochemical evidence of recurrence (i.e., rising thyroglobulin)
despite a negative TBI scan. This behavior suggests dedifferentiation and
increased aggressivity of the original tumor [11]. In such cases, restaging
with PET/CT has an overall sensitivity of up to 90% in detecting occult disease
[8] (Figure 10.3; see Plate 10.3C in the color insert). According to the PET

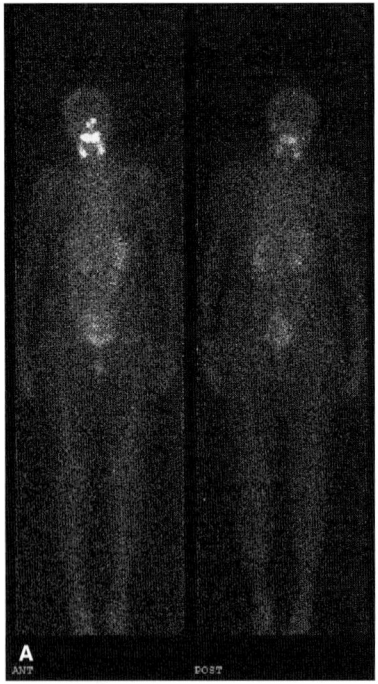

Figure 10.3. Dedifferentiated thyroid
cancer. (A) Whole-body ^{131}I post-
therapy scan of a patient with
resected papillary thyroid cancer. The
patient's thyroglobulin is 78 ng/ml
(normal range for an athyrotic patient
is less than 5 ng/ml). Physiologic
radioiodide uptake is seen within
the nasopharynx and oropharynx;
however, focal radioiodide activity in
the right and left neck is consistent
with metastatic adenopathy. From
prior imaging, the patient was known
to have multiple pulmonary nodules
which are not seen on this study.

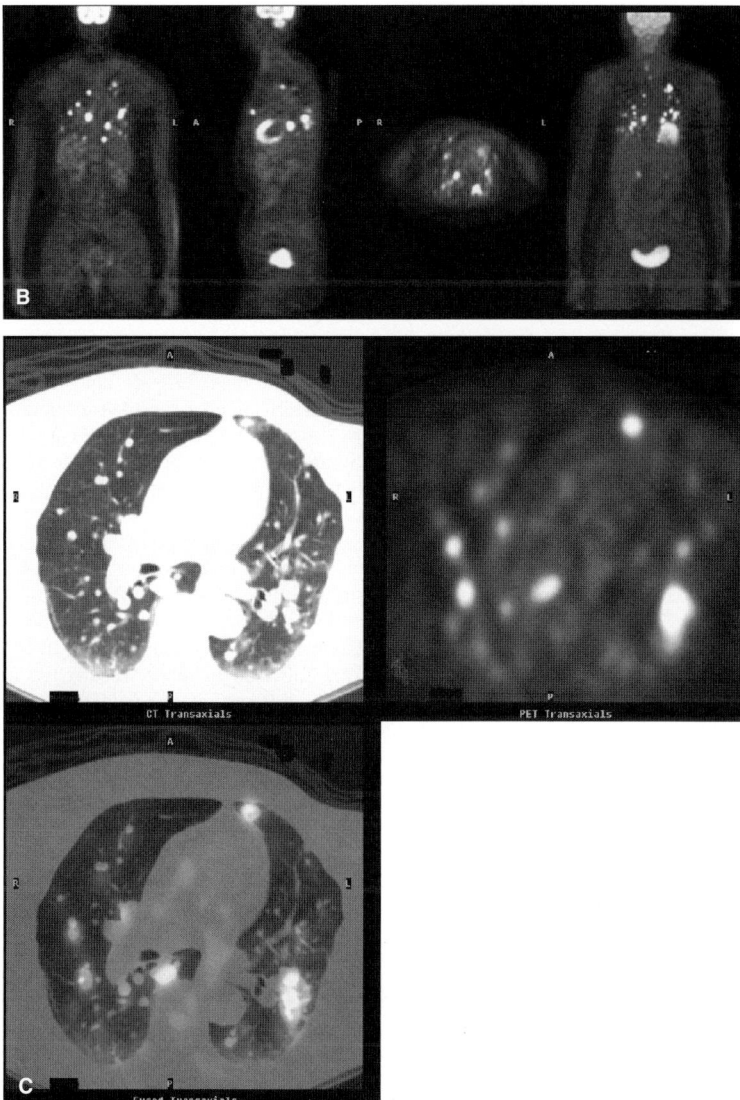

Figure 10.3. *Continued.* (**B** and **C**) Images from an FDG-PET/CT demonstrate multiple hypermetabolic foci within the lungs consistent with widespread pulmonary metastases. These represent dedifferentiated papillary thyroid cancer tumor deposits which have ceased to accumulate iodide but are now FDG avid. (See part C only in color insert.)

indication established by the CMS for thyroid cancer, only thyroid cancers of follicular origin that have been previously treated by thyroidectomy and radioiodine ablation and have a rising serum thyroglobulin (greater than 10 ng/ml) but a negative iodine-131 whole-body scan are covered by the CMS at this time [12].

Positron Emission Tomography and Medullary Thyroid Cancer

Medullary thyroid cancer (MTC) arises from the parafollicular cells of the thyroid gland. Unlike those of follicular cell origin, these cells do not produce thyroid hormone, but instead secrete calcitonin. They also secrete carcinoembryonic antigen (CEA). There are many different etiologies of MTC, with approximately 80% occurring sporadically around the 5th or 6th decade. The remainder are either familial or associated with multiple endocrine neoplasia syndromes (i.e., MEN 2A and MEN 2B).

Like well-differentiated thyroid cancer, MTC is often first detected as a painless, palpable thyroid nodule. These lesions are treated surgically with thyroidectomy, central neck dissection, and additional right or left neck nodal dissection as indicated. Because of their different cell origin, neither total body radioiodine scanning nor radioiodine ablation plays a role in managing MTC. Fortunately, just as thyroglobulin levels are followed to detect recurrence in patients with well-differentiated thyroid malignancies, calcitonin and CEA levels are assayed periodically in patients with MTC.

When calcitonin and/or CEA levels rise, FDG-PET has the best chance of detecting the site(s) of recurrence [13]. Several studies have compared FDG-PET with both other nuclear medicine agents such as ^{99m}technetium dimercaptosuccinic acid (DMSA), indium ^{111}In pentetreotide (OctreoScan®), and iodine ^{123}I metaiodobenzylguanidine (MIBG), as well as other imaging techniques such as CT and MRI to detect metastatic disease. In these studies, FDG-PET has distinguished itself as the single most sensitive and specific modality, with sensitivities ranging from 76% to 96%, and specificities ranging from 78% to 80% [13–17]. One study reported that FDG-PET may even be successful in lesion localization when the calcitonin level is below 20 pg/ml in individual cases [14]. As FDG-PET/CT is used increasingly in these cases, the powerful morphologic data gained with hybrid studies is likely to raise sensitivity even higher and be useful in guiding possible reoperation [14–18].

Although FDG-PET does have superior sensitivity in detecting MTC relative to other nuclear medicine techniques, this does not mean that those techniques have no place in the management of these patients. In particular, MIBG has high specificity for MTC, but a low sensitivity of only 30% [19]. Scanning with MIBG is nonetheless useful, especially if the patient may have a pheochromocytoma as part of MEN 2A or MEN 2B. Furthermore, when MTC demonstrates increased uptake with MIBG scanning, there is the potential for treatment with high-dose ^{131}I MIBG [19].

Limitations of Positron Emission Tomography in Thyroid Cancer

There are certain limitations to FDG-PET in the scanning of patients with thyroid cancer. False-positive uptake within the neck can occur from thyroid adenoma, vocal cord(s), and brown fat. False-positive uptake in distant sites can be caused by a number of factors ranging from inflammation to unrelated neoplasm. In such cases, the more clinical information the imager has at the time of interpretation (e.g. a history of prior granulomatous disease), the more accurate the interpretation of the scan is likely to be.

False-negative scans tend to occur with microscopic or small macroscopic disease. This limitation is shared with other malignancies and is the result of current limitations in image resolution. With PET/CT hybrid scanning, both specificity and sensitivity are expected to increase because of the dramatically improved morphological correlation relative to PET alone.

Horizons

Although FDG is the most widely used PET radiopharmaceutical – by far – there is active research underway to develop novel radiopharmaceuticals which may be better suited to particular cancer types. In the case of medullary thyroid cancer, one such compound that shows promise is radiolabeled dihydroxyphenylalanine (^{18}F-DOPA), which has been evaluated for a variety of neuroendocrine tumors. However, much more work is needed to better define its role in thyroid cancer [20].

References

1. What are the key statistics for thyroid cancer? American Cancer Society (www.cancer.org); 2005 Accessed February 2005.
2. Greene FL, Page DL, Fleming ID, et al. AJCC Cancer Staging Manual, sixth edition. New York: Springer-Verlag; 2002.
3. Mackenzie EJ, Mortimer RH. 6: Thyroid nodules and thyroid cancer. Med J Aust 2004;180(5):242–247.
4. Baloch ZW, LiVolsi VA. Fine-needle aspiration of thyroid nodules: past, present, and future. Endocr Pract 2004;10(3):234–241.
5. Kim CE, Joyce JM, Patel N, Lichter J. Fortuitous detection of papillary carcinoma of the thyroid with 18F FDG positron emission tomography in a patient with non-Hodgkin lymphoma. Clin Nucl Med 2003;28(9):782–783.
6. Kresnik E, Gallowitsch HJ, Mikosch P, et al. Fluorine-18-fluorodeoxyglucose positron emission tomography in the preoperative assessment of thyroid nodules in an endemic goiter area. Surgery 2003;133(3):294–299.

7. Ramos CD, Chisin R, Yeung HW, Larson SM, Macapinlac HA. Incidental focal thyroid uptake on FDG positron emission tomographic scans may represent a second primary tumor. Clin Nucl Med 2001;26(3):193–197.

8. Schoder H, Yeung HW. Positron emission imaging of head and neck cancer, including thyroid carcinoma. Semin Nucl Med 2004;34(3):180–197.

9. Van den Bruel A, Maes A, De Potter T, et al. Clinical relevance of thyroid fluorodeoxyglucose-whole body positron emission tomography incidentaloma. J Clin Endocrinol Metab 2002;87(4):1517–1520.

10. Fernandes JK, Day TA, Richardson MS, Sharma AK. Overview of the management of differentiated thyroid cancer. Curr Treat Options Oncol 2005;6(1):47–57.

11. Sarkar SD, Savitch I. Management of thyroid cancer. Appl Radiol 2004; November: 34–45.

12. Medicare Coverage Homepage: Centers for Medicare and Medicaid Services (www.cms.hhs.gov/coverage/); 2004 Accessed December 2004.

13. de Groot JW, Links TP, Jager PL, Kahraman T, Plukker JT. Impact of 18F-fluoro-2-deoxy-D-glucose positron emission tomography (FDG-PET) in patients with biochemical evidence of recurrent or residual medullary thyroid cancer. Ann Surg Oncol 2004;11(8):786–794.

14. Bockisch A, Brandt-Mainz K, Gorges R, Muller S, Stattaus J, Antoch G. Diagnosis in medullary thyroid cancer with [18F]FDG-PET and improvement using a combined PET/CT scanner. Acta Med Austriaca 2003;30(1):22–25.

15. Diehl M, Risse JH, Brandt-Mainz K, et al. Fluorine-18 fluorodeoxyglucose positron emission tomography in medullary thyroid cancer: results of a multicentre study. Eur J Nucl Med 2001;28(11):1671–1676.

16. Szakall S, Jr., Esik O, Bajzik G, et al. 18F-FDG PET detection of lymph node metastases in medullary thyroid carcinoma. J Nucl Med 2002;43(1):66–71.

17. Brandt-Mainz K, Muller SP, Gorges R, Saller B, Bockisch A. The value of fluorine-18 fluorodeoxyglucose PET in patients with medullary thyroid cancer. Eur J Nucl Med 2000;27(5):490–496.

18. Gotthardt M, Battmann A, Hoffken H, et al. 18F-FDG PET, somatostatin receptor scintigraphy, and CT in metastatic medullary thyroid carcinoma: a clinical study and an analysis of the literature. Nucl Med Commun 2004;25(5):439–443.

19. Rufini V, Salvatori M, Garganese MC, Di Giuda D, Lodovica Maussier M, Troncone L. Role of nuclear medicine in the diagnosis and therapy of medullary thyroid carcinoma. Rays 2000;25(2):273–282.

20. Hoegerle S, Altehoefer C, Ghanem N, Brink I, Moser E, Nitzsche E. 18F-DOPA positron emission tomography for tumour detection in patients with medullary thyroid carcinoma and elevated calcitonin levels. Eur J Nucl Med 2001;28(1):64–71.

11. PET in Other Malignancies

Ronald B. Workman, Jr. and R. Edward Coleman

The previous chapters have discussed the well-documented diagnostic accuracy of PET and PET/CT in imaging a wide variety of common malignancies. FDG-PET can also make a valuable contribution in evaluating a wide range of less common entities. This chapter focuses on those cancers that, although less common, are nonetheless effectively imaged by FDG-PET. Some common tumors such as prostate cancer are not reliably FDG avid, and instances in which FDG-PET is less useful are also presented. More than just tumor avidity for FDG is necessary to see widespread clinical acceptance of FDG-PET scanning in these cases. Clinically useful information must also be provided.

Cancer of Unknown Primary Syndrome

Metastatic cancer of unknown primary (CUP) syndrome is a difficult clinical entity to manage. It is relatively common, accounting for approximately 3–4% of all malignant neoplasms. In a recent meta-analysis, FDG-PET showed a high sensitivity (87%) and intermediate specificity (71%) in detecting the primary tumor in patients with CUP [1]. Many of the studies evaluating the accuracy of PET obtained for the CUP syndrome did not include patients that had been studied thoroughly prior to the performance of the PET scan. In patients who have been evaluated extensively before having the PET scan, the likelihood that PET can find the primary cancer is quite limited. The one exception is in the patient who presents with squamous cell cancer metastatic to a lymph node in the neck. In this circumstance, PET detects the primary cancer in at least 30% of the patients. Because PET is a whole-body imaging modality, it can provide additional biopsy targets which may not be clinically or radiographically apparent otherwise. Histopathologic analysis of biopsies from different deposits may improve the likelihood of establishing a primary diagnosis in such cases. Furthermore, the distribution pattern of metastases can be readily assessed by PET which may offer clues to the primary tumor (Figure 11.1).

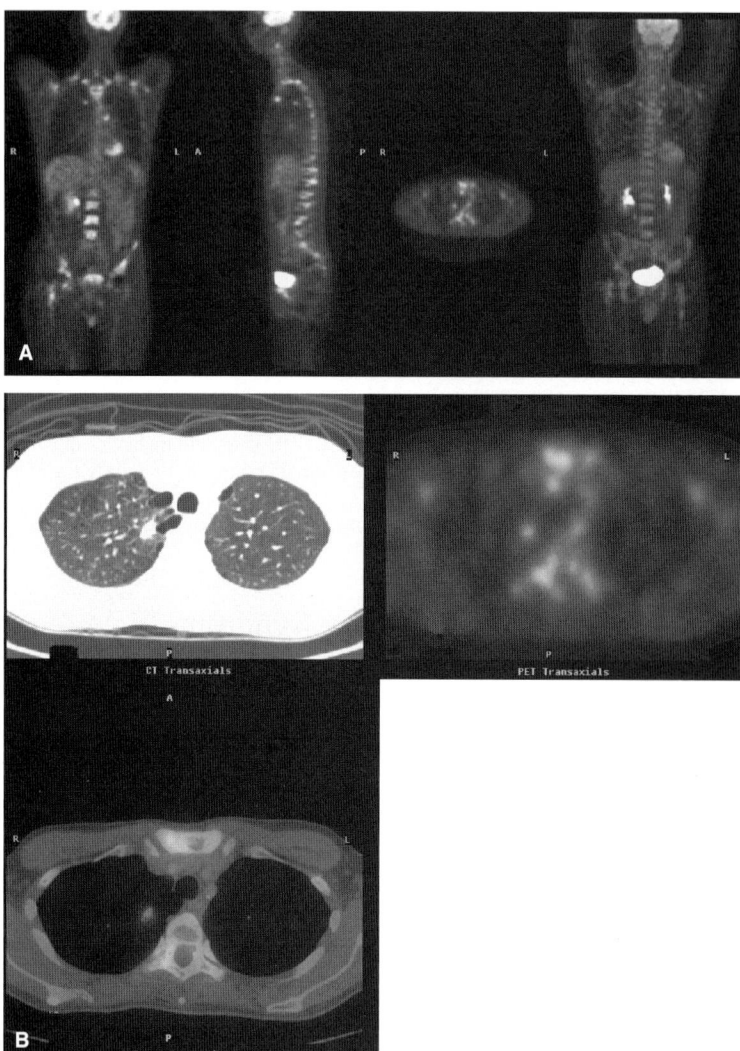

Figure 11.1. Carcinoma of unknown primary. This patient presented with diffuse skeletal metastatic disease and lymph node enlargement within the neck, mediastinum, and bihilar regions. Initial bone marrow biopsy revealed metastatic adenocarcinoma, site uncertain. FDG-PET/CT was performed which demonstrated widespread disease in the axial and appendicular skeleton as well as lymph nodes within the neck, mediastinum, and hila (A). A hypermetabolic spiculated right upper lobe nodule was also found (B) (and (C) with bone windows). Further specialized immunohistochemical stains were then performed which were positive for cytokeratin 7 and TTF-1, suggestive of lung primary.

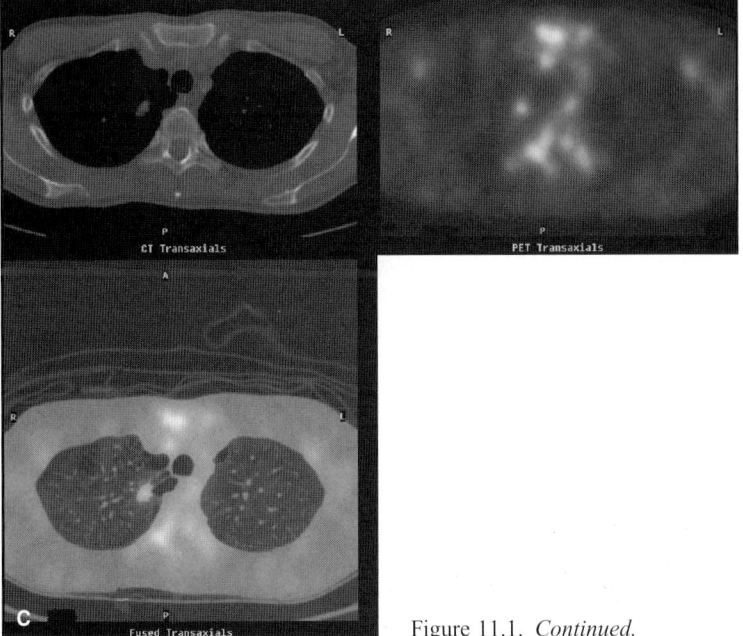

Figure 11.1. *Continued.*

Gynecologic Cancers

Cervical Cancer

Deaths from cervical cancer have fallen substantially since the use of the Pap test. Even with effective screening, however, approximately 10,370 women were diagnosed with invasive cervical cancer in the United States and approximately 3700 died in 2005. FDG-PET is an excellent staging and restaging modality in cases of cervical cancer. In a recent retrospective study of 41 patients with cervical cancer, 9 PET studies were performed for initial staging and 52 were performed for restaging. PET identified the primary disease in all 9 patients for initial staging, and also distinguished those with localized disease from those with metastatic disease with 100% accuracy. For restaging cervical cancer, FDG-PET had a sensitivity of 82% and a specificity of 97% (accuracy of 92%) for evaluation of local recurrence. For evaluating distant disease in these patients, PET was 100% sensitive and 90% specific (accuracy of 94%). These results were achieved without the use of bowel preparations, diuretics, or Foley catheters [2]. False-positive results can be seen with inflammatory adenopathy, hormonally stimulated endometrium, uterine fibroids, and focal adjacent bowel activity. The use of PET/CT hybrid systems is likely to improve specificity in such cases. PET and PET/CT have been shown to provide independent prognostic information in these patients (Figures 11.2 and 11.3).

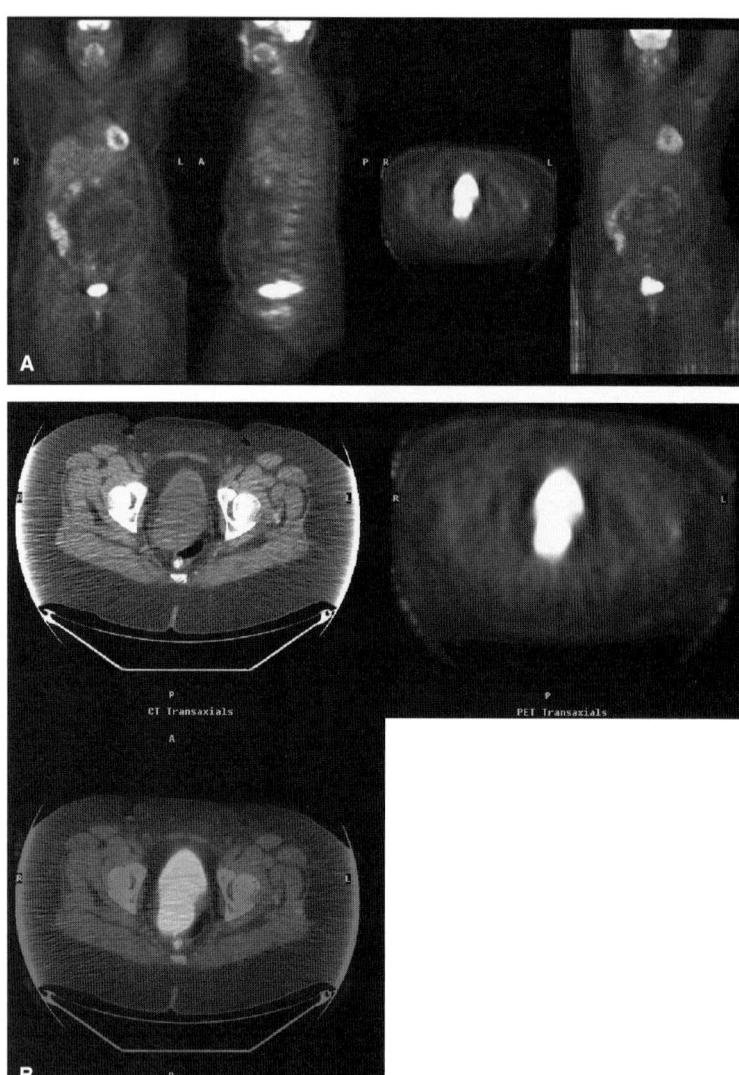

Figure 11.2. Cervical cancer. This patient presented with vaginal bleeding. On physical examination, a large mass was palpated at the cervix, and subsequent biopsy revealed invasive large cell keratinizing squamous cell carcinoma of the cervix. Staging FDG-PET/CT scan (**A**, **B**, and **C**) demonstrated a large hypermetabolic mass just posterior to the bladder consistent with cervical cancer. There was also a 1.5-cm hypermetabolic para-aortic node (white arrow) consistent with metastatic disease.

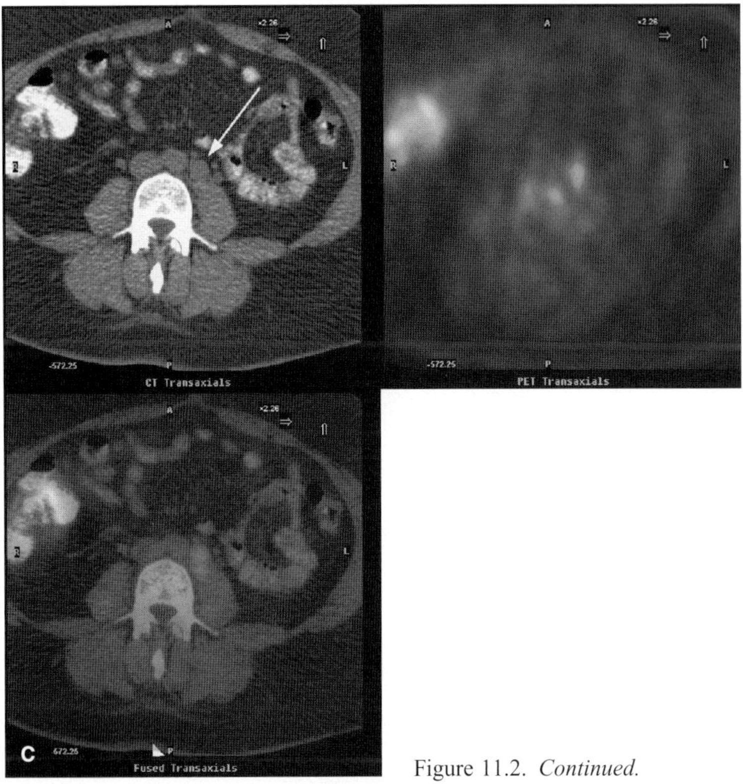

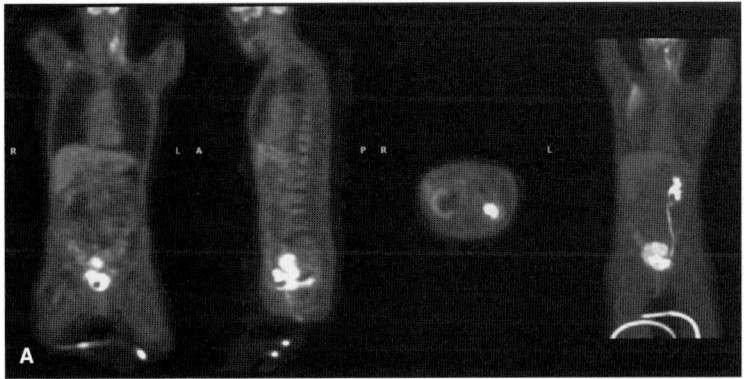

Figure 11.2. *Continued.*

Figure 11.3. Cervical cancer. This patient has a large pelvic mass with left hydronephrosis and hydroureter. The right kidney is not seen by PET **(A)**. Notice also the physiologic muscular activity within the left sternocleidomastoid and right pectoralis muscles.

Continued.

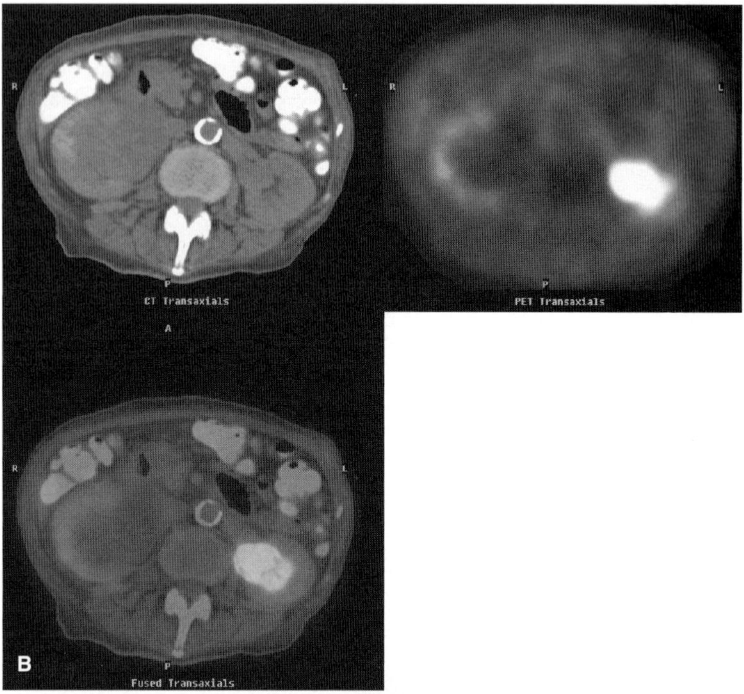

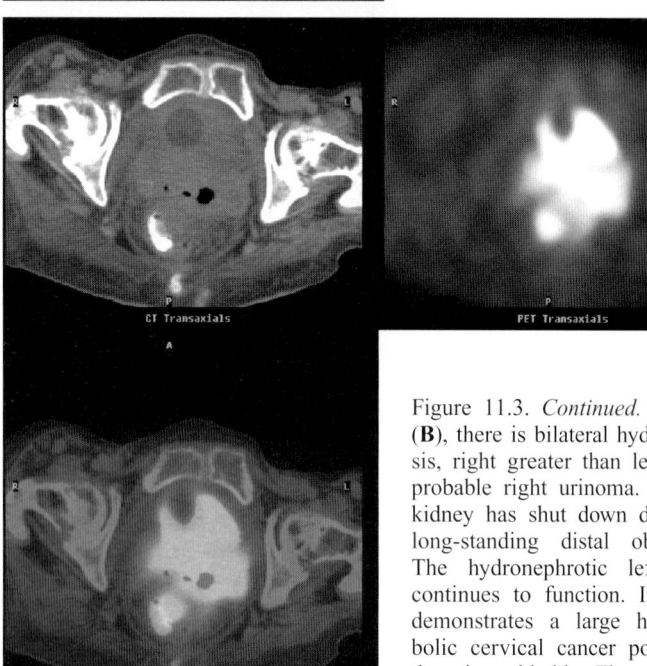

Figure 11.3. *Continued.* In image (**B**), there is bilateral hydronephrosis, right greater than left, with a probable right urinoma. The right kidney has shut down due to the long-standing distal obstruction. The hydronephrotic left kidney continues to function. Image (**C**) demonstrates a large hypermetabolic cervical cancer posterior to the urinary bladder. There is a Foley catheter within the bladder lumen.

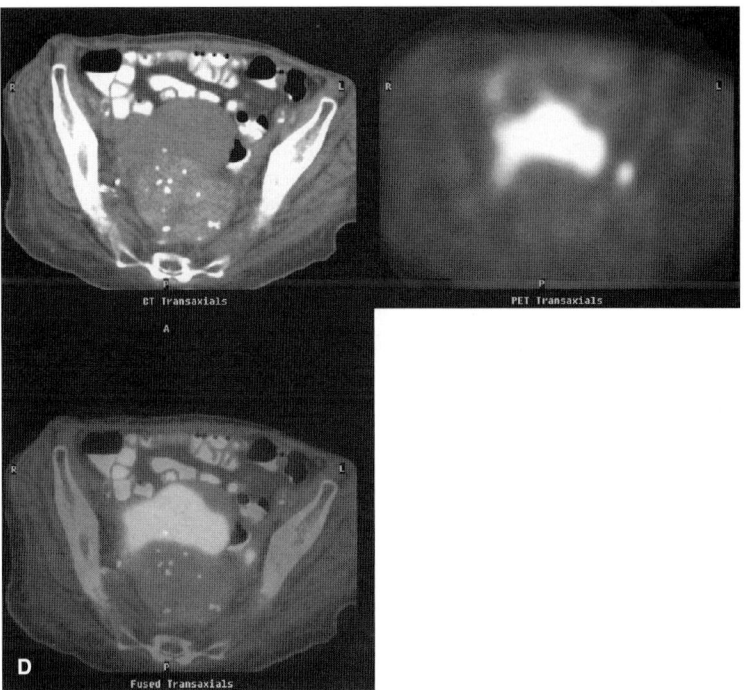

Figure 11.3. *Continued.* Imaging more superiorly **(D)** demonstrates a mass within the uterus containing stippled calcifications. This mass is not hypermetabolic and represents a degenerative uterine leiomyoma.

For a breakdown of the Tumor, Node, Metastasis (TNM) staging classification in cervical cancer, see Table 11.1 [3]. Note that definitions for the T categories correspond to the stages accepted by the Fédération Internationale de Gynécologie et d'Obstétrique (FIGO).

Ovarian Cancer

Ovarian cancer is a particularly challenging malignancy to treat because it is frequently advanced at presentation. In restaging after primary treatment, some researchers suggest that the best use of FDG-PET is when anatomic imaging shows an abnormality or when CA-125 levels rise above 30 U/ml [4,5]. As for PET/CT, recent research has shown an advantage in sensitivity of 86% versus 74% for CT alone in detecting viable tumor after primary therapy [6]. In

Table 11.1. TNM staging classification for cervical cancer

Primary tumor (T)

TNM categories	FIGO stages	
TX		Primary tumor cannot be assessed
T0		No evidence of primary tumor
Tis	0	Carcinoma in situ
T1	I	Cervical carcinoma confined to uterus (extension to corpus should be disregarded)
T1a	IA	Invasive carcinoma diagnosed only by microscopy. Stromal invasion with a maximum depth of 5.0 mm measured from the base of the epithelium and a horizontal spread of 7.0 mm or less. Vascular space involvement, venous or lymphatic, does not affect classification
T1a1	IA1	Measured stromal invasion 3.0 mm or less in depth and 7.0 mm or less in horizontal spread
T1a2	IA2	Measured stromal invasion more than 3.0 mm and not more than 5.0 mm with a horizontal spread 7.0 mm or less
T1b	IB	Clinically visible lesion confined to the cervix or microscopic lesion greater than T1a/IA2
T1b1	IB1	Clinically visible lesion 4.0 cm or less in greatest dimension
T1b2	IB2	Clinically visible lesion more than 4.0 cm in greatest dimension
T2	II	Cervical carcinoma invades beyond uterus but not to pelvic wall or to lower third of vagina
T2a	IIA	Tumor without parametrial invasion
T2b	IIB	Tumor with parametrial invasion
T3	III	Tumor extends to pelvic wall and/or involves lower third of vagina, and/or causes hydronephrosis or non-functioning kidney
T3a	IIIA	Tumor involves lower third of vagina, no extension to pelvic wall
T3b	IIIB	Tumor extends to pelvic wall and/or causes hydronephrosis or non-functioning kidney
T4	IVA	Tumor invades mucosa of bladder or rectum, and/or extends beyond true pelvis (bullous edema is not sufficient to classify tumor as T4)

Table 11.1. *Continued.*

Regional lymph nodes (N)
NX   Regional lymph nodes cannot be assessed
N0   No regional lymph node metastasis
N1   Regional lymph node metastasis

Distant metastasis (M)
MX   Distant metastasis cannot be assessed
M0   No distant metastasis
M1   Distant metastasis

Stage grouping

Stage 0	Tis	N0	M0
Stage I	T1	N0	M0
Stage IA	T1a	N0	M0
Stage IA1	T1a1	N0	M0
Stage IA2	T1a2	N0	M0
Stage IB	T1b	N0	M0
Stage IB1	T1b1	N0	M0
Stage IB2	T1b2	N0	M0
Stage II	T2	N0	M0
Stage IIA	T2a	N0	M0
Stage IIB	T2b	N0	M0
Stage III	T3	N0	M0
Stage IIIA	T3a	N0	M0
Stage IIIB	T1	N1	M0
	T2	N1	M0
	T3a	N1	M0
	T3b	Any N	M0
Stage IVA	T4	Any N	M0
Stage IVB	Any T	Any N	M1

Source: Used with permission of the American Joint Committee on Cancer (AJCC), Chicago, Illinois. The original source for this material is the *AJCC Cancer Staging Manual*, Sixth Edition (2002), published by Springer-Verlag, New York, www.springeronline.com.

the case of peritoneal carcinomatosis, FDG-PET is not particularly sensitive; however, it has been shown to be more sensitive than CT alone (57% vs. 42%) [7]. As more work is done, it is becoming apparent that fused PET/CT in these difficult cases can improve tumor localization, help differentiate physiologic from pathologic activity, and add to diagnostic confidence by having both functional and anatomic data in one study [8] (Figure 11.4).

For a breakdown of the TNM staging classification in ovarian cancer, see Table 11.2. Note that definitions for the T categories correspond to the stages accepted by the Fédération Internationale de Gynécologie et d'Obstétrique (FIGO) [3].

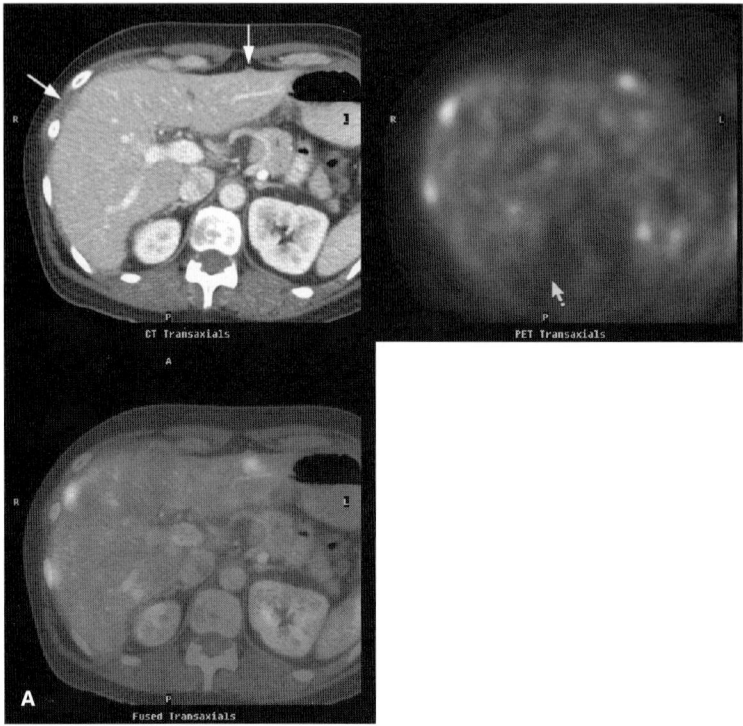

Figure 11.4. Ovarian cancer with peritoneal carcinomatosis. This patient with ovarian cancer underwent debulking and chemotherapy. Preoperatively, her CA-125 level was 1339 units/ml (normal <35 units/ml). Following surgery and chemotherapy, levels dropped to 16.5 units/ml. When levels again began to rise (107 units/ml), the patient underwent FDG-PET/CT. Maximum intensity projection (MIP) image (A) demonstrates multiple scattered foci of increased activity within the peritoneum, the most conspicuous of which are noted along the liver surface (white arrows). A prominent lymph node is also seen at the anterior midline, approximately 8 cm superior to the umbilicus (B). This is consistent with peritoneal carcinomatosis.

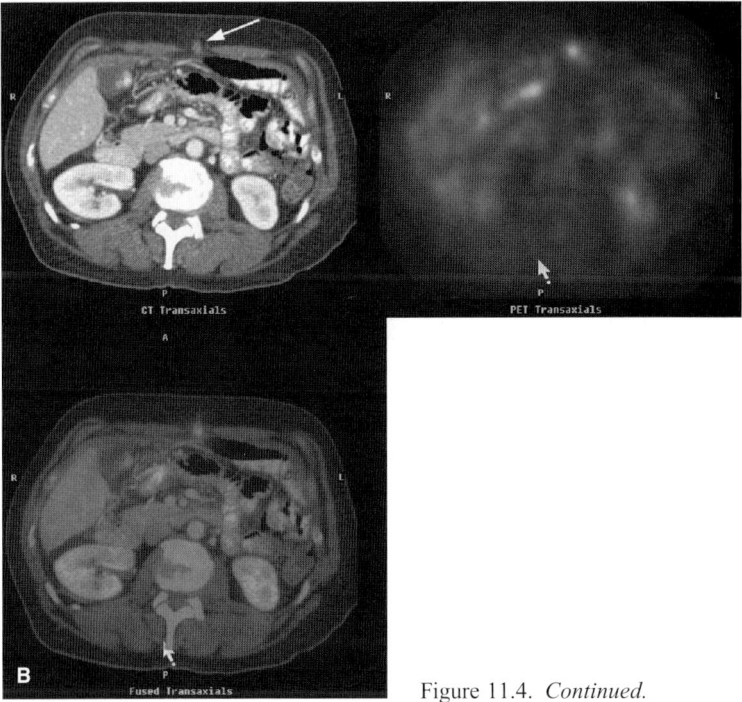

Figure 11.4. *Continued.*

Table 11.2. TNM staging classification for ovarian cancer

Primary tumor (T)

TNM categories	FIGO stages	
TX		Primary tumor cannot be assessed
T0		No evidence of primary tumor
T1	I	Tumor limited to ovaries (one or both)
T1a	IA	Tumor limited to one ovary; capsule intact, no tumor on ovarian surface. No malignant cells in ascites or peritoneal washings
T1b	IB	Tumor limited to both ovaries; capsules intact, no tumor on ovarian surface. No malignant cells in ascites or peritoneal washings
T1c	IC	Tumor limited to one or both ovaries with any of the following: capsule ruptured, tumor on ovarian surface, malignant cells in ascites or peritoneal washings

Continued.

Table 11.2. *Continued.* TNM staging classification for ovarian cancer

T2	II	Tumor involves one or both ovaries with pelvic extension and/or implants
T2a	IIA	Extension and/or implants on uterus and/or tube(s). No malignant cells in ascites or peritoneal washings
T2b	IIB	Extension to and/or implants on other pelvic tissues. No malignant cells in ascites or peritoneal washings
T2c	IIC	Pelvic extension and/or implants (T2a or T2b) with malignant cells in ascites or peritoneal washings
T3	III	Tumor involves one or both ovaries with microscopically confirmed peritoneal metastasis outside the pelvis
T3a	IIIA	Microscopic peritoneal metastasis beyond pelvis (no macroscopic tumor)
T3b	IIIB	Macroscopic peritoneal metastasis beyond pelvis 2 cm or less in greatest dimension
T3c	IIIC	Peritoneal metastasis beyond pelvis more than 2 cm in greatest dimension and/or regional lymph node metastasis

Regional lymph nodes (N)
NX   Regional lymph nodes cannot be assessed
N0   No regional lymph node metastasis
N1   Regional lymph node metastasis

Distant metastasis (M)
MX   Distant metastasis cannot be assessed
M0   No distant metastasis
M1   Distant metastasis (excludes peritoneal metastasis)

Stage grouping

Stage I	T1	N0	M0
Stage IA	T1a	N0	M0
Stage IB	T1b	N0	M0
Stage IC	T1c	N0	M0
Stage II	T2	N0	M0
Stage IIA	T2a	N0	M0
Stage IIB	T2b	N0	M0
Stage IIC	T2c	N0	M0
Stage III	T3	N0	M0
Stage IIIA	T3a	N0	M0
Stage IIIB	T3b	N0	M0
Stage IIIC	T3c	N0	M0
	Any T	N1	M0
Stage IV	Any T	Any N	M1

Source: Used with permission of the American Joint Committee on Cancer (AJCC), Chicago, Illinois. The original source for this material is the *AJCC Cancer Staging Manual*, Sixth Edition (2002), published by Springer-Verlag, New York, www.springeronline.com.

Gastric Cancer

Gastric cancer is the second leading cause of cancer deaths worldwide, accounting for approximately 700,000 deaths in 2002 [9]. Gastric cancer is generally more common in less developed countries, although it is the leading cause of cancer death in Japan and South Korea. There is a heavy association with eating smoked, salted, and fermented foods as well as with *Helicobacter pylori* infection. Like other gastrointestinal cancers, its onset can be insidious and its symptoms can be ignored or dismissed by being falsely attributed to other, benign, causes. CT, endoscopic ultrasound (EUS), and esophagogastroduodenoscopy (EGD) are the usual imaging modalities employed in assessing patients with gastric cancer.

In 2005, researchers in Korea looked at the role of FDG-PET in preoperative staging of gastric adenocarcinoma in 68 patients. For primary tumor detection, PET demonstrated sensitivity of 94%, with a mean standardized uptake value (SUV) of 7.0 (range: 0.9–27.7). PET scan had similar accuracy compared to CT for diagnosing local and distant lymph node metastases as well as peritoneal involvement. In assessing local lymph node status, however, PET had a higher specificity than CT (92% vs. 62%, $P = 0.000$). Moreover, PET had additional diagnostic value in 10 (15%) of 68 patients by upstaging 4 (6%) and downstaging 6 (9%) patients. FDG-PET combined with CT was more accurate for preoperative staging than either modality alone (66% vs. 51%, 66% vs. 47%, respectively; $P = 0.002$) [10]. The response to preoperative chemotherapy can be predicted by FDG-PET early in the treatment course [11]. There is a poorer prognosis with higher SUV tumors likely due to increased tumor aggressiveness and early metastasis in such cases [12]. Limitations include confusion with sometimes high physiologic stomach uptake and low cellularity tumor subtypes, such as signet ring and mucinous. For a breakdown of the TNM staging classification in gastric cancer, see Table 11.3 [3].

Table 11.3. TNM staging classification for gastric cancer

Primary tumor (T)	
TX	Primary tumor cannot be assessed
T0	No evidence of primary tumor
Tis	Carcinoma in situ: intraepithelial tumor without invasion of the lamina propria
T1	Tumor invades lamina propria
T2	Tumor invades muscularis propria or subserosa
T2a	Tumor invades muscularis propria
T2b	Tumor invades subserosa
T3	Tumor penetrates serosa (visceral peritoneum) without invasion of adjacent structures
T4	Tumor invades adjacent structures
Regional lymph nodes (N)	
NX	Regional lymph node(s) cannot be assessed
N0	No regional lymph node metastasis

Continued.

Table 11.3. *Continued.* TNM staging classification for gastric cancer

N1	Metastasis in 1 to 6 regional lymph nodes		
N2	Metastasis in 7 to 15 regional lymph nodes		
N3	Metastasis in more than 15 regional lymph nodes		

Distant metastasis (M)
MX	Distant metastasis cannot be assessed		
M0	No distant metastasis		
M1	Distant metastasis		

Stage grouping
Stage 0	Tis	N0	M0
Stage IA	T1	N0	M0
Stage IB	T1	N1	M0
	T2a/b	N0	M0
Stage II	T1	N2	M0
	T2a/b	N1	M0
	T3	N0	M0
Stage IIIA	T2a/b	N2	M0
	T3	N1	M0
	T4	N0	M0
Stage IIIB	T3	N2	M0
Stage IV	T4	N1–3	M0
	T1–3	N3	M0
	Any T	Any N	M1

Source: Used with permission of the American Joint Committee on Cancer (AJCC), Chicago, Illinois. The original source for this material is the *AJCC Cancer Staging Manual*, Sixth Edition (2002), published by Springer-Verlag, New York, www.springeronline.com.

Hepatocellular Cancer

Patients with chronic hepatitis B, hepatitis C, or alcoholic cirrhosis carry a high risk of developing hepatocellular carcinoma (HCC). Some risk also exists with exposure to aflatoxins and long-term anabolic steroid use. Patients at high risk can be followed with serum markers such as α-fetoprotein (AFP), CT, ultrasound, and MRI. Unfortunately, HCC is an example of a tumor that is not reliably visualized by FDG-PET. There is a sensitivity of about 60% for PET in these cases due to the increased levels of glucose-6-phosphatase in HCC cells. As discussed in Chapter 1, elevated levels of this enzyme can result in "escape" of FDG from the tumor cells. The sensitivity is higher in higher-grade (less well-differentiated) tumors. Furthermore, some studies have shown that FDG-PET may be helpful in detecting unsuspected metastatic disease in patients with HCC, and in following patients who have had hepatic-directed therapy such as chemoembolization and radiofrequency ablation [13,14] (Figure 11.5). For a breakdown of the TNM staging classification in hepatocellular carcinoma, see Table 11.4 [3].

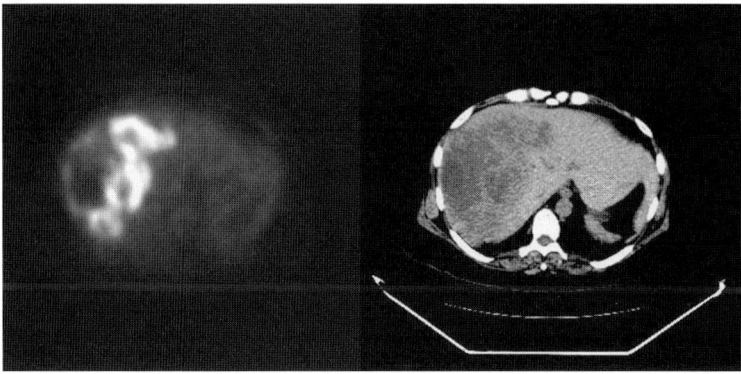

Figure 11.5. Hepatocellular carcinoma (HCC). While FDG-PET is relatively insensitive for HCC, this patient was diagnosed with a poorly differentiated variant which is more likely to be PET positive. Note the large heterogeneous HCC within the right lobe of the liver which demonstrates marked FDG uptake. Areas of hypometabolism within this mass suggest necrosis.

Table 11.4. TNM staging classification for hepatocellular carcinoma

Primary tumor (T)
TX	Primary tumor cannot be assessed
T0	No evidence of primary tumor
T1	Solitary tumor without vascular invasion
T2	Solitary tumor with vascular invasion or multiple tumors none more than 5 cm
T3	Multiple tumors more than 5 cm or tumor involving a major branch of the portal or hepatic vein(s)
T4	Tumor(s) with direct invasion of adjacent organs other than the gall-bladder or with perforation of visceral peritoneum

Regional lymph nodes (N)
NX	Regional lymph nodes cannot be assessed
N0	No regional lymph node metastasis
N1	Regional lymph node metastasis

Distant metastasis (M)
MX	Distant metastasis cannot be assessed
M0	No distant metastasis
M1	Distant metastasis

Continued.

Table 11.4. *Continued.* TNM staging classification for hepatocellular carcinoma

Stage grouping			
Stage I	T1	N0	M0
Stage II	T2	N0	M0
Stage IIIA	T3	N0	M0
Stage IIIB	T4	N0	M0
Stage IIIC	Any T	N1	M0
Stage IV	Any T	Any N	M1

Source: Used with permission of the American Joint Committee on Cancer (AJCC), Chicago, Illinois. The original source for this material is the *AJCC Cancer Staging Manual*, Sixth Edition (2002), published by Springer-Verlag, New York, www.springeronline.com.

Multiple Myeloma

Multiple myeloma is a malignancy of plasma cells. Approximately 15,980 people were diagnosed in the United States in 2005. Age is the primary risk factor. Skeletal survey with radiographs, CT, and MRI can be used to detect myeloma. Bone scan is insensitive. The data that are available discussing the role of FDG-PET in multiple myeloma are positive. One study evaluated the FDG-PET scans performed on 13 patients with multiple myeloma and determined a sensitivity of 85% in detecting myelomatous involvement with a specificity of 92%. Limitations occurred with lesions below the spatial resolution of PET, and a false positive was called in a patient recently status post radiation therapy. Although more work is needed, this and other studies have concluded that FDG-PET can detect early marrow involvement, assess the extent of active disease at presentation, and monitor therapy response [15,16].

Additionally, some authors have also evaluated the utility of FDG-PET in working up multiple myeloma patients with clinically significant infection. They have found that FDG-PET is a useful tool in diagnosing and managing such patients, even in cases of severe neutropenia/lymphopenia. The majority of infections involved the respiratory tract (e.g., pneumonias), the musculoskeletal system (e.g., bone, joint, and soft tissue infections), and the gastrointestinal system (e.g., colitis, diverticulitis). PET identified infection in many cases not identified by other methods, determined extent of infection, and led to modification of therapy in a large number of cases [17].

Pancreatic Cancer

Pancreatic cancer has long been a difficult malignancy to manage. Disease is often advanced before symptoms lead patients to seek medical attention, especially in pancreatic tail lesions. Curative resection and chemotherapy can be attempted in cases of limited disease, but often therapy is directed more at palliation. FDG-PET may be helpful in detecting unexpected distant metastatic disease prior to attempted curative resection. One recent study from the surgical literature determined that FDG-PET/CT changed management in 16% of patients with pancreatic cancer who were deemed resectable after routine staging [18]. False negatives arise due to the often poor cellularity of these tumors; false positives can be seen in cases of acute or chronic pancreatitis [19] (Figures 11.6 and 11.7; see also Plate 11.7D in color insert). For a breakdown of the TNM staging classification in pancreatic cancer, see Table 11.5 [3].

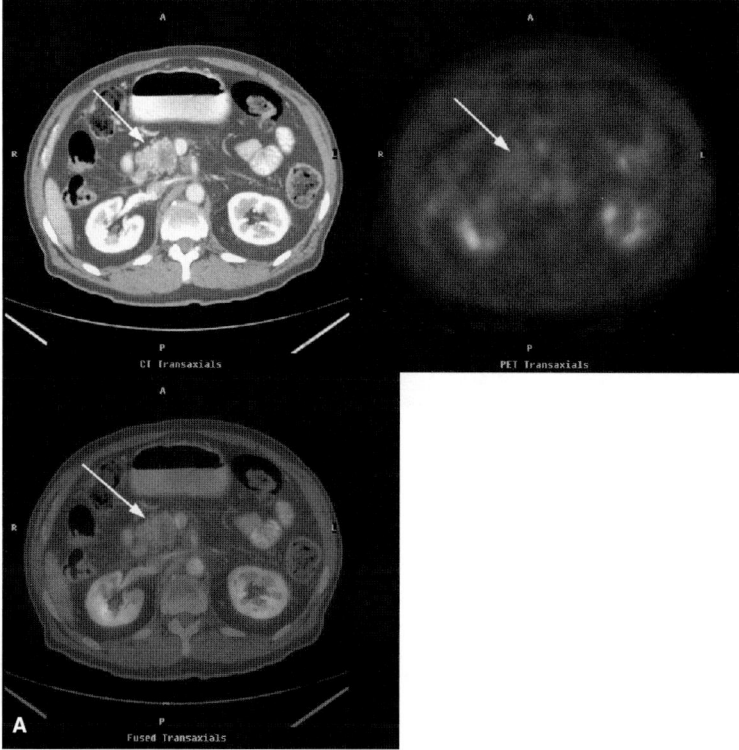

Figure 11.6. Pancreatic cancer. There is a low attenuation pancreatic head mass which has low-to-moderate hypermetabolism (white arrow) **(A)**. There are also innumerable cavitary lung lesions of varying size which are only faintly visible by FDG-PET **(B)**. CT-guided biopsy of the pancreatic head mass revealed a well-differentiated mucinous adenocarcinoma. One of the right lower lobe lung lesions was also biopsied and demonstrated metastatic mucinous adenocarcinoma. Well-differentiated and mucinous neoplasms can easily be missed by FDG-PET due to their low glycolytic activity and poor cellularity.

Continued.

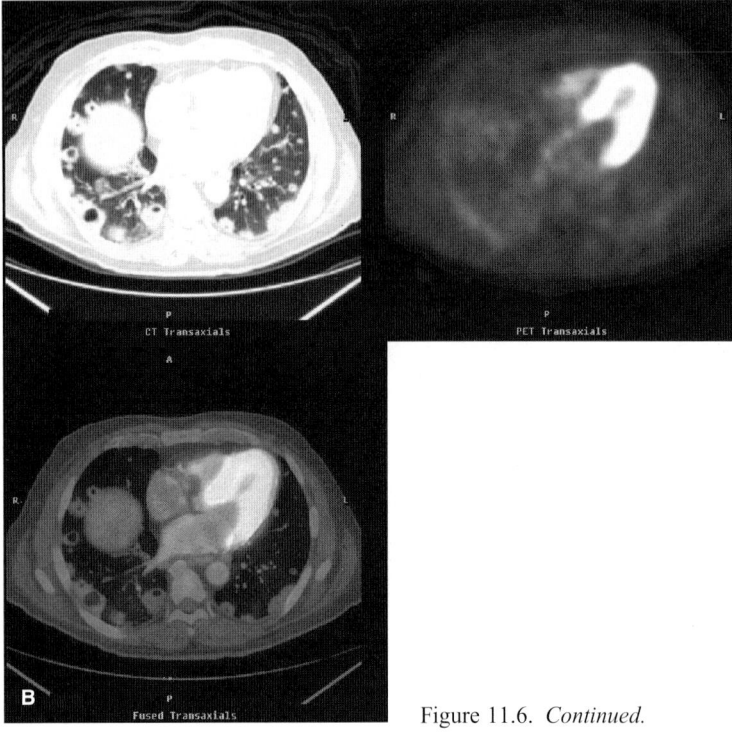

Figure 11.6. *Continued.*

Figure 11.7. Pancreatic cancer with second lung primary. This patient presented with painless jaundice. Work-up revealed not only a pancreatic head mass, but also right lower lobe nodules and hilar and mediastinal adenopathy. Biopsy of both the pancreatic and lung lesions revealed two separate adenocarcinoma primaries. Images (**A, B, C**, and **D**) demonstrate the findings at FDG-PET/CT. The patient had a CA-19.9 of 138 units/ml (normal <40 units/ml). (See part D only in color insert.)

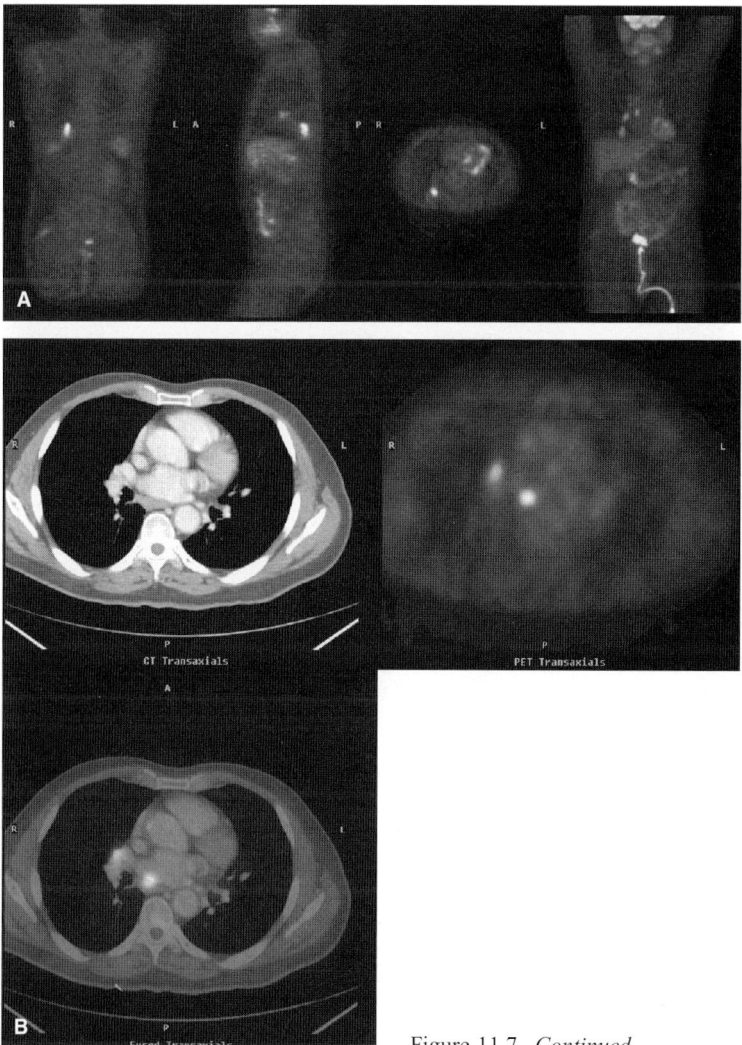

Figure 11.7. *Continued.*

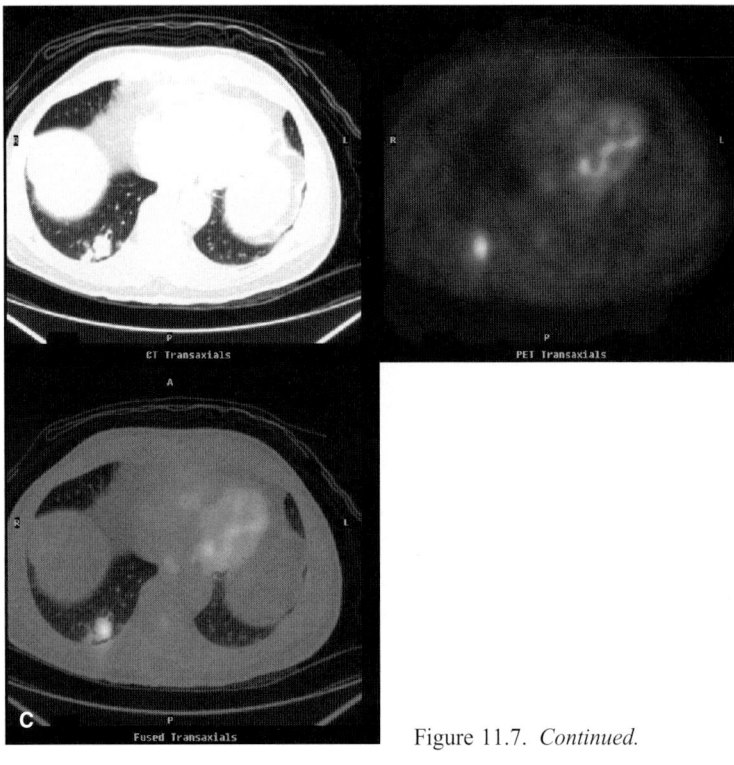

Figure 11.7. *Continued.*

Table 11.5. TNM staging classification for pancreatic cancer

Primary tumor (T)
TX   Primary tumor cannot be assessed
T0   No evidence of primary tumor
Tis   Carcinoma in situ
T1   Tumor limited to the pancreas, 2 cm or less in greatest dimension
T2   Tumor limited to the pancreas, more than 2 cm in greatest dimension
T3   Tumor extends beyond the pancreas but without involvement of the
        celiac axis or the superior mesenteric artery
T4   Tumor involves the celiac axis or the superior mesenteric artery
        (unresectable primary tumor)

Regional lymph nodes (N)
NX   Regional lymph nodes cannot be assessed
N0   No regional lymph node metastasis
N1   Regional lymph node metastasis

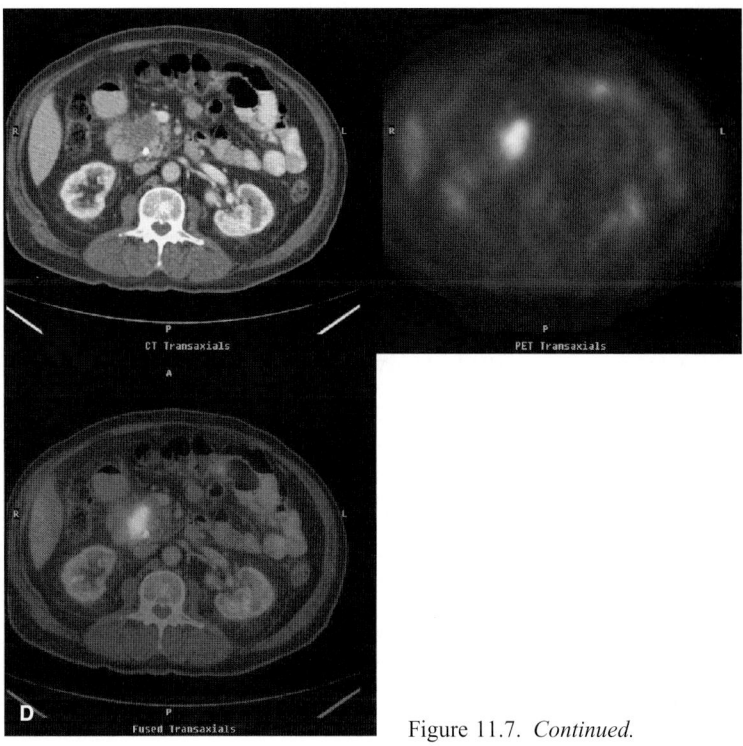

Figure 11.7. *Continued.*

Table 11.5. *Continued.*

Distant metastasis (M)
MX   Distant metastasis cannot be assessed
M0   No distant metastasis
M1   Distant metastasis

Stage grouping			
Stage 0	Tis	N0	M0
Stage IA	T1	N0	M0
Stage IB	T2	N0	M0
Stage IIA	T3	N0	M0
Stage IIB	T1	N1	M0
	T2	N1	M0
	T3	N1	M0
Stage III	T4	Any N	M0
Stage IV	Any T	Any N	M1

Source: Used with permission of the American Joint Committee on Cancer (AJCC), Chicago, Illinois. The original source for this material is the *AJCC Cancer Staging Manual*, Sixth Edition (2002), published by Springer-Verlag, New York, www.springeronline.com.

Prostate Cancer

Prostate cancer is the most common cancer in men, excluding skin cancers such as basal and squamous cell, afflicting about 1 in 6. It is the second leading cause of cancer death in American men, with about 30,350 deaths in 2005. Yearly screening beginning at age 45 or 50 with digital rectal examination and prostate-specific membrane antigen (PSA) assay allows most cancers to be caught early (e.g., local and locoregional disease). Treatment is also effective, and 99% of prostate cancer patients live at least 5 years after diagnosis.

FDG-PET is not recommended in evaluating most patients with prostate cancer. This is due to the frequently low glycolytic rate of prostate cancer cells as well as the proximity of the prostate to physiologic excreted activity within the genitourinary tract. FDG-PET may be helpful in evaluating those patients with more aggressive, less well-differentiated tumors. The group at Memorial Sloan-Kettering has shown that patients with recurrent, hormone-resistant prostate cancer frequently have FDG-avid disease, and FDG-PET may be useful in identifying the site causing the rising PSA in these patients. While FDG-PET is not as useful in most prostate cancer cases compared to other malignancies, there is much excitement about the use of newer PET radiopharmaceuticals which target cell membrane synthesis such as ^{18}F-fluorocholine (FCH) and ^{11}C-choline PET [20–22]. A prospective investigation of FCH-PET/CT published in 2005 demonstrated limited effectiveness in differentiating benign hyperplasia from prostate cancer in patients undergoing initial staging scans; however, restaging scans using FCH showed promise in detecting local recurrence and lymph node metastases [23]. Much additional work is needed. For a breakdown of the TNM staging classification in prostate cancer, see Table 11.6 [3].

Table 11.6. TNM staging classification for prostate cancer

Primary tumor (T)	
TX	Primary tumor cannot be assessed
T0	No evidence of primary tumor
T1	Clinically inapparent tumor neither palpable nor visible by imaging
T1a	Tumor incidental histologic finding in 5% or less of tissue resected
T1b	Tumor incidental histologic finding in more than 5% of tissue resected
T1c	Tumor identified by needle biopsy (e.g., because of elevated PSA)
T2	Tumor confined within prostate
T2a	Tumor involves one-half of one lobe or less
T2b	Tumor involves more than one-half of one lobe but not both lobes
T2c	Tumor involves both lobes
T3	Tumor extends through the prostate capsule
T3a	Extracapsular extension (unilateral or bilateral)
T3b	Tumor invades seminal vesicle(s)
T4	Tumor is fixed or invades adjacent structures other than seminal vesicles: bladder neck, external sphincter, rectum, levator muscles, and/or pelvic wall

Table 11.6. *Continued.*

Regional lymph nodes (N)
NX   Regional lymph nodes cannot be assessed
N0   No regional lymph node metastasis
N1   Regional lymph node metastasis

Distant metastasis (M)
MX   Distant metastasis cannot be assessed
M0   No distant metastasis
M1   Distant metastasis
M1a   Non-regional lymph node(s)
M1b   Bone(s)
M1c   Other site(s) with or without bone disease

Histologic grade (G)
GX   Grade cannot be assessed
G1   Well differentiated (slight anaplasia) (Gleason 2–4)
G2   Moderately differentiated (moderate anaplasia) (Gleason 5–6)
G3–4 Poorly differentiated/undifferentiated (marked anaplasia) (Gleason
        7–10)

Stage grouping				
Stage I	T1a	N0	M0	G1
Stage II	T1a	N0	M0	G2, 3–4
	T1b	N0	M0	Any G
	T1c	N0	M0	Any G
	T1	N0	M0	Any G
	T2	N0	M0	Any G
Stage III	T3	N0	M0	Any G
Stage IV	T4	N0	M0	Any G
	Any T	N1	M0	Any G
	Any T	Any N	M1	Any G

Source: Used with permission of the American Joint Committee on Cancer (AJCC), Chicago, Illinois. The original source for this material is the *AJCC Cancer Staging Manual*, Sixth Edition (2002), published by Springer-Verlag, New York, www.springeronline.com.

Renal Cell Cancer

The American Cancer Society estimated that there would be about 36,160 new cases of renal cell cancer (RCC) diagnosed in the United States in the year 2005. Of these, about 50% were confined to the kidney, 25% demonstrated regional spread, and the remaining 25% had metastasized to distant sites. The overall survival at 5 years is 60% with 90% 5-year survival for local disease, 60% for regional disease, and only 9% for metastatic disease. The classic triad of flank pain, palpable mass, and hematuria does not occur in the majority of cases. When it does occur, disease is usually advanced since these tumors can become quite large before being symptomatic. Urinalysis is very non-specific.

Renal protocol CT and MRI can detect small tumors, but these tests are not indicated unless the patient is symptomatic or at high risk (such as patients with positive family history, von Hippel–Lindau disease, chronic dialysis, etc.).

Early work in 1996 by Hoh and colleagues demonstrated 100% accuracy for PET in detecting local recurrence and metastases compared to 88% for CT. PET was also found to better differentiate between viable tumor and fibrosis within the post-nephrectomy renal fossa [24]. A more recent and larger study in 2004 looked at 66 patients with RCC who had a total of 90 FDG-PET scans. Those authors reported FDG-PET sensitivity of 60% and specificity of 100% for primary RCC tumors compared to 92% sensitivity and 100% specificity for CT. For retroperitoneal lymph node metastases and/or renal bed recurrence, PET was 75% sensitive and 100% specific, with corresponding sensitivity and specificity for CT of 93% and 98%, respectively. PET had a sensitivity of 75% and a specificity of 97% for pulmonary metastases compared to 91% and 73%, respectively, for chest CT. PET was 77% sensitive and 100% specific for bone metastases, compared to 94% and 87% for combined CT and bone scan. In 39 scans (32 patients) PET failed to detect RCC lesions identified by conventional imaging [25]. FDG-PET's role in evaluating RCC is continuing to evolve, but it seems to be most useful in staging and restaging those with known RCC. Diagnosis of RCC remains in the realm of anatomic imaging with CT and MRI, although PET can be used to complement those studies with equivocal findings. For a breakdown of the TNM staging classification in renal cell cancer, see Table 11.7 [3].

Table 11.7. TNM staging classification for renal cell cancer

Primary tumor (T)

TX	Primary tumor cannot be assessed
T0	No evidence of primary tumor
T1	Tumor 7 cm or less in greatest dimension, limited to the kidney
T1a	Tumor 4 cm or less in greatest dimension, limited to the kidney
T1b	Tumor more than 4 cm but not more than 7 cm in greatest dimension, limited to the kidney
T2	Tumor more than 7 cm in greatest dimension, limited to the kidney
T3	Tumor extends into major veins or invades adrenal gland or perinephric tissues but not beyond Gerota's fascia
T3a	Tumor directly invades adrenal gland or perirenal and/or renal sinus fat but not beyond Gerota's fascia
T3b	Tumor grossly extends into the renal vein or its segmental (muscle-containing) branches, or vena cava below the diaphragm
T3c	Tumor grossly extends into vena cava above diaphragm or invades the wall of the vena cava
T4	Tumor invades beyond Gerota's fascia

Regional lymph nodes (N)

NX	Regional lymph nodes cannot be assessed
N0	No regional lymph node metastasis
N1	Metastasis in a single regional lymph node
N2	Metastasis in more than one regional lymph node

Table 11.7. *Continued.*

Distant metastasis (M)	
MX	Distant metastasis cannot be assessed
M0	No distant metastasis
M1	Distant metastasis

Stage grouping			
Stage I	T1	N0	M0
Stage II	T2	N0	M0
Stage III	T1	N1	M0
	T2	N1	M0
	T3	N0	M0
	T3	N1	M0
	T3a	N0	M0
	T3a	N1	M0
	T3b	N0	M0
	T3b	N1	M0
	T3c	N0	M0
	T3c	N1	M0
Stage IV	T4	N0	M0
	T4	N1	M0
	Any T	N2	M0
	Any T	Any N	M1

Source: Used with permission of the American Joint Committee on Cancer (AJCC), Chicago, Illinois. The original source for this material is the *AJCC Cancer Staging Manual*, Sixth Edition (2002), published by Springer-Verlag, New York, www.springeronline.com.

Sarcoma

FDG-PET has primarily been used in the evaluation of carcinomas, and much work is still needed to better define its place in the work-up of patients with soft tissue sarcoma. A recent meta-analysis has shown that FDG-PET has excellent ability to distinguish high/intermediate-grade soft tissue sarcomas from benign tumors, but it is less effective in discriminating low-grade from benign lesions [26]. In another study, FDG-PET showed promise in restaging patients with an extensive history of surgery and radiation therapy [27] (Figure 11.8); see also Plate 11.8B in color insert). For a breakdown of the TNM staging classification in soft tissue sarcoma, see Table 11.8 [3].

There has been much excitement over the use of FDG-PET in following patients with gastrointestinal stromal tumors (GIST), also referred to as spindle cell sarcomas. The malignant behavior of GIST is driven by activation of the c-kit gene, and treatment with a tyrosine kinase inhibitor effectively blocks this activation. PET is very accurate in assessing GIST response to tyrosine kinase inhibitor therapy with imatinib mesylate (Glivec or Gleevec) [28] (Figure 11.9).

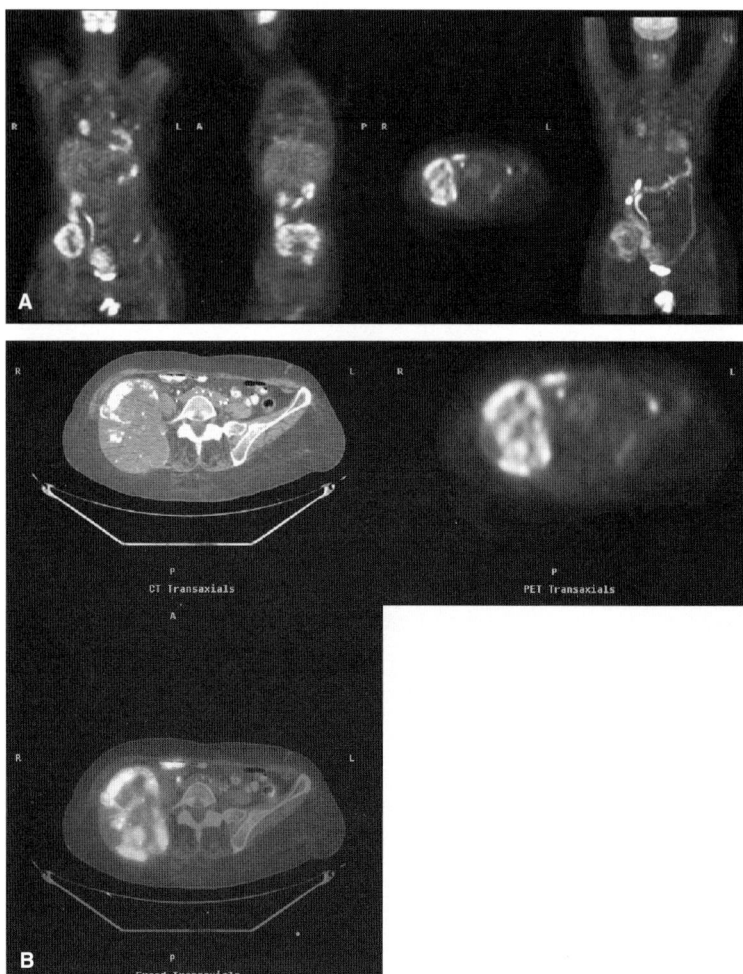

Figure 11.8. Radiation-induced chondrosarcoma with pulmonary metastases. This is a patient who underwent whole pelvic irradiation with multiple boosts for cervical cancer dating back two decades. She subsequently developed urinary incontinence and a right ureteral stricture requiring stent placement. During work-up for urinary incontinence surgery, the patient was found to have a large destructive mass involving her right ilium. Innumerable bilateral pulmonary nodules were also discovered. Clinicians elected to perform an FDG-PET/CT scan. Whole-body images **(A)** demonstrate a large hypermetabolic mass in the right hemipelvis. The right ureter is also prominent. Multiple hypermetabolic pulmonary lesions are also seen consistent with metastatic disease. Axial images through the pelvis **(B)** demonstrate a large mass with focal chondroid differentiation arising within the right iliac wing. Biopsy revealed chondrosarcoma, likely radiation induced. (See part B only in color insert.)

Table 11.8. TNM staging classification for soft tissue sarcoma

Primary tumor (T)

TX	Primary tumor cannot be assessed
T0	No evidence of primary tumor
T1	Tumor 5 cm or less in greatest dimension
	T1a – superficial tumor
	T1b – deep tumor
T2	Tumor more than 5 cm in greatest dimension
	T2a – superficial tumor
	T2b – deep tumor

Regional lymph nodes (N)

NX	Regional lymph nodes cannot be assessed
N0	No regional lymph node metastasis
N1	Regional lymph node metastasis

Distant metastasis (M)

MX	Distant metastasis cannot be assessed
M0	No distant metastasis
M1	Distant metastasis

Histologic grade (G)

GX	Grade cannot be assessed
G1	Well differentiated
G2	Moderately differentiated
G3	Poorly differentiated
G4	Undifferentiated

Stage grouping

Stage I	T1a, 1b, 2a, 2b	N0	M0
Stage II	T1a, 1b, 2a	N0	M0
Stage III	T2b	N0	M0
Stage IV	Any T	N1	M0
	Any T	N0	M1

Source: Used with permission of the American Joint Committee on Cancer (AJCC), Chicago, Illinois. The original source for this material is the *AJCC Cancer Staging Manual*, Sixth Edition (2002), published by Springer-Verlag, New York, www.springeronline.com.

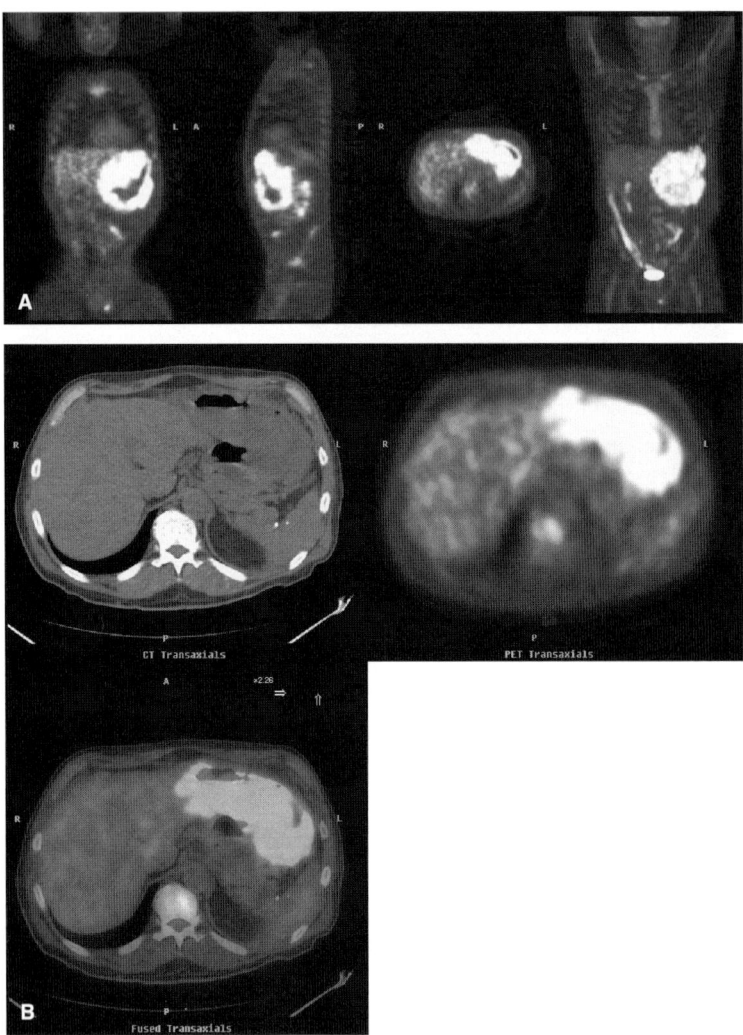

Figure 11.9. Gastrointestinal stromal tumor (GIST). This patient presented with complaints of vague abdominal pain and anorexia. Endoscopy with biopsy revealed GIST, and the patient underwent an FDG-PET/CT scan (A) and (B) which demonstrates marked gastric wall thickening with corresponding hyper-metabolism. The patient was treated with Gleevec and demonstrated marked interval improvement (C) and (D). The rim of moderate hypermetabolism noted in (D) was felt to be inflammatory change around an area of necrosis.

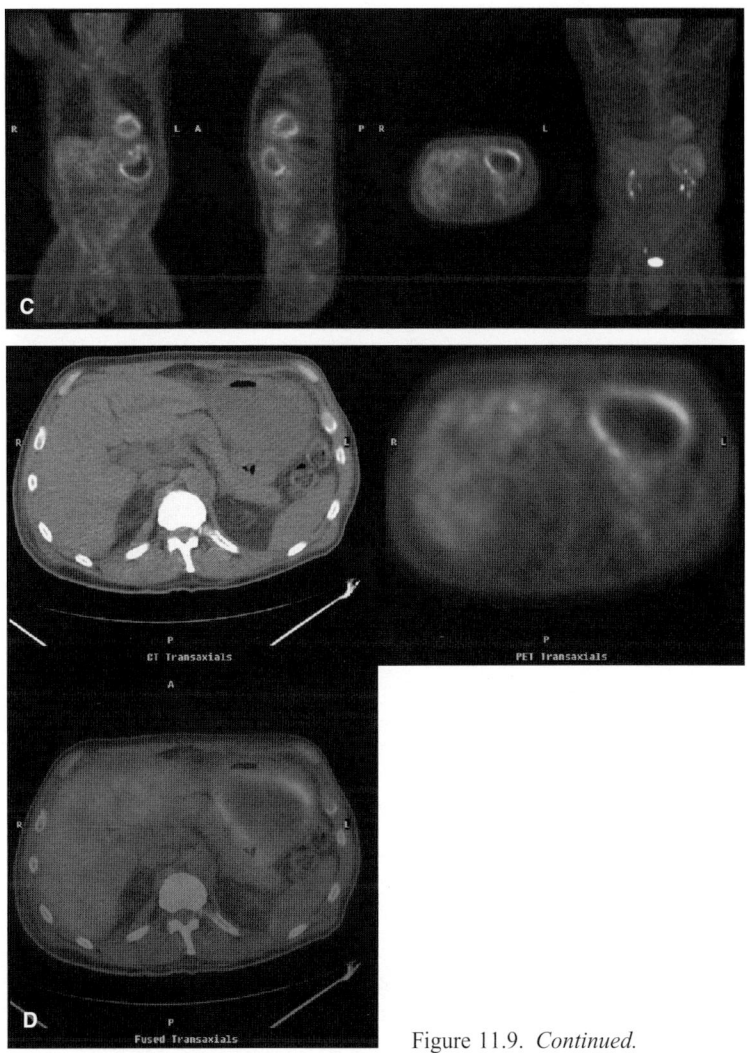

Figure 11.9. *Continued.*

Testicular Cancer

A man's lifetime risk of acquiring testicular cancer is about 1 in 300. Fortunately, it is one of the most curable forms of cancer, and the lifetime risk of dying from the disease is about 1 in 5000. Men who have had cryptorchidism are at slightly higher risk, and white men are 5–10 times more likely than black men to be afflicted [29]. Public awareness has improved the frequency of self-examination, and diagnosis is usually made early. Classically, the initial complaint is of a painless lump in the testicle. This can be well evaluated without using ionizing radiation by scrotal ultrasound. FDG-PET does not have a role in testicular cancer diagnosis.

FDG-PET is establishing itself as a useful tool in staging and restaging patients with testicular neoplasms. In staging, there is no clear advantage over CT in detecting disease in clinical stage I seminoma patients. However, as lymph nodes increase in size, and as a patient moves toward stage II disease, PET may be helpful in determining whether enlarged node(s) are benign or malignant [30]. In stage I non-seminomatous germ cell tumors (NSGCT), FDG-PET has been shown to be effective in detecting early metastatic disease with a sensitivity of 88% for small retroperitoneal deposits – a result that was superior to conventional imaging with CT [31]. PET is less accurate in NSGCT where there may be a teratomatous component. FDG-PET was also shown to be superior to CT and tumor markers at predicting viable residual tumor in post-chemotherapy seminoma patients [32]. For a breakdown of the TNM staging classification in testicular cancer, see Table 11.9 [3].

Table 11.9. TNM staging classification for testicular cancer

Primary tumor (T)*	
pTX	Primary tumor cannot be assessed
pT0	No evidence of primary tumor
pTis	Intratubular germ cell neoplasia (carcinoma in situ)
pT1	Tumor limited to the testis and epididymis without vascular/lymphatic invasion; tumor may invade into the tunica albuginea but not the tunica vaginalis
pT2	Tumor limited to the testis and epididymis with vascular/lymphatic invasion, or tumor extending through the tunica albuginea with involvement of the tunica vaginalis
pT3	Tumor invades the spermatic cord with or without vascular/lymphatic invasion
pT4	Tumor invades the scrotum with or without vascular/lymphatic invasion
Regional lymph nodes (N)	
NX	Regional lymph nodes cannot be assessed
N0	No regional lymph node metastasis
N1	Metastasis with a lymph node mass 2 cm or less in greatest dimension; or multiple lymph nodes, none more than 2 cm in greatest dimension

Table 11.9. *Continued.*

N2	Metastasis with a lymph node mass more than 2 cm but not more than 5 cm in greatest dimension; or multiple lymph nodes, any one mass greater than 2 cm but not more than 5 cm in greatest dimension
N3	Metastasis with a lymph node mass more than 5 cm in greatest dimension

Distant metastasis (M)

MX	Distant metastasis cannot be assessed
M0	No distant metastasis
M1	Distant metastasis
M1a	Non-regional nodal or pulmonary metastasis
M1b	Distant metastasis other than non-regional lymph nodes and lungs

Serum tumor markers (S)

SX	Marker studies not available or not performed
S0	Marker study levels within normal limits
S1	LDH < 1.5 × upper limit of normal and hCG (mIU/ml) <5000 and AFP (ng/ml) <1000
S2	LDH 1.5–10 × normal or hCG 5000–50,000 or AFP 1000–10,000
S3	LDH > 10 × normal or hCG > 50,000 or AFP > 10,000

Stage grouping

Stage 0	pTis	N0	M0	S0
Stage I	pT1–4	N0	M0	SX
Stage IA	pT1	N0	M0	S0
Stage IB	pT2	N0	M0	S0
	pT3	N0	M0	S0
	pT4	N0	M0	S0
Stage IS	Any pT	N0	M0	S1–3
Stage II	Any pT	N1–3	M0	SX
Stage IIA	Any pT	N1	M0	S0
	Any pT	N1	M0	S1
Stage IIB	Any pT	N2	M0	S0
	Any pT	N2	M0	S1
Stage IIC	Any pT	N3	M0	S0
	Any pT	N3	M0	S1
Stage III	Any pT	Any N	M1	SX
Stage IIIA	Any pT	Any N	M1a	S0
	Any pT	Any N	M1a	S1
Stage IIIB	Any pT	N1–3	M0	S2
	Any pT	Any N	M1a	S2
Stage IIIC	Any pT	N1–3	M0	S3
	Any pT	Any N	M1a	S3
	Any pT	Any N	M1b	Any S

* The extent of primary tumor is usually classified after radical orchidectomy, thus a pathologic stage denoted "p" is assigned.

References

1. Delgado-Bolton RC, Fernandez-Perez C, Gonzalez-Mate A, Carreras JL. Meta-analysis of the performance of 18F-FDG PET in primary tumor detection in unknown primary tumors. J Nucl Med 2003;44(8):1301–1314.

2. Wong TZ, Jones EL, Coleman RE. Positron emission tomography with 2-deoxy-2-[(18)F]fluoro-D-glucose for evaluating local and distant disease in patients with cervical cancer. Mol Imaging Biol 2004;6(1):55–62.

3. Greene FL, Page DL, Fleming ID, et al. AJCC Cancer Staging Manual, sixth edition. New York: Springer-Verlag; 2002.

4. Menzel C, Dobert N, Hamscho N, et al. The influence of CA 125 and CEA levels on the results of (18)F-deoxyglucose positron emission tomography in suspected recurrence of epithelial ovarian cancer. Strahlenther Onkol 2004;180(8):497–501.

5. Takekuma M, Maeda M, Ozawa T, Yasumi K, Torizuka T. Positron emission tomography with 18F-fluoro-2-deoxyglucose for the detection of recurrent ovarian cancer. Int J Clin Oncol 2005;10(3):177–181.

6. Picchio M, Sironi S, Messa C, et al. Advanced ovarian carcinoma: usefulness of [(18)F]FDG-PET in combination with CT for lesion detection after primary treatment. Q J Nucl Med 2003;47(2):77–84.

7. Turlakow A, Yeung HW, Salmon AS, Macapinlac HA, Larson SM. Peritoneal carcinomatosis: role of (18)F-FDG PET. J Nucl Med 2003;44(9):1407–1412.

8. Pannu HK, Bristow RE, Cohade C, Fishman EK, Wahl RL. PET-CT in recurrent ovarian cancer: initial observations. Radiographics 2004;24(1):209–223.

9. What are the key statistics for stomach cancer?: American Cancer Society (www.cancer.org); 2005 Accessed October 2005.

10. Chen J, Cheong JH, Yun MJ, et al. Improvement in preoperative staging of gastric adenocarcinoma with positron emission tomography. Cancer 2005;103(11):2383–2390.

11. Ott K, Fink U, Becker K, et al. Prediction of response to preoperative chemotherapy in gastric carcinoma by metabolic imaging: results of a prospective trial. J Clin Oncol 2003;21(24):4604–4610.

12. Mochiki E, Kuwano H, Katoh H, Asao T, Oriuchi N, Endo K. Evaluation of 18F-2-deoxy-2-fluoro-D-glucose positron emission tomography for gastric cancer. World J Surg 2004;28(3):247–253.

13. Jeng LB, Changlai SP, Shen YY, Lin CC, Tsai CH, Kao CH. Limited value of 18F-2-deoxyglucose positron emission tomography to detect hepatocellular carcinoma in hepatitis B virus carriers. Hepatogastroenterology 2003;50(54):2154–2156.

14. Wudel LJ, Jr., Delbeke D, Morris D, et al. The role of [18F]fluorodeoxyglucose positron emission tomography imaging in the evaluation of hepatocellular carcinoma. Am Surg 2003;69(2):117–124; discussion 124–126.

15. Bredella MA, Steinbach L, Caputo G, Segall G, Hawkins R. Value of FDG PET in the assessment of patients with multiple myeloma. AJR Am J Roentgenol 2005; 184(4):1199–1204.

16. Jadvar H, Conti PS. Diagnostic utility of FDG PET in multiple myeloma. Skeletal Radiol 2002;31(12):690–694.

17. Mahfouz T, Miceli MH, Saghafifar F, et al. 18F-Fluorodeoxyglucose positron emission tomography contributes to the diagnosis and management of infections in patients with multiple myeloma: a study of 165 infectious episodes. J Clin Oncol 2005; 23(31):7857–7863.

18. Heinrich S, Goerres GW, Schafer M, et al. Positron emission tomography/computed tomography influences on the management of resectable pancreatic cancer and its cost-effectiveness. Ann Surg 2005;242(2):235–243.

19. Higashi T, Saga T, Nakamoto Y, et al. Diagnosis of pancreatic cancer using fluorine-18 fluorodeoxyglucose positron emission tomography (FDG PET) – usefulness and limitations in "clinical reality". Ann Nucl Med 2003;17(4):261–279.

20. Coleman R, DeGrado T, Wang S, et al. 9:30–9:45. Preliminary evaluation of F-18 fluorocholine (FCH) as a PET tumor imaging agent. Clin Positron Imaging 2000;3(4):147.

21. de Jong IJ, Pruim J, Elsinga PH, Vaalburg W, Mensink HJ. Visualization of prostate cancer with 11C-choline positron emission tomography. Eur Urol 2002;42(1):18–23.

22. Price DT, Coleman RE, Liao RP, Robertson CN, Polascik TJ, DeGrado TR. Comparison of [18 F]fluorocholine and [18 F]fluorodeoxyglucose for positron emission tomography of androgen dependent and androgen independent prostate cancer. J Urol 2002;168(1):273–280.

23. Schmid DT, John H, Zweifel R, et al. Fluorocholine PET/CT in patients with prostate cancer: initial experience. Radiology 2005;235(2):623–628.

24. Hoh CK, Seltzer MA, Franklin J, deKernion JB, Phelps ME, Belldegrun A. Positron emission tomography in urological oncology. J Urol 1998;159(2):347–356.

25. Kang DE, White RL, Jr., Zuger JH, Sasser HC, Teigland CM. Clinical use of fluorodeoxyglucose F 18 positron emission tomography for detection of renal cell carcinoma. J Urol 2004;171(5):1806–1809.

26. Ioannidis JP, Lau J. 18F-FDG PET for the diagnosis and grading of soft-tissue sarcoma: a meta-analysis. J Nucl Med 2003;44(5):717–724.

27. Johnson GR, Zhuang H, Khan J, Chiang SB, Alavi A. Roles of positron emission tomography with fluorine-18-deoxyglucose in the detection of local recurrent and distant metastatic sarcoma. Clin Nucl Med 2003;28(10):815–820.

28. Stroobants S, Goeminne J, Seegers M, et al. 18FDG-Positron emission tomography for the early prediction of response in advanced soft tissue sarcoma treated with imatinib mesylate (Glivec). Eur J Cancer 2003;39(14):2012–2020.

29. How many men get testicular cancer?: American Cancer Society (www.cancer.org); 2005 Accessed October 2005.

30. Albers P, Bender H, Yilmaz H, Schoeneich G, Biersack HJ, Mueller SC. Positron emission tomography in the clinical staging of patients with Stage I and II testicular germ cell tumors. Urology 1999;53(4):808–811.

31. Lassen U, Daugaard G, Eigtved A, Hojgaard L, Damgaard K, Rorth M. Whole-body FDG-PET in patients with stage I non-seminomatous germ cell tumours. Eur J Nucl Med Mol Imaging 2003;30(3):396–402.

32. De Santis M, Becherer A, Bokemeyer C, et al. 2-18fluoro-deoxy-D-glucose positron emission tomography is a reliable predictor for viable tumor in postchemotherapy seminoma: an update of the prospective multicentric SEMPET trial. J Clin Oncol 2004;22(6):1034–1039.

12. PET/CT in Cardiology

Michael W. Hanson and Salvador Borges-Neto

The high incidence of cardiovascular disease and the resultant morbidity associated with the sequelae of acute cardiovascular events continue to be major issues of medical concern. To assist in the clinical evaluation of patients with known or suspected cardiovascular disease, several methodologies of investigation have been developed to detect the presence of disease and to provide an assessment for prognosis, effects of therapy, and risk stratification of patients. These diagnostic modalities include exercise and/or pharmacologic stress testing, nuclear cardiac imaging, echocardiography, cardiac catheterization/coronary angiography, and magnetic resonance imaging. These patients frequently require an anatomic, physiologic, and functional assessment of their cardiovascular status to determine optimal clinical management. Nuclear cardiac imaging techniques lend themselves more to physiologic and functional assessments. Techniques used in nuclear cardiology can be broadly divided into those that rely on standard single photon emitting radiopharmaceuticals (e.g. multigated blood pool imaging, first pass radionuclide ventriculography, and planar and/or single photon emission computed tomographic (SPECT) myocardial perfusion and metabolic imaging) and those that rely on positron emitting radiopharmaceuticals (e.g. rubidium-82, nitrogen-13 ammonia, and oxygen-15 water for myocardial perfusion imaging and ^{18}F fluorodeoxyglucose for metabolic imaging).

Cardiovascular nuclear imaging for the assessment of myocardial blood flow has been available for over 30 years. The clinical use of thallium-201 for myocardial perfusion imaging was approved in 1973. The two technetium-99m labeled radiopharmaceuticals currently in use for myocardial perfusion imaging were both approved in the 1990s. The predominant cardiac applications of nuclear imaging during this time have been evaluation of myocardial perfusion and assessment of myocardial viability. These investigations have traditionally been performed in conventional nuclear cardiology with planar and/or SPECT imaging in most clinical practices. Although PET imaging techniques for the assessment of myocardial perfusion and viability were also developed many years ago [1,2], the utilization of cardiac PET imaging has suffered predominantly from the lack of widespread availability of PET scanners and radiopharmaceuticals, expense of the technology with limited reimbursement, and limited approval of cardiac PET radiopharmaceuticals by regulatory agencies. However, in recent years, there has been significant improvement of these limitations. The recent proliferation of PET scanners has made them more widely available, thus allowing greater patient access to this technology. In addition, ^{13}N ammonia has been added to ^{82}Rb as an approved radiopharmaceutical for myocardial perfusion imaging for reimbursement by the Centers for Medicare and Medicaid

Services. Cardiac PET imaging with ^{18}F fluorodeoxyglucose (FDG) is also approved for reimbursement for the assessment of myocardial viability. Another factor of importance for myocardial viability imaging has been the development of regional delivery systems for same day shipment of ^{18}F FDG, which precludes the need for on-site cyclotrons and radiopharmacies for the production of ^{18}F FDG. A recent major improvement related to cardiac PET imaging is the development of the combined PET/CT scanner. In a single study, with the use of intravenous contrast, stress testing and PET imaging, patients with known or suspected coronary artery disease can undergo anatomic assessment of coronary anatomy, evaluation of stress-induced ischemia (or evaluation of coronary flow reserve) and evaluation of left ventricular function.

Cardiac imaging with PET offers selected advantages over cardiac imaging with planar or SPECT modalities. PET imaging provides a high degree of diagnostic accuracy. In comparison to conventional planar or SPECT imaging, PET provides a higher temporal and spatial resolution, and a well-established methodology for attenuation correction. PET images can be analyzed qualitatively or semi-quantitatively. Unlike conventional cardiac imaging, PET studies can also provide absolute quantification of myocardial blood flow and ^{18}F FDG utilization.

Overall, the combination of the technological advantages of PET imaging, relative to SPECT imaging, the progress and improvements in the availability of PET scanners and PET radiopharmaceuticals, the ability to assess coronary anatomy, myocardial perfusion, and ventricular function with a combined PET/CT scanner, and the progress in reimbursement policies should lead to an increase in myocardial assessment by cardiac PET imaging.

Positron Emission Tomography Assessment of Myocardial Ischemia

Tracers for Myocardial Perfusion Imaging in Positron Emission Tomography

There are primarily three tracers that are currently used to assess myocardial perfusion with PET imaging, each of which has certain advantages and disadvantages. These tracers include oxygen-15 water, nitrogen-13 ammonia, and rubidium-82 chloride.

Oxygen-15 labeled water is a nearly ideal, freely diffusible tracer for the evaluation of myocardial perfusion, relative to its linear uptake in relation to increasing myocardial blood flow. Its uptake and clearance are related directly to perfusion and unrelated to metabolic considerations. However, image quality can be adversely affected because of the presence of ^{15}O water in the blood pool; the myocardial perfusion image must be corrected for this vascular activity, which is accomplished by obtaining a blood pool image with ^{15}O labeled carbon monoxide [3]. In addition, the very brief physical half-life of ^{15}O of only 2.1

minutes requires its production from an on-site cyclotron, which limits its avail-ability. Research studies have been performed with ^{15}O water, but the issues of limited availability and somewhat demanding and cumbersome methodology have precluded its use for routine clinical studies.

Nitrogen-13 ammonia is a PET tracer that is extracted from the blood and distributed in the myocardium in relation to blood flow. Its uptake and reten-tion, however, are dependent on metabolic processes in the myocardium. It demonstrates high single pass extraction of approximately 90% and subsequent long retention in the myocardium, which results in high contrast images, rela-tive to blood pool activity. Unlike ^{15}O water, uptake of ^{13}N ammonia is non-linear and plateaus at blood flows greater than around 2 ml/gram per minute. Its uptake and retention depends on conversion of ammonia to glutamine [4]. The availability of ^{13}N ammonia is also somewhat limited due to the 10-minute physical half-life of ^{13}N, which must also be produced by an on-site cyclotron. Where available, however, the overall favorable characteristics of this agent make it suitable for routine clinical studies, which can be performed relatively efficiently.

Rubidium-82 chloride is also a PET tracer that is extracted from the blood and distributed in the myocardium in relation to blood flow. Rubidium-82 is similar to thallium-201 in that it acts as a potassium analogue. Its myocardial extraction is approximately 65% at normal resting blood flow, and like ^{13}N ammonia is also non-linear at higher flow rates. Unlike ^{15}O and ^{13}N, ^{82}Rb is pro-duced from a free-standing generator (strontium-82 parent), which avoids the need for an on-site cyclotron and radiopharmacy, thereby making this radio-pharmaceutical more readily and widely available. The half-life of ^{82}Rb is only 76 seconds, which, in general, allows for a shorter imaging time for a rest and stress perfusion study than is required for ^{13}N ammonia.

Most clinical PET studies are performed with either ^{13}N ammonia (Figure 12.1) or ^{82}Rb chloride. Both of these tracers have been found to be highly accu-rate for evaluating patients with known or suspected coronary artery disease [5–12]. The overall averages of reported sensitivity and specificity of myocar-dial PET perfusion imaging with ^{82}Rb or ^{13}N ammonia for the detection of coro-nary artery disease are 94% and 95%, respectively (Table 12.1) [13].

Comparison of Positron Emission Tomography and Single Photon Emission Computed Tomographic Myocardial Perfusion Imaging

In comparing PET and SPECT for myocardial perfusion imaging, there are several issues to be considered. If patients are able, the preferred modality for stress testing for myocardial perfusion imaging is physical exercise, while phar-macologic stress testing with either vasodilators (i.e., adenosine or dipyridamole) or catecholamine stimulation (i.e., dobutamine) is considered an alternative modality. Any of these modalities lend themselves well to SPECT imaging tech-nology. For PET imaging, pharmacologic stress is usually preferred, although

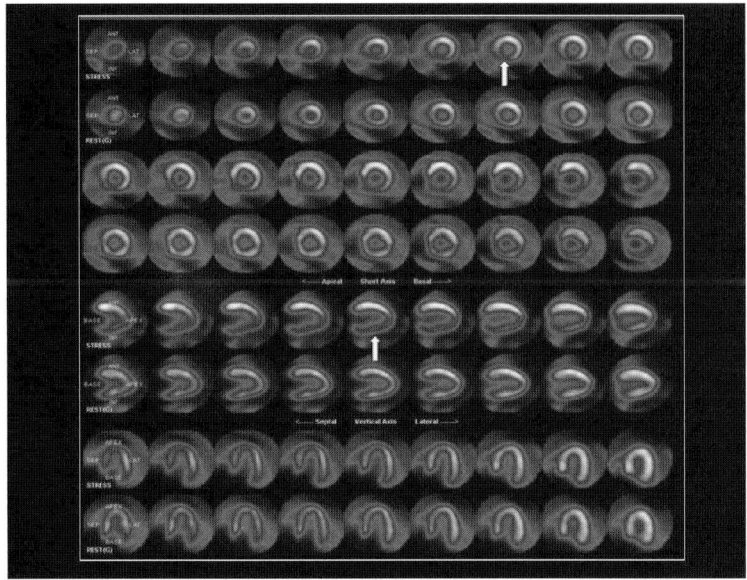

Figure 12.1. [13]N ammonia PET scan on a 70-year-old man with recurring chest pain, which demonstrates reversible ischemia in the inferior and inferoapical segments of the left ventricle (arrows).

exercise is feasible, particularly in conjunction with ^{13}N ammonia. PET offers advantages in spatial resolution and in accepted methodology for attenuation correction, which in turn, can result in improvement in specificity in patients being evaluated for known or suspected coronary artery disease. The higher photon

Table 12.1. Detection of coronary artery disease with ^{13}N ammonia and [82]Rb chloride

Radiopharmaceutical	Investigator	n	Sensitivity	Specificity
[13]N ammonia	Yonekura [5]	49	97%	100%
[13]N ammonia	Schelbert [6]	32	97%	100%
[13]N ammonia	Tamaki [7]	46	98%	–
[82]Rb	Gould [8]	50	95%	100%
[82]Rb	Williams [9]	146	98%	100%
[82]Rb	Demer [10]	193	82%	95%
[82]Rb	Stewart [11]	81	84%	88%
[82]Rb	Go [12]	132	95%	82%
Total		729	94%	95%

Source: Adapted from Schwaiger, Ziegler, Bengel [13], by permission of Lippincott Williams and Wilkins.

energy of PET tracers and the attenuation correction capability of PET imaging offer advantages over SPECT for evaluating obese patients. In addition to improvement in image quality, a myocardial perfusion study in an obese patient that would require a two-day protocol with SPECT imaging due to body habitus can frequently be completed in one day with PET imaging. Overall, there is high sensitivity and specificity for detection of coronary artery disease with PET perfusion imaging.

In comparing rubidium-82 PET and thallium-201 SPECT in the same patient population (132 patients without previous therapeutic interventions), Go et al. demonstrated a higher sensitivity with PET (95% vs. 79%) and a slightly higher specificity with PET (82% vs. 76%) [12], while Stewart et al. demonstrated no significant difference in sensitivity (84% vs. 84%) with a higher specificity for PET (88% vs. 53%) [11].

Finally, one of the major advantages of PET is the ability to measure myocardial blood flow in absolute terms (ml/gram per minute), which cannot be determined by SPECT imaging.

Assessment of Myocardial Viability

Recent estimates suggest that there are 4–5 million people in the United States who have chronic heart failure, with 400,000 new cases and one million hospitalizations occurring each year; as many as 70% of these patients may have underlying coronary artery disease as the cause of their left ventricular dysfunction [14]. The left ventricular ejection fraction (LVEF) is a major prognostic indicator for survival in patients who have coronary artery disease, particularly in patients who have severe depression of LVEF [15]. Patients who have left ventricular dysfunction as a result of coronary artery disease may demonstrate improvement of their left ventricular ejection fraction after a revascularization procedure [16]. Surgical revascularization has shown a significant survival benefit, as compared to medical therapy in patients with coronary artery disease and depressed left ventricular function; a 7-year survival rate of 63% has been shown for patients who had revascularization, as compared to a 34% survival rate after medical therapy [17]. The improved survival may relate, at least partially, to an improvement in left ventricular ejection fraction. However, revascularization presents a high clinical risk for intervention in these patients [18]. Therefore, it is clinically important to prospectively determine whether a patient has evidence of reversible left ventricular dysfunction prior to submitting the patient to a revascularization procedure, and to identify those patients who are likely to benefit most from revascularization. The most benefit appears to occur in those patients who have moderate to severe left ventricular dysfunction and evidence of significant viability. A recent study has shown an 80% reduction in annual mortality among patients with viable myocardium identified by non-invasive testing who were treated with revascularization, while there was no significant difference in mortality between revascularization and medical therapy in patients who did not demonstrate viable myocardium. In addition, patients with viable myocardium demonstrated a direct relationship between the magnitude of benefit from revascularization and the severity of left ventricular dysfunction [19].

Table 12.2. Detection of ventricular functional recovery after revascularization: weighted mean values from pooled analysis of reported non-invasive imaging studies

Modality	Sensitivity	Specificity	Positive predictive value	Negative predictive value
Echocardiography (low-dose dobutamine)	82%	79%	78%	83%
[201]Tl rest-redistribution	86%	59%	69%	80%
[18]F FDG-PET	93%	58%	71%	86%

Source: From Bax, Poldermans, Elhendy et al. [20], by permission of *Current Problems in Cardiology*.

In patients with coronary artery disease, dysfunctional myocardium can occur from variable etiologies that result in segmental wall motion abnormalities and diminished left ventricular function. A completed myocardial infarction may result in left ventricular dysfunction due to a segmental scar that represents irreversible, non-viable myocardial tissue. An acute, reversible ischemic event ("stunned" myocardium) or chronic myocardial ischemia ("hibernating" myocardium) may also result in left ventricular dysfunction with segmental wall motion abnormalities, but the affected myocardial segment may contain myocardial tissue whose function can be improved by revascularization, and is thus characterized as viable myocardium. Diagnostic studies that can define left ventricular dysfunction, but examine only wall motion at rest, cannot distinguish whether a wall motion abnormality is caused by potentially reversible or irreversible myocardial damage. Therefore, several imaging modalities have been devised or modified to assess myocardial viability (Table 12.2). These techniques rely on the ability to stimulate improvement in myocardial contractility or the ability to interrogate certain physiologic aspects of the myocardium to distinguish viable from non-viable tissue.

Echocardiography

Echocardiography is a technique that can assess wall motion at rest. In order to assess for viability, echocardiography requires a stress agent, which most often is dobutamine; vasodilator stress, such as dipyridamole, is less often employed. Viability is determined by assessing for stress-induced myocardial contractile reserve. As dobutamine is administered in increasing dosage, tissue that is viable demonstrates improvement in contractility at a lower dose, but becomes dysfunctional again at higher doses as the heart is further stressed. From a pooled analysis of reported studies in the medical literature, the weighted mean sensitivity and specificity of low-dose dobutamine echocardiography for predicting functional recovery after revascularization were 82% and 79%, respectively [20].

Magnetic Resonance Imaging

Cinegraphic magnetic resonance imaging (MRI) is similar to echocardiography in allowing real-time evaluation of cardiac wall motion, which then allows assessment of contractile reserve with dobutamine in a manner similar to echocardiography. In the prediction of functional recovery on an individual patient basis, dobutamine-induced systolic wall thickening evaluated by MRI has demonstrated a sensitivity of 89% and a specificity of 94% whereas assessment of preserved end diastolic wall thickness demonstrated a sensitivity of 92% and a specificity of 56% [21]. MRI can also assess myocardial viability after administration of gadolinium-DTPA contrast. Areas of completed myocardial infarction demonstrate a region of hyper-enhancement of contrast on delayed imaging. In a recent study comparing contrast-enhanced MRI to ^{18}F FDG-PET, the sensitivity and specificity of MRI for detecting myocardium characterized as non-viable by PET were 96% and 84%, respectively [22].

Thallium-201 Scintigraphy

Thallium-201 is used to assess perfusion and cell membrane integrity as markers of viability. The uptake of ^{201}Tl requires an intact and functional cell membrane. The redistribution of ^{201}Tl on delayed images in myocardial segments that demonstrated a defect on initial images is compatible with viable myocardium in that segment. From a pooled analysis of reported studies in the medical literature, the weighted mean sensitivity and specificity of thallium rest-redistribution imaging for detecting improvement in regional contractible function after revascularization were 86% and 59%, respectively [20].

Positron Emission Tomography

The most common method for evaluating myocardial viability with PET is assessing myocardial perfusion in conjunction with assessment of regional myocardial metabolism. Perfusion can be assessed with either ^{13}N ammonia or rubidium-82 chloride. Metabolism is assessed by the uptake of ^{18}F FDG, a glucose analogue that is transported into the myocardial cell and becomes metabolically trapped after intracellular phosphorylation. Image analysis relies on evaluation of the match or mismatch of segmental perfusion and metabolism. From pooled analysis of reported studies, the weighted mean sensitivity and specificity of ^{18}F FDG-PET for detecting improvement in regional contractile function after revascularization were 93% and 58%, respectively [20].

There are some nuances of cardiac PET imaging that need consideration prior to imaging, most of which relate to dietary status and blood levels of glucose and fatty acids. Under normal resting conditions, the myocardium uses free fatty acids and glucose as major sources of energy. In ischemic myocardium, however, oxidative metabolism of free fatty acids is decreased and glucose becomes the preferred substrate for energy source. The ability of the myocardium to metabolize glucose, even though it may be inadequate for normal myocardial contractility (depending on the severity of ischemia), is indicative of viable myocardium.

Because normal myocardium uses predominantly free fatty acids and ischemic myocardium may use predominantly glucose as their respective energy substrates under normal resting conditions, one consideration for myocardial viability imaging would be to administer ^{18}F FDG in a fasting state to identify ischemic viable myocardium. The rationale of this protocol would be that ischemic viable myocardium would take up ^{18}F FDG, while normal or infarcted, non-viable myocardium would take up little, if any ^{18}F FDG. However, in that setting, overall image quality has been shown to be suboptimal for definitive evaluation [23]. The uptake of FDG into the myocardium is very dependent on dietary conditions, as particularly related to plasma levels of glucose, insulin and free fatty acids. Elevated levels of free fatty acids inhibit myocardial uptake of FDG, whereas increased levels of glucose and insulin facilitate myocardial uptake of FDG [24]. Therefore, optimizing the relative concentrations of these metabolic substrates is desired for optimal FDG cardiac imaging, and various techniques have been devised to accomplish this goal. Patients with diabetes mellitus, however, do present a challenge to obtain optimal image quality. The most demanding protocol involves the use of a euglycemic hyperinsulinemic clamping technique, which regulates these various substrates and frequently results in optimal image quality [25]. However, this procedure is time-consuming and difficult to apply in the general clinical setting. An alternative that is most frequently used in clinical practice is an oral glucose loading technique, often accompanied by the administration of intravenous regular insulin on a sliding scale, dependent upon the patient's response to the oral administration of usually 25–50 grams of oral glucose. Another alternative that has been proposed is the oral administration of acipimox, which is a derivative of nicotinic acid [26]. This agent inhibits peripheral lipolysis, which reduces the plasma level of free fatty acids, thereby indirectly stimulating cardiac uptake of glucose, and thus FDG-18. This technique has resulted in good image quality that is reported as comparable to the optimal euglycemic hyperinsulinemic technique [26].

The protocol for viability assessment includes a resting myocardial perfusion study (usually using ^{13}N ammonia or [82]Rb), followed by a glucose loaded ^{18}F FDG metabolic study. Myocardial segments that have been shown to be dysfunctional on wall motion analysis are then analyzed for perfusion and metabolic findings. The analysis involves evaluating the studies for areas of matched or mismatched findings (Table 12.3).

In general, viable ischemic myocardium demonstrates mismatched increased FDG activity in areas of decreased perfusion, while non-viable myocardium demonstrates matched areas of decreased FDG activity and decreased perfusion (Figure 12.2). These findings allow identification of myocardium that may benefit from revascularization. In general, any segment of the myocardium that demonstrates preservation of ^{18}F FDG uptake that is greater than 50% of normal is considered viable.

Viability studies with ^{18}F FDG-PET have been analyzed from several perspectives to determine the ability of the studies to predict clinically useful information [27]. In addition to predicting improvement of regional left ventricular function after revascularization, ^{18}F FDG-PET has also been predictive of

Table 12.3. Wall motion and PET scan findings (perfusion and ^{18}F FDG metabolism) as related to myocardial status

Myocardium	Wall motion	Perfusion	^{18}F FDG uptake
Normal	Normal	Normal	Normal
Stunned	Decreased	Normal	Normal or increased
Hibernating	Decreased	Decreased	Normal or increased
Infarcted scar	Decreased	Decreased	Decreased

improvement in global LV function after revascularization. Cardiac FDG-PET has also been shown to be predictive of improvement in heart failure symptoms and exercise capacity. Viability assessment with FDG has also been shown to have a significant clinical impact on patient management. Based on results of an FDG-PET viability study, patient therapy can be redirected between medical and

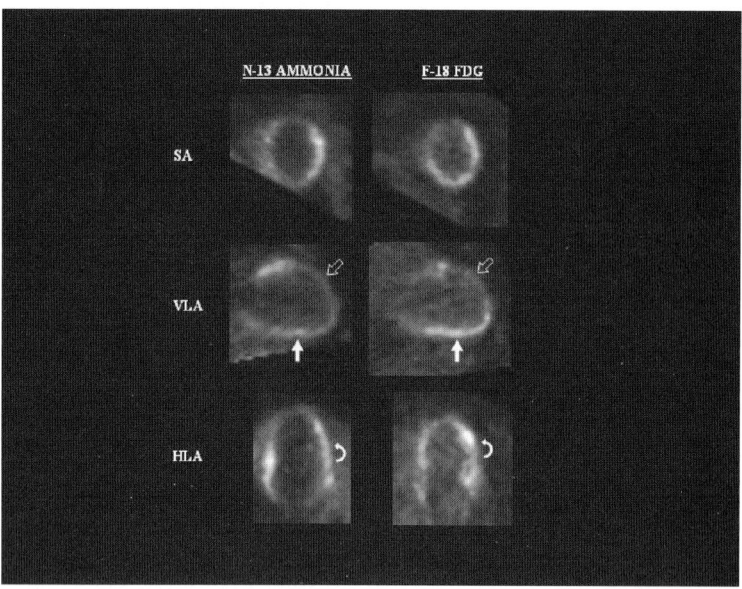

Figure 12.2. Myocardial viability study (^{13}N ammonia perfusion and ^{18}F FDG metabolism) of a 53-year-old man with coronary artery disease and ischemic cardiomyopathy being considered for coronary artery bypass graft surgery. There is a completed transmural infarct with non-viable myocardium (matched defect with severely diminished perfusion and FDG metabolism) in the anterior segment (open arrows) and segmental ischemic viable myocardium (mismatched defect with diminished perfusion, but preserved FDG metabolism) in the inferior segment (closed arrows). Normal viable myocardium (matched normal perfusion and FDG metabolism) is demonstrated in the lateral segment (curved arrows).

surgical therapy, and between heart transplant and revascularization. Therefore, patients that would be suitable for myocardial viability studies would include patients with left ventricular dysfunction and low ejection fractions as a result of sequelae of coronary artery disease who are under consideration for revascularization or cardiac transplantation.

Horizons: Positron Emission Tomography/Computed Tomography Angiography/Calcium Scoring

Scintigraphic myocardial perfusion imaging evaluates the physiology of myocardial blood flow at the cellular level, as various tracers are deposited in the myocardium in proportion to the blood flow to any given region. The usual adjunctive study to scintigraphy is the invasive coronary angiogram that is performed with contrast injection directly into the coronary arteries to evaluate the degree of potential stenosis of the epicardial coronary artery supplying a region of detected ischemia. Vice versa, myocardial perfusion scintigraphy can be utilized to determine the physiologic significance of epicardial stenoses identified on preceding coronary angiography. Currently, there is extensive interest in PET/multidetector CT scanners, which can provide a non-invasive functional and anatomical cardiac evaluation in a single setting. While the PET scanner component of these hybrid cameras can evaluate myocardial perfusion and metabolism, the CT scanner component can detect calcified and non-calcified atherosclerotic coronary artery disease, and identify suspected flow-limiting coronary artery stenoses. Thus, this combined study can provide the location and composition of atherosclerotic lesions and their physiologic significance, relative to myocardial perfusion.

The logistics for performing combined PET/CT will vary depending upon the PET radiopharmaceutical employed and the method of performing the stress test (i.e., exercise or pharmacologic stress agents). Patients are screened and prepared as per routine protocol for stress testing. Special attention to heart rate is required for optimal acquisition of the CT angiogram. For a typical ^{13}N ammonia vasodilator stress PET/CT scan, beta-blocker therapy is not withheld. If the patient is not taking an oral beta-blocker, or if the resting heart rate prior to scanning is greater than 65 beats per minute, and the resting blood pressure is greater than 90/60, oral and/or intravenous beta-blocker medication (e.g. metoprolol) can be administered prior to the CT angiogram. For exercise stress testing, beta-blocker therapy is withheld per protocol prior to the PET/CT scan. If the resting heart rate is greater than 65 beats per minute, and the resting blood pressure is greater than 90/60, a shorter-acting beta-blocker (e.g. esmolol) can be administered. After establishing an optimal heart rate of around 55–60 beats per minute, the CT angiogram is performed as the initial study. An initial non-contrast thoracic CT scan is acquired for cardiac localization. Circulation time is evaluated by giving a small bolus of intravenous contrast and determining the time to peak intensity of contrast in the root of the aorta. Subsequently, a gated contrast-enhanced scan is acquired from the ascending aorta to just below the diaphragm.

The myocardial perfusion study is acquired after the CT angiogram. The rest perfusion study, which is preceded by a CT scan for attenuation correction, is acquired with ^{13}N ammonia, and can be gated for evaluation of left ventricular ejection fraction. The patient is then stressed as per exercise or pharmacologic protocol, followed by the stress myocardial perfusion scan and a repeat CT scan that is acquired for attenuation correction of the stress perfusion images (Figure 12.3). The combined ^{13}N ammonia stress PET/CT scan can be completed in approximately 90–120 minutes (Figure 12.4).

Calcification of the coronary artery is present in most atherosclerotic lesions, and is more likely to be found in advanced disease. CT can detect the presence of calcium in the coronary arteries, and can also quantify the extent of calcium that is detected, which can be reported in a standard scoring format (the Agatston score). Identification of coronary calcium is a sensitive, though not specific, marker for the presence of obstructive coronary artery disease (Figure 12.5). Published data from Shaw et al. suggest that the presence of coronary calcium provides independent incremental information, in addition to traditional risk factors, in predicting all-cause mortality [28]. Non-calcified atherosclerotic plaque, whether or not it is associated with hemodynamically significant luminal stenosis, can also be delineated by CT.

Active research is being conducted to evaluate the ability of CT coronary angiography to non-invasively detect the presence and extent of coronary artery

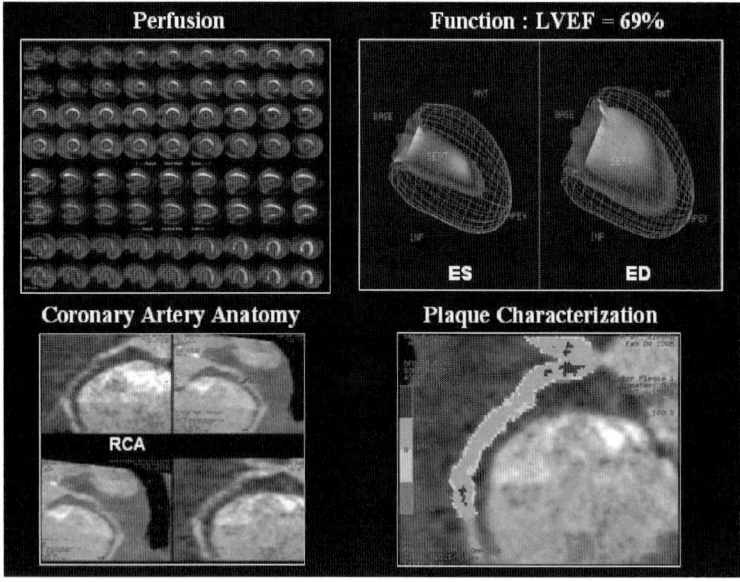

Figure 12.3. Combined PET/CT scan demonstrates inferior wall ischemia on the myocardial perfusion image. The left ventricular ejection fraction (LVEF) is normal (69%). Atherosclerotic disease is demonstrated in the proximal right coronary artery (RCA), the composition of which can be characterized by analysis of plaque density.

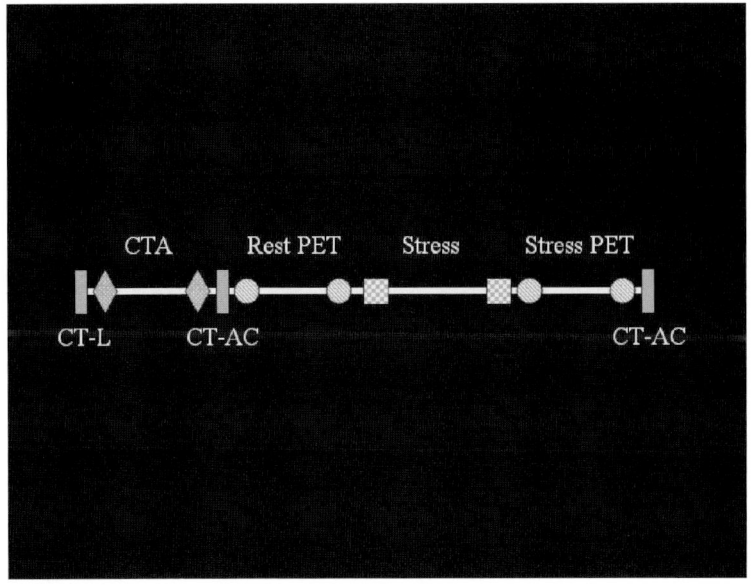

Figure 12.4. Methodology for acquisition of PET/CT scan. CT-L = localizing CT scan; CT-AC = attenuation correction CT scan; CTA = CT angiogram.

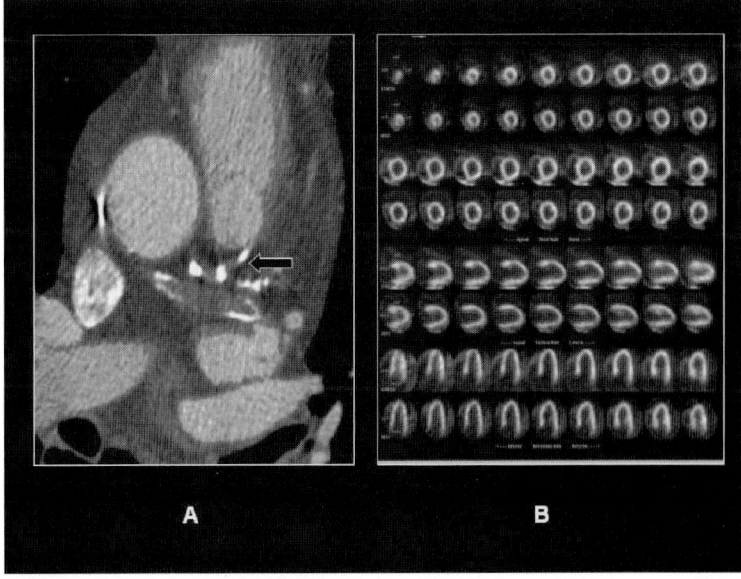

Figure 12.5. Dense calcification is noted in the coronary arteries (arrow) **(A)**. The ¹³N ammonia myocardial perfusion study **(B)** does not demonstrate any evidence of myocardial ischemia.

stenosis. The sensitivity for detection of coronary artery disease with CT can vary depending on several factors, including the location of disease (e.g. proximal versus distal vessel) and the CT scanner employed (e.g. 4-slice versus 16-slice or 64-slice scanners). Leber et al. have reported on the diagnostic accuracy of a 64-slice CT scanner to identify and quantify atherosclerotic coronary lesions in comparison to catheter-based angiography and intravascular ultrasound [29]. In this study, 59 patients with stable angina pectoris were included who had coronary angiography performed within 2 days of the contrast-enhanced CT angiogram. A subset of 18 patients had intravascular ultrasound of 32 vessels performed as part of the catheterization procedure. The 64-slice CT scanner obtained diagnostic image quality of the entire coronary artery tree (American Heart Association 15-segment model for proximal, mid and distal segments) in 55/59 patients. For all segments, sensitivity for the detection of stenosis <50% was 79%, stenosis >50% was 73%, and stenosis >75% was 80%. Specificity for all three groups was 97%. Sensitivity for the detection of stenoses that subsequently required revascularization, however, was 89%. In comparison with intravascular ultrasound, the overall sensitivity and specificity of CT for the detection of coronary lesions were 84% and 91%, respectively.

Although the full impact of PET/CT on the clinical management of patients with known or suspected coronary artery disease remains to be determined, this exciting new technology provides an attractive modality for the simultaneous non-invasive evaluation of the status of the coronary arteries, myocardial perfusion and/or metabolism, and evaluation of left ventricular function (Figure 12.6).

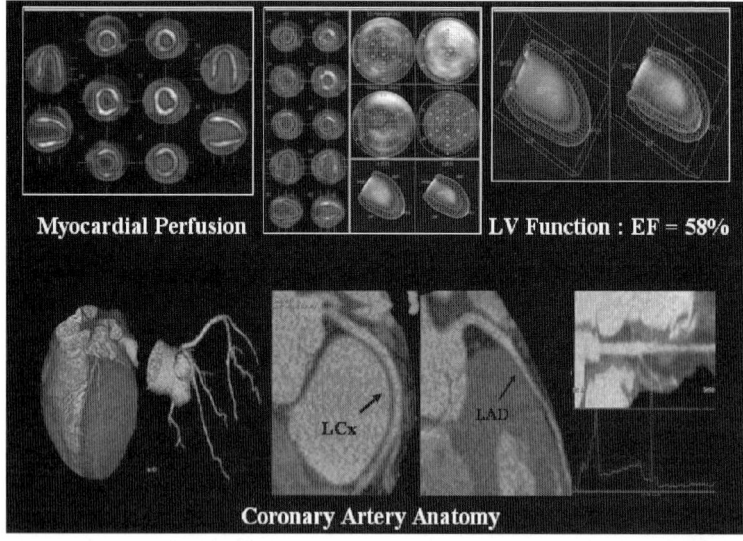

Figure 12.6. In a non-invasive, single setting, combined PET/CT demonstrates myocardial perfusion, evaluation of left ventricular function, and coronary artery anatomy, which can be displayed in various planar and three-dimensional displays.

References

1. Schelbert HR, Phelps ME, Hoffman EJ, et al. Regional myocardial perfusion assessed with N-13 labeled ammonia and positron emission computerized axial tomography. Am J Cardiol 1979;43:209–218.
2. Tillisch J, Brunken R, Marshall R, et al. Reversibility of cardiac wall motion abnormalities predicted by positron emission tomography. N Engl J Med 1986;314: 884–888.
3. Bergmann SR, Fox KA, Raud AL, et al. Quantification of regional myocardial blood flow in vivo with $H_2^{15}O$. Circulation 1984;70:724–733.
4. Bergmann SR. Quantification of myocardial perfusion with positron emission tomography. In: Bergmann SR, Sobel BE, editors. Positron Emission Tomography of the Heart. Mount Kisco, NY: Futura; 1992:97–127.
5. Yonekura Y, Tamaki N, Senda M, et al. Detection of coronary artery disease with 13N-ammonia and high-resolution positron-computed tomography. Am Heart J 1987;113: 645–654.
6. Schelbert H, Phelps M, Huang S, et al. N-13 ammonia as an indicator of myocardial blood flow. Circulation 1981;63:1259–1272.
7. Tamaki N, Yonekura Y, Senda M, et al. Myocardial positron computed tomography with 13N-ammonia at rest and during exercise. Eur J Nucl Med 1985;11: 246–251.
8. Gould K, Goldstein R, Mullani N. Economic analysis of clinical positron emission tomography of the heart with rubidium-82. J Nucl Med 1989;30(5):707–717.
9. Williams B, Jansen D, Wong L, et al. Positron emission tomography for the diagnosis of coronary artery disease: a non-university experience and correlation with coronary angiography. J Nucl Med 1989;30:845.
10. Demer LL, Gould KL, Goldstein RA, et al. Assessment of coronary artery disease severity by positron emission tomography. Comparison with quantitative arteriography in 193 patients. Circulation 1989;79:825–835.
11. Stewart R, Schwaiger M, Molina E, et al. Comparison of rubidium-82, positron emission tomography and thallium-201 SPECT imaging for detection of coronary artery disease. Am J Cardiol 1991;67:1303–1310.
12. Go RT, Marwick TH, MacIntyre WJ, et al. A prospective comparison of rubidium-82 PET and thallium-201 SPECT myocardial perfusion imaging utilizing a single dipyridamole stress in the diagnosis of coronary artery disease. J Nucl Med 1990;31: 1899–1905.
13. Schwaiger M, Ziegler SI, Bengel FM. Assessment of myocardial blood flow with positron emission tomography. In: Pohost GM, O'Rourke RA, Berman DS, et al., editors. Imaging in Cardiovascular Disease. Philadelphia: Lippincott, Williams and Wilkins; 2000:195–212.
14. Gheorghiade M, Bonow RO. Chronic heart failure in the United States. A manifestation of coronary artery disease. Circulation 1998;97:282–289.
15. The Multicenter Post Infarction Research Groups. Risk stratification and survival after myocardial infarction. N Engl J Med 1993;309:331–336.

216   M.W. Hanson and S. Borges-Neto

16. Bonow RO, Dilsizian V. Thallium-201 for assessing myocardial viability. Semin Nucl Med 1991;21:230–241.
17. Pigott JD, Kouchoukos NT, Oberman A, et al. Late results of surgical and medical therapy for patients with coronary artery disease and depressed left ventricular function. J Am Coll Cardiol 1985;5:1036–1045.
18. Baker DW, Jones R, Hodges J, et al. Management of heart failure III. The role of revascularization in treatment of patients with moderate or severe left ventricular systolic dysfunction. JAMA 1994;272:1528–1534.
19. Allman KC, Shaw LJ, Hachamovitch R, et al. Myocardial viability testing and impact of revascularization on prognosis in patients with coronary artery disease and left ventricular dysfunction: a meta-analysis. J Am Coll Cardiol 2002;39:1151–1158.
20. Bax JJ, Poldermans D, Elhendy A, et al. Sensitivity, specificity, and predictive accuracies of various non invasive techniques for detecting hibernating myocardium. Curr Probl Cardiol 2001;26:147–186.
21. Baer FM, Theissen P, Schneider CA, et al. Dobutamine magnetic resonance imaging predicts contractile recovery of chronically dysfunctional myocardium after successful revascularization. J Am Coll Cardiol 1998;31:1041–1048.
22. Kuhl HP, Beek AM, van deer Weerdt AP, et al. Myocardial viability in chronic ischemic heart disease. Comparison of contrast-enhanced magnetic resonance imaging with ^{18}F-Fluorodeoxyglucose positron emission tomography. J Am Coll Cardiol 2003;41:1341–1348.
23. Berry JJ, Baker JA, Pieper KS, et al. The effect of metabolic milieu on cardiac PET imaging using fluorine-18-deoxyglucose and nitrogen-13-ammonia in normal volunteers. J Nucl Med 1991;32:1518–1525.
24. Nuutila P, Koivisto VA, Knuuti J, et al. Glucose-free fatty acid cycle operates in human heart and skeletal muscle in vivo. J Clin Invest 1992;89:1767–1774.
25. Knuuti J, Nuutila P, Ruotsalainen U, et al. Euglycemic hyperinsulinemic clamp and oral glucose load in stimulating myocardial glucose utilization during positron emission tomography. J Nucl Med 1992;33:1255–1262.
26. Knuuti MJ, Yki-Jarvinen H, Voipio-Pulkki LM, et al. Enhancement of myocardial [fluorine-18] fluorodeoxyglucose uptake by a nicotinic acid derivative. J Nucl Med 1994;35:989–998.
27. Bax JJ, Patton JA, Poldermans D, et al. 18-Fluorodeoxyglucose imaging with positron emission tomography and single photon emission computed tomography: cardiac applications. Semin Nucl Med 2000;30:281–298.
28. Shaw LJ, Raggi P, Schisterman E, et al. Prognostic value of cardiac risk factors and coronary artery calcium screening for all cause mortality. Radiology 2003;228:826–833.
29. Leber AW, Knez A, Von Ziegler F, et al. Quantification of obstructive and nonobstructive coronary lesions by 64-slice computed tomography: a comparative study with quantitative coronary angiography and intravascular ultrasound. J Am Coll Cardiol 2005;46:147–154.

13. PET in Neurology

Ronald B. Workman, Jr., Terence Z. Wong, and R. Edward Coleman

Neuro-oncology

Approximately 18,500 new cases of central nervous system (CNS) malignancy were diagnosed in 2005 in the United States, with an estimated 12,760 deaths attributable to these neoplasms [1]. Although the incidence of primary neoplasm of the brain and spinal cord is low relative to other cancers, the mortality remains high with 2.2% of the overall cancer mortality due to CNS tumors. Furthermore, the overall 5-year survival has only improved from 22% in the mid-1970s to 32% in the mid-1990s [2].

Brain tumors occur in the young and old, but the average age at diagnosis for all primary brain tumors is approximately 54 years. In adults, the most common primary brain tumors are gliomas and meningiomas, with gliomas constituting about half of all brain tumors and having a slight male predisposition. Lower-grade gliomas, such as oligodendrogliomas, tend to occur in younger patients, and higher-grade gliomas, such as glioblastoma multiforme (GBM), tend to occur in older individuals. Prognosis is highly correlated with patient age and tumor grade, and the 2-year survival rates for those with GBM range from 30% for younger patients (i.e., those less than 20 years) to only 2% for those older than 65 years. Meningiomas represent about 20% of all brain tumors, occur more frequently in females and the elderly, and are extra-axial. Prognosis is good for these tumors, with an 81% overall 5-year survival; however, this decreases to 55% overall 5-year survival if the tumors have undergone malignant degeneration [2]. Primary CNS lymphomas constitute about 4% of primary brain tumors and tend to occur in the immunocompromised patient.

In pediatric patients, CNS tumors comprise approximately 16% of all malignancies, and are the most frequently occurring solid tumors. Roughly half of these tumors are astrocytomas, with medulloblastoma, primitive neuroectodermal tumors (PNET), other gliomas, and ependymomas following in frequency. Younger patients typically have a better prognosis than older patients, and the overall 5-year survival for children with brain tumors is 67%. Pediatric brain tumors are notoriously challenging to treat, with morbidity and local recurrence being a long-term problem.

The etiology of brain tumors has both genetic and environmental components. Research has shown that over-expression of the gene coding for platelet-derived growth factor (PDGF), which results in increased proliferation and migration of glioma cells, coupled with a defect in the tumor-suppressing p53 gene may constitute a cooperative tumorigenic effect [3]. There are also hereditary syndromes such as tuberous sclerosis and neurofibromatosis that carry a high incidence of brain tumors. Despite these observations, only about 2–10% of patients with brain tumors have an identified genetic predisposition, and only approximately 5% of gliomas are familial [2]. Previous exposure to radiation therapy has been shown to be a strong risk factor in the subsequent development of primary brain tumors. Some studies have also pointed to other environmental factors such as heavy metal and petrochemical exposure as causing an increased risk [4]. Immune suppression, either due to HIV or immunosuppressive medication, has been shown to confer an increased risk in the development of primary CNS lymphoma [2]. Recent years have seen a dramatic increase in the number of individuals using cellular phones; however, there has been no clear link made between the electromagnetic radiation exposure from cellular phone use and the development of primary brain tumors. With the exception of primary CNS lymphoma, the incidence of brain tumors has remained relatively stable over the time that cellular phones have been in use [5].

Classification of Brain Tumors

There are a wide variety of CNS tumors, and their classification is complex. The World Health Organization (WHO) organizes primary brain tumors according to their cell of origin. The most common class of brain tumors is that of neuroepithelial lineage, and it includes the astrocytomas, oligodendrogliomas, ependymomas, and mixed gliomas. Less common are tumors of the choroid plexus, pineal parenchymal tumors, embryonal tumors, and primitive neuroectodermal tumors. Other CNS tumors include pituitary adenomas, craniopharyngiomas, primary CNS lymphomas, and extra-axial tumors such as meningiomas [6]. Tumor grade is typically assigned based on an assessment of conventional histologic features such as the degree of cellular atypia, mitotic activity, necrosis, endothelial proliferation, invasion, and sometimes an analysis of gene expression profiles.

Currently, no TNM staging scheme is recommended for CNS tumors. The WHO has devised a tumor-grading scheme ranging from I to IV, with grades I and II representing low-grade neoplasms, and grades III and IV assigned to high-grade lesions. Low-grade tumors include pilocytic astrocytomas (I) and well-differentiated astrocytomas and oligodendrogliomas (II). High-grade tumors include anaplastic astrocytomas and anaplastic oligodendrogliomas (III). The most common primary brain cancer of adults, glioblastoma multiforme (GBM), is also the most aggressive, has the highest grade (IV), and has the worst prognosis. The high-grade gliomas (III and IV) can be further described as either primary or secondary malignant astrocytomas [7]. Primary malignant astrocytomas occur in older patients with no history of prior low-grade tumor. Secondary malignant astrocytomas arise from further malignant degeneration of pre-existing low-grade gliomas and tend to occur in younger patients. The occurrence of secondary malignant astrocytomas in younger patients is the main reason behind the previously mentioned prolonged morbidity and high late mortality often seen in children.

Brain tumors are microscopically heterogeneous, and the more dedifferentiated cell populations within a tumor tend to grow more aggressively than other,
better differentiated, cells. This cellular heterogeneity results in a tumor which
has varying grades within it and helps account for the disease progression seen
when low-grade tumors become high grade after a period of time.

Conventional Imaging of Brain Tumors

Computed tomography (CT) and especially magnetic resonance imaging
(MRI) are the mainstays of any comprehensive diagnostic work-up of neurological disease. MRI provides superb anatomic detail by allowing exceptional
spatial resolution and delineation of gray and white matter structures. The most
sensitive imaging modality for the detection of brain tumors can be found with
standard T1- and T2-weighted MR images. The administration of intravenous
contrast assesses the integrity of the blood–brain barrier and further raises the
sensitivity of MRI because many tumors, particularly those which are higher
grade, show a corresponding increase in contrast enhancement. Lower-grade
tumors may have low or minimal contrast enhancement, but typically do show
increased signal on T2-weighted images. Often, MRI provides additional clinically useful information such as the presence and/or degree of mass effect, hemorrhage, edema, and necrosis, which often accompany brain tumors [8].

MRI and CT provide anatomic information. The degree of contrast enhancement can also provide information about the grade of tumor; however, this is
limited. Because brain tumors are heterogeneous and often grow in an infiltra-
tive manner, accurate information regarding tumor grade is essential. Limitations in MRI may arise in the post-therapeutic setting in which patients treated
with resection followed by radiotherapy show enhancement that may be caused
by post-therapy changes (i.e., radionecrosis) or residual tumor [9]. To address
these limitations, much work is being done with nuclear medicine techniques,
particularly positron emission tomography (PET), as a way to gain invaluable
information regarding tumor grade. For increased diagnostic accuracy, the
anatomic information provided by MRI or CT can be combined, or *registered*,
with the metabolic information provided by nuclear medicine techniques. At our
institution, we routinely register ^{18}F-2-fluoro-2-deoxy-D-glucose (FDG) PET
and MRI images for evaluation of patients with brain tumors. This technique is
discussed in a separate section at the end of this chapter.

Positron Emission Tomography Imaging of Brain Tumors

Since the early 1990s, the use of PET in imaging brain tumors has become
the standard of care at many medical centers across the United States. The value
of FDG-PET in evaluating brain tumors is the correlation between FDG uptake
and tumor grade. Physiologic background FDG uptake is low in white matter,

and high in gray matter. For an example of a normal FDG-PET brain scan, see Figure 13.1. When evaluating the metabolic activity of a brain tumor, comparison of the FDG uptake within the tumor to contralateral homologous (and presumably more normal) brain allows a relatively simple and rapid qualitative assessment of grade. By this method, low-grade tumors have FDG accumulation similar to or less than normal white matter, and high-grade tumors have activity that is similar to or greater than normal gray matter [8].

The FDG uptake in low- and high-grade tumors relative to normal white and gray matter has also been studied quantitatively. In 1995, Delbeke et al. studied 58 patients with brain tumors; 32 had biopsy-proven high-grade disease (WHO III and IV), and 26 had biopsy-proven low-grade tumor (WHO I and II). Regions of interest were used to assign tumor-to-white matter (T/WM) and tumor-to-gray matter (T/GM) ratios in an effort to determine an appropriate threshold value to distinguish high from low grade. They found that T/WM ratios greater than 1.5 and T/GM ratios greater than 0.6 were indicative of high-grade disease with a sensitivity of 94% and a specificity of 77% [10]. These findings support the qualitative approach described above in which FDG uptake in low-grade tumors resembles white matter and uptake in high-grade tumors resembles gray matter.

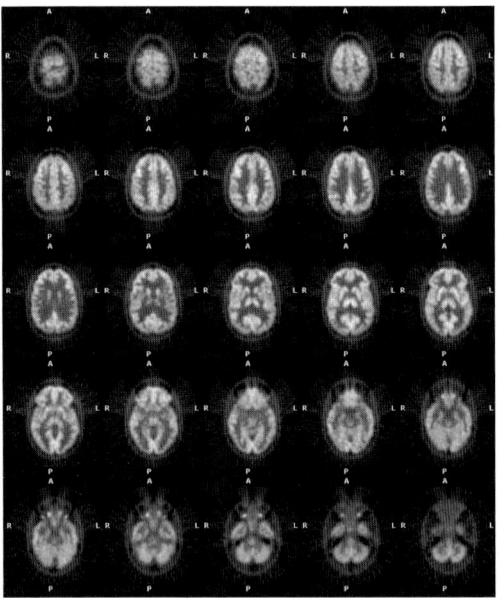

Figure 13.1. Normal FDG-PET brain scan. Transaxial FDG-PET images of a normal brain. Notice the increased activity of gray matter, both in cortical and deep gray structures, compared to relatively hypometabolic white matter. In this patient you can also see physiologic FDG uptake in the extraocular muscles.

As mentioned previously, glial tumors have notoriously heterogeneous pathology. This was quantified when Paulus and Peiffer studied the histologic features of 1000 samples from 50 brain tumors (20 samples per tumor to simulate multiple biopsies). They observed that different grades were detected in 82% of tumors, and a majority (62%) of the gliomas contained low- and high-grade features (WHO grades II, III, and IV) [11]. This heterogeneity accounts for the sampling error and under-staging often encountered in managing brain tumors. The emergence of high-grade disease within a previously low-grade lesion cannot be detected by MRI, but with FDG-PET, hypermetabolic areas are more likely to have the highest grade and can be specifically targeted for stereotactic biopsy, thereby improving the chances of accurately staging the tumor [12–15].

The degree of FDG uptake in brain tumors also carries prognostic significance. One study of 29 patients with treated and untreated primary brain tumors found that patients with hypermetabolic tumors had a substantially worse prognosis than those with hypometabolic tumors [16]. Another study of 45 patients with high-grade tumors showed that those with high metabolic activity had a mean survival of 5 months compared to a mean survival of 19 months for those with less metabolically active tumors [17]. Patients with low-grade tumors who then develop hypermetabolic foci also have a poorer prognosis [18,19].

For accurate interpretation of findings in FDG-PET and MRI scans, the PET images must be correlated with areas of enhancement on MRI to differentiate post-therapy changes from residual tumor, which may be indistinguishable by MRI alone. Post-surgical changes do not result in hypermetabolism, although there typically is a rim of enhancement on the MRI along the surgical resection cavity [20].

In patients who receive high-dose radiotherapy, the resulting radionecrosis is usually hypometabolic; however, hypermetabolism can be observed occasionally. This mechanism is thought to be due to inflammatory changes brought on by accumulation of metabolically active macrophages at therapy sites. This intermediate, or moderate, degree of uptake may be seen in other areas such as the thorax, which can be subject to radiation-induced changes following treatment for pulmonary malignancies. While the typical post-radiotherapy hypermetabolism is uniform and intermediate, in some cases there can be nodular characteristics and/or hypermetabolism that approaches or even exceeds gray matter activity. In these scenarios, radionecrosis cannot be differentiated from high-grade tumor recurrence. In 1997, Barker et al. evaluated at 55 patients with high-grade tumors that underwent surgery and radiation therapy who had suspected recurrence because of enlarging areas of enhancement on MRI. Those who had FDG uptake equal to or exceeding gray matter had a significantly poorer prognosis than those without corresponding hypermetabolism [21]. In 2001, Chao et al. studied 47 patients with primary and metastatic brain tumors who underwent stereotactic biopsy. The results revealed 75% sensitivity and 81% specificity for detecting recurrent tumor as opposed to radionecrosis [22] (Figure 13.2). Seizures, either clinical or subclinical, during the uptake phase can result in false-positive FDG-PET brain study results [23]. Patients with documented or suspected seizure disorders can be scanned with EEG monitoring to minimize the impact on specificity.

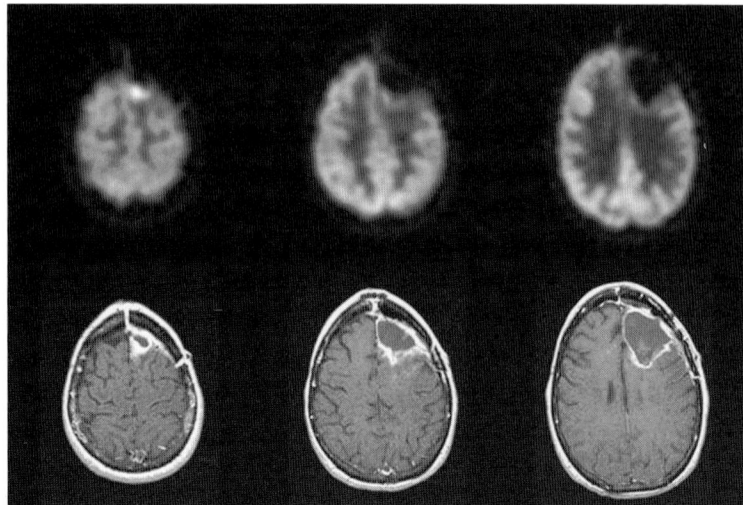

Figure 13.2. A 44-year-old man with a history of surgical removal of an anaplastic astrocytoma from the left frontal lobe. Recent MRI shows increasing enhancement at the surgical margin. Registered FDG-PET and contrast-enhanced MRI show abnormal FDG accumulation in the enhancing lesion that is greater than gray matter on the vertex image, suggesting recurrent tumor.

At our institution, we are investigating high-dose brachytherapy with iodine-131 (^{131}I) labeled monoclonal antibodies directed against the glycoprotein tenascin expressed by gliomas. Patients receiving this treatment have undergone resection and placement of an indwelling reservoir that allows controlled access to the resection cavity [24]. The beta emission from the ^{131}I results in a very high local radiation dose delivered to the tumor cavity. The FDG-PET images from patients who have had brachytherapy may have a uniform rim of intermediate level hypermetabolism along the resection margin. The development of hypermetabolic nodularity along this rim suggests recurrence [25].

The majority of the work with FDG-PET and brain tumors involves the astrocytic tumors; however, the correlation between FDG uptake and malignancy generally applies to other CNS tumors as well. Although usually benign, meningiomas can become aggressive and recur, and a positive correlation has been shown between glucose metabolism and aggressive behavior in these tumors [26]. CNS lymphomas are typically very FDG avid, and FDG-PET can accurately differentiate patients with CNS lymphoma from infectious etiologies like toxoplasmosis [27] (Figure 13.3). Juvenile pilocytic astrocytomas are markedly enhancing low-grade tumors with a favorable prognosis; however, because of their metabolically active fenestrated epithelial cells, they typically have hypermetabolism, which resembles gray matter [28].

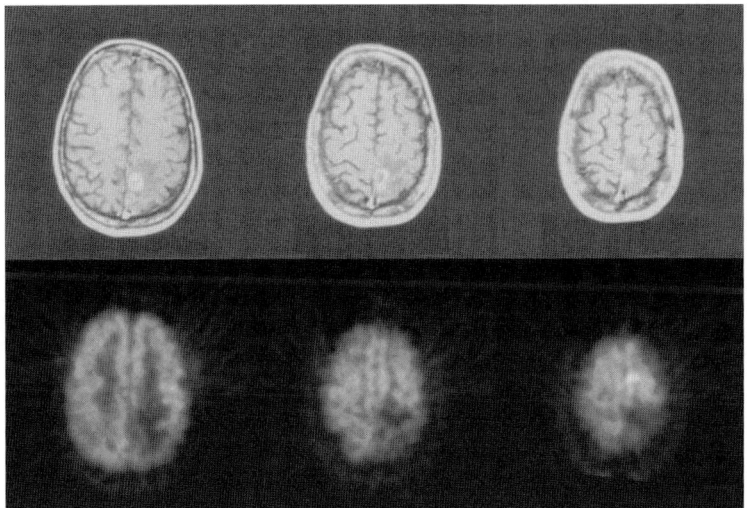

Figure 13.3. A 33-year-old man with acquired immunodeficiency disease who presented with headache, fever, chills, and right leg weakness. MRI reveals an enhancing lesion in the left parietal region. Registered FDG-PET and contrast-enhanced MRI show FDG uptake in the enhancing rim at a level between white and gray matter suggesting an inflammatory process like toxoplasmosis. CNS lymphoma usually has uptake greater than gray matter. The patient responded to therapy for toxoplasmosis.

Positron Emission Tomography and Brain Metastases

Far and away the most common brain tumor is a metastasis, frequently from either a lung or breast primary given their high prevalence. In one recent study of 40 patients by Rohren et al, 38 had metastatic disease by MRI, with only 23 (61%) of these being identified by PET [29]. Because it is relatively insensitive in detecting cerebral metastases, FDG-PET brain scanning is not recommended in screening for cerebral metastases. If there is a high clinical suspicion for cerebral metastatic disease, contrast-enhanced MRI of the brain is recommended.

Horizons: Other Positron Emission Tomography Radiotracers

Just as there is an increased glucose demand by cancer cells, amino acid transport is also increased. Radiolabeled amino acid PET imaging using carbon-11 (^{11}C) has been used clinically primarily with ^{11}C-methionine (MET) and ^{11}C-tyrosine [30]. A major advantage over FDG-PET imaging is the low background amino acid uptake, and MET-PET in particular has 1.2 to 3.5 times greater uptake in tumor than in normal brain. MET-PET is better than FDG-PET in delineating tumor margins and in differentiating between tumor and radionecrosis because amino acid uptake is less influenced by inflammation [30,31]. In 1998, Sasaki et al. showed that MET-PET is more sensitive than ^{201}Tl SPECT or FDG-PET in detecting low-grade astrocytomas, and is able to reliably distinguish between low- and high-grade tumors [32]. Chung et al. recently looked at MET-PET in the evaluation of brain lesions with low level FDG uptake and found 89% sensitivity in detecting low-grade tumors, with 100% specificity in identifying benign processes [33]. MET-PET may have a role in distinguishing low-grade tumors from entities in which FDG-PET is inconclusive such as inflammation from radionecrosis, infection, or benign tumors. One of the major limitations to the use of ^{11}C in clinical practice is its very short physical half-life ($t_{1/2}$ = 20 minutes) which requires the presence of a cyclotron on-site. Some preliminary studies have been performed with ^{18}F-ethyl-tyrosine, and the initial results are promising.

Some encouraging work is being performed with thymidine analogues such as FMAU (1-(2′-deoxy-2′-[^{18}F]-beta-D-arabinofuranosyl) thymine) and FLT ([^{18}F] 3′-deoxy-3′-fluorothymidine) as a way to image cellular proliferation via DNA synthesis [34,35]. ^{18}F-fluorocholine, and ^{11}C-choline have also been used to image brain tumors, and the initial results are promising. The low accumulation of these tracers in normal brain provides better tumor-to-normal brain ratios than are available with FDG.

PET imaging using radiopharmaceuticals labeled with the positron emitter oxygen-15 (^{15}O) has been used to study cerebral blood volume, blood flow, and oxygen utilization [36,37]. Because cerebral perfusion to a particular area is related to cortical activation, PET studies using H_2^{15}O can be obtained while the patient is performing various purposeful tasks, thereby helping to localize eloquent cortical regions to be avoided during surgery. Like ^{11}C, the use of ^{15}O is significantly limited because of its very short physical half-life ($t_{1/2}$ = 2 minutes).

Dementia

Dementia is a condition of deteriorating mental faculties, particularly memory and cognitive function, and can also be associated with personality changes such as paranoia, aggression, or depression. The most common type of dementia is Alzheimer's disease (AD), and an estimated 4.5 million Americans are afflicted. Approximately 70% of patients with dementia have AD. Increasing age is the greatest risk factor, affecting 1 in 10 people by age 65 and nearly half of those aged 85 or over. Most cases are sporadic and attack later in life; however, rare, familial forms of the disease can strike individuals in their 30s or 40s [38]. The number of AD cases is expected to grow significantly in the near future, with projections of 11.3–16 million by 2050 [39]. Those with AD will live an average of 8 years or as many as 20 years after diagnosis, with an estimated national direct and indirect cost of caring for those with AD of at least $100 billion annually [40–42]. This monumental financial burden is paralleled by the devastating emotional strain on family members and loved ones.

The precise cause for AD has not been determined, but ongoing research has suggested a variety of conditions that appear to play a role in development of the disease. The APOE 4 gene is associated with higher risk, and the presence of beta amyloid deposits in the form of plaques and neurofibrillary tangles within affected brain tissue (particularly cholinergic cells) is a common histopathologic feature. Identifying other genes and mechanisms that contribute to the development of AD is an area of active investigation.

Fluorodeoxyglucose-Positron Emission Tomography in Dementia

The diagnosis of AD can be made with high accuracy once complete clinical, neuropsychiatric, and imaging assessments have been obtained. It is estimated that finding a treatment that could delay onset by 5 years would reduce the number of individuals with AD by almost 50% in 50 years [43]. If neuroprotective measures can be taken in this early, asymptomatic period, progression to severe dementia can be delayed. Therefore, it is highly desirable to diagnose patients early, when they present with mild cognitive impairment rather than when clinical dementia arises. Not only can this mitigate the burden on families and society, but it can also extend patients' quality of life as well as enable them to maintain a more active role in setting their affairs in order. It is in this capacity that FDG-PET finds its niche (Table 13.1).

The classic FDG-PET finding in AD is bilateral posterior temporoparietal and posterior cingulate hypometabolism; however, there can be hemispheric asymmetry (Figure 13.4). In contrast to other dementia types, glucose metabolism is normal in the basal ganglia, primary motor and visual cortex, and the cerebellum. Posterior temporoparietal hypometabolism in patients with mild cognitive impairment is being shown to be predictive of developing AD [44–47]. Sensitivity of FDG-PET in AD is in the range of 90–95%, but specificity is slightly less at 65–75%, due to overlap with other neurodegenerative disorders [48].

Other dementing neurodegenerative entities include diffuse Lewy body disease (frequently seen with Parkinson's disease), frontotemporal dementia (Pick's disease), vascular (or multi-infarct) dementia, and Creutzfeldt–Jakob disease. There are certain characteristics of FDG distribution which allow refinement of the differential diagnosis when evaluating a patient with dementia of unknown type. FDG-PET scans of patients with diffuse Lewy body disease can be very similar to those of patients with AD. However, in dementia with Lewy bodies the primary visual cortex is often hypometabolic, but spared in AD [49]. Frontotemporal dementia is characterized by bifrontal or bifrontotemporal

Table 13.1. Checklist to determine whether FDG-PET dementia evaluation is indicated and covered by Medicare*

---

1. Does the patient have diminished memory and other cognitive deficits that have been present for at least 6 months, and that now impair her or his ability to function as he or she normally would (professionally, socially, or with respect to activities of daily living)?
   Yes (continue to 2)
   No (PET scan is not covered*)
2. Based on history, physical examination, and blood tests, is evidence present for any of the following correctable conditions?
   Depression? Substance abuse? Malnourishment? Medication effects? Cardiopulmonary compromise? Anemia? Hypoxemia? Infection? Thyroid dysfunction? Renal or hepatic disorder? Glucose or electrolyte/calcium dysregulation?
   Yes (continue to 3)
   No (continue to 4)
3. After treatment of the previously listed conditions, do the deficits still persist?
   Yes (continue to 4)
   No (PET scan is not indicated)
4. Does the patient suffer from Alzheimer's disease in the judgment of a physician experienced in the diagnosis and assessment of dementia who evaluated this patient, aided by (a) cognitive scales or neuropsychological tests, (b) corroborating history from a well-acquainted informant, or (c) laboratory tests (including serum B12 and TSH levels) and structural imaging (MRI or CT)?
   Yes (the physician judges the presence of Alzheimer's disease to be certain. PET scan is not covered*)
   No (the physician judges the absence of Alzheimer's disease to be certain. PET scan is not covered*)
   Uncertain (the physician judges that it is uncertain whether the patient suffers from Alzheimer's disease. Continue to 5)
5. Does the patient exhibit symptoms (e.g. early onset or prominence of social disinhibition, awkwardness, difficulties with language, loss of executive function) such that frontotemporal dementia is suspected as an alternative cause of the patient's cognitive deficits?
   Yes (continue to 6)
   No (PET scan is not covered*)
6. Is it reasonable to expect that information obtained through FDG-PET will help with diagnosis and management of the patient?
   Yes (continue to 7)
   No (PET scan is not covered)
7. Has the patient previously undergone SPECT or FDG-PET for the same indication?
   Yes (the results were conclusive and the patient's condition has not substantially changed. PET scan is not covered)
   Yes (but the results were not conclusive and at least a year has elapsed. Continue to 8)

Table 13.1. *Continued.*

Yes (but there have been important changes in scope or severity of the
patient's cognitive deficits since then. Continue to 8)
No (continue to 8)

8. An FDG-PET scan is considered "reasonable and necessary" by CMS. The
patient should be referred to a facility accredited to operate nuclear
medicine equipment and the scan should be read by an expert with
experience interpreting PET scans for the evaluation of dementia.

---

* *Note*: PET scans not covered by Medicare according to these criteria may be covered
in the context of a CMS-approved clinical trial.
Source: From Silverman D. Alzheimer's dementia checklist. *Academy of Molecular
Imaging Newsletter* Fall 2004, with permission.

hypometabolism [50] (Figure 13.5). While this pattern is distinct with regard to
AD, other psychiatric conditions can cause frontal lobe dysfunction and hypometabolism [51]. Vascular dementia is characterized by global hypometabolism
which does not spare the deep gray structures as well as focal cortical defeats.
Finally, the uncommon entity known as Creutzfeldt–Jakob disease is a rapidly
debilitating and irreversible disease caused by infectious proteins known as
prions. The rapid clinical course of this illness differs from the other causes of
dementia, and some data with FDG-PET has demonstrated profound multifocal
hypometabolism in the cerebrum and cerebellum with relative sparing of the
temporal cortex, and, to a lesser extent, the deep gray structures [52].

In the Fall 2004 issue of the *Academy of Molecular Imaging Newsletter*, a
dementia evaluation checklist was published to help clinicians determine
whether FDG-PET is indicated and covered by Medicare. For your convenience,
that checklist is included here (Table 13.1).

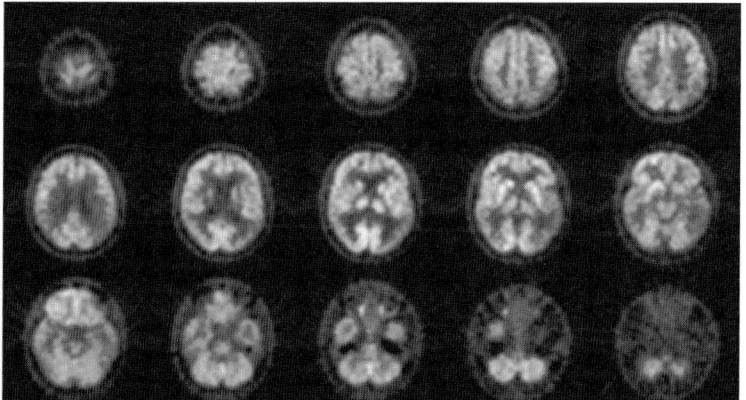

Figure 13.4. Transaxial FDG-PET images in a patient with Alzheimer's disease
demonstrating decreased activity in the posterior parietal lobes bilaterally.

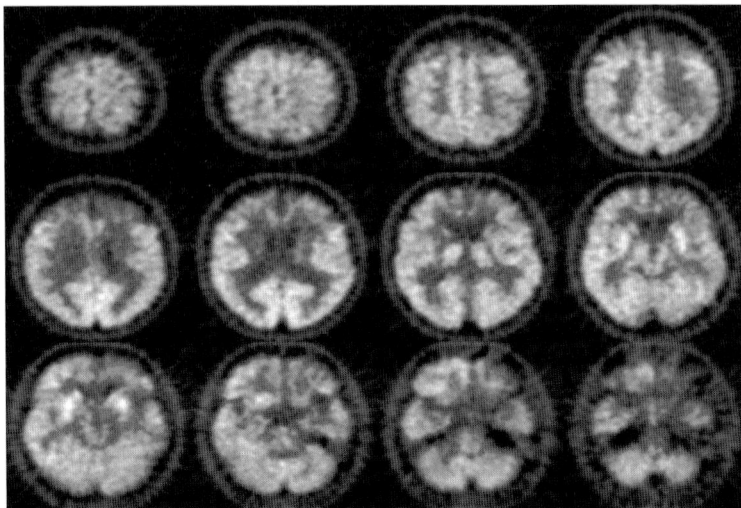

Figure 13.5. Transaxial FDG-PET images in a patient with frontotemporal dementia demonstrating decreased activity in the frontal lobes bilaterally.

Quantitative programs are now available for evaluating the FDG-PET brain scans (Figure 13.6, see Plate 13.6, in the color insert). These programs compare the distribution for FDG with a normal database, which is similar in principle to image analysis programs that are used in nuclear cardiology. These programs are now becoming available, and their utility has yet to be determined. The initial impression is that the programs are particularly helpful to an inexperienced interpreter, but provide less benefit to someone who has a lot of experience in interpreting PET scans in demented patients.

Horizons

Much work is being done with radiolabeled piperidine analogues (^{11}C-labeled *N*-methyl-4-piperidyl-acetate and *N*-methyl-4-piperidyl-propionate), which serve as substrates for acetylcholine esterase in cholinergic cells. While degeneration of cholinergic neurons is a sine qua non of AD, it is not a feature of other types of dementia. Therefore, use of these radiopharmaceuticals may become helpful in cases where the type of dementia is unclear. Another avenue of research is with radiolabeled molecules, which bind to beta amyloid deposits in the affected neurons of patients with AD. One such radiopharmaceutical is FDDNP (2-(1-(6-[(2-[18F] fluoroethyl)(methyl)amino]-2-naphthyl)ethylidene) malononitrile). These new agents are in clinical trials and are promising for being accurate in the detection of AD.

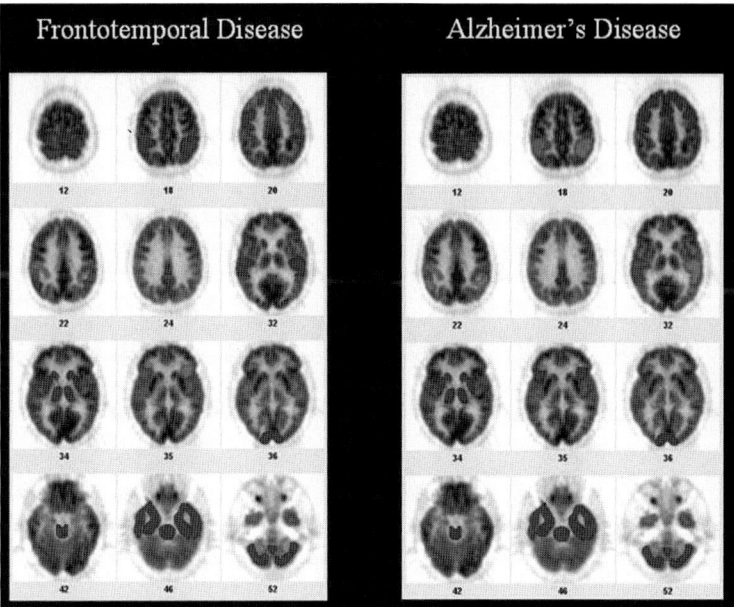

Figure 13.6. NeuroQ analysis of patients with frontotemporal disease and Alzheimer's disease. The areas of most significant abnormality compared to normal controls are highlighted in red. In the patient with frontotemporal dementia, the major abnormality is in the frontal and frontotemporal areas, whereas the abnormality in the patient with Alzheimer's disease is mainly in the posterior parietal areas extending into the temporal lobes. (See color insert.)

Epilepsy

Epilepsy is one of the most common neurological disorders, and is characterized by recurring episodes of excessive neuronal discharge. These episodes manifest as seizures, which result in sensory, motor, and/or psychic disturbance. Loss of consciousness can also occur. Incidence is estimated to be 181,000 annually and is highest under 2 and over 65 years of age. The prevalence is approximately 2.5 million with an annual direct and indirect cost of approximately $12.5 billion.

There are special populations which have heightened risk of developing epilepsy. Thirty-three percent of those who have had a single, unprovoked seizure will go on to develop epilepsy, and 22% of stroke and head trauma patients will develop the disorder. Other high-risk populations include those with Alzheimer's disease, cerebral palsy, mental retardation, and children of those with epilepsy [53].

The spectrum of disease is broad, with most people able to live reasonably normal, uncomplicated lives on medication. Others, however, are severely compromised or devastated by the disorder. For the roughly 10% of cases that are refractory to medical management, surgical referral for excision of epileptogenic foci is the next step.

Fluorodeoxyglucose-Positron Emission Tomography in Epilepsy

FDG-PET brain scanning is indicated for patients with intractable epilepsy who are under consideration for surgical treatment. The most common type of focal epilepsy that is refractory to medical therapy is temporal lobe epilepsy. In one recent study of 113 patients with temporal lobe epilepsy, the sensitivity and specificity of FDG-PET was 89% and 91%, respectively [54]. Cortical dysgenesis resulting in heterotopia, mesial temporal sclerosis, and low-grade neoplasms located in the mesial temporal cortex/hippocampus are the most frequent culprits behind the disorder.

Because the majority of scans are performed in the interictal state (i.e., no seizure activity for 24 hours or more), the most frequent and characteristic finding at FDG-PET is a zone of hypometabolism in the affected cortex. The zone of hypometabolism is often much larger than the area of actual pathologic involvement [55]. In approximately 10% of cases, bilateral temporal hypometabolism is seen and is usually associated with more generalized, rather than focal, seizure activity. Unfortunately, postoperative seizure remission is markedly worse in these circumstances compared to unilateral temporal lobe epilepsy cases [56].

While focal hypometabolism is consistently found on an interictal scan, a hypermetabolic focus suggests an ictal scan. Seizure patients are typically monitored by EEG during the FDG uptake phase to document their seizure status on the day of imaging.

FDG-PET is accurate in identifying temporal lobe involvement in patients with epilepsy, but when abnormalities are in the frontal lobe or in the parietal lobe, the sensitivity is less than that seen in temporal lobe epilepsy cases (on the order of 50–75% for both) [57,58].

Horizons

The zone of hypometabolism during an interictal FDG-PET scan is more often larger than the actual epileptogenic lesion detected by MRI or at a pathologic evaluation. To more accurately identify the size of the abnormal focus causing the seizures, radiopharmaceuticals which target gamma-aminobutyric acid (GABA) receptors in neurons, such as ^{11}C-labeled flumazenil (FMZ), have been used to more finely localize the epileptogenic site. FMZ-PET has also been shown to be effective in localizing a seizure focus in the absence of a structural abnormality on MRI, and may improve surgical outcome in selected patients [50–61].

Positron Emission Tomography Imaging Protocol

Some elements of the FDG-PET brain scanning protocol are similar to the whole-body protocol discussed in Chapter 1. Some elements, however, are unique. Patients scheduled to undergo an FDG-PET brain study are asked to avoid any caloric intake for at least 4 hours prior to scanning, and a blood glucose level is obtained just prior to FDG injection. Frequently, patients with brain tumors are on corticosteroids, which can result in insulin resistance and hyperglycemia. Hyperglycemia leads to competitive inhibition of FDG uptake and can result in decreased differentiation between gray and white matter on the PET images. However, it has been shown that steroids do not significantly affect metabolism within brain tumors [62]. For adults, we typically inject 370 MBq (10 mCi) of FDG intravenously and instruct the patient to rest quietly for 30–40 minutes during the uptake phase. Patients are told to keep their eyes open, and we do not use ear occlusion; however, the uptake phase takes place in an environment where auditory and visual stimuli are minimized to avoid extraneous cortical activation. An 8-minute emission acquisition is obtained with three-dimensional mode with one table position, and the data are reconstructed using filtered back projection. Attenuation correction is calculated rather than measured, which eliminates the need for a separate transmission scan. By using 3D acquisition and calculated attenuation correction, scan time is minimized. Not only does this improve throughput, but it also reduces motion-induced artifacts. Often, pediatric patients or patients with altered mental status who may have difficulty obeying commends may require even shorter scan time, which can be accomplished with dynamic imaging.

In patients undergoing FDG-PET scanning for epilepsy, EEG monitoring is often performed to document whether seizure activity is occurring at the time of the scan. For reasons discussed above, clinical information regarding the patient's seizure status, that is, ictal versus interictal, is extremely important to the interpreting nuclear medicine physician or radiologist. We administer the FDG at least 2 hours after a clinical seizure in a patient who is having frequent seizures. The impact of seizure on a subsequent FDG-PET scan is unknown, but probably relates to both the duration and frequency of seizures.

The registration of FDG-PET brain images with a recent MRI (sometimes referred to as co-registration) takes place routinely at our institution when imaging brain tumors and is occasionally used for seizure disorder patients (Figure 13.7). Wong et al. describe scenarios where registration may not be necessary, such as when the tumors have high-grade activity which exceeds that of gray matter, or when the tumors are located well within white matter [8]. Both of these scenarios may avoid confusing tumor activity with physiologic gray matter activity. However, in the majority of cases where an anatomic abnormality is within or very near cortical or deep gray structures, PET alone cannot satisfactorily characterize such a lesion. It is in these cases where image registration

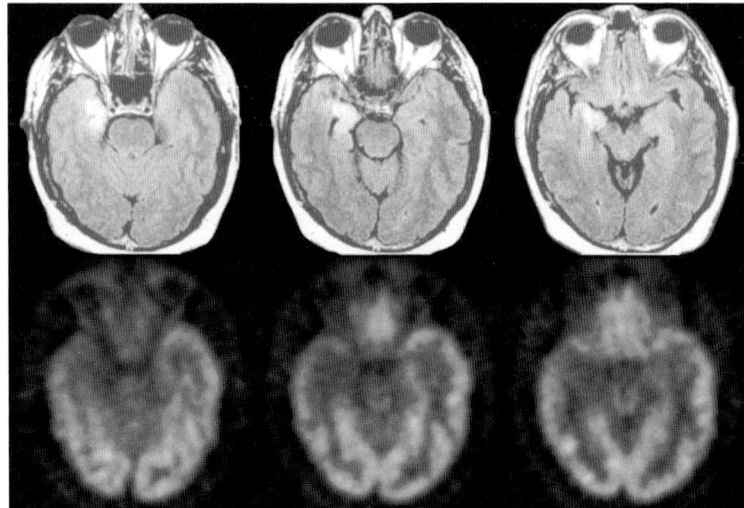

Figure 13.7. A 26-year-old man with seizure disorder not responding to therapy. MRI shows a non-enhancing mass in the right temporal lobe. The registered FLAIR sequence images and FDG-PET images show that the right temporal lobe is hypometabolic. The PET scan cannot differentiate mesial temporal sclerosis from a low-grade tumor.

is essential. Registration is not usually performed in patients who are undergoing PET brain scanning for dementia or epilepsy.

For registration to occur, digital images are gathered either by direct transfer in the case of in-house imaging, from recordings on digital media, or in the case of hardcopies, following digitization by a high resolution film digitizer. The registered images can then be interpreted one slice at a time at any point along a continuum ranging from 100% MRI to 100% PET. As an aid in interpretation, a mouse arrow, or any other pointing device, can be placed near an area of interest on MRI and physicians can toggle between 100% MRI and 100% PET or move along the continuum between the two modalities to evaluate the metabolic activity of the area in question.

References

1. What are the key statistics for brain and spinal cord tumors? American Cancer Society (www.cancer.org); 2005 Accessed February 2005.
2. Wrensch M, Minn Y, Chew T, Bondy M, Berger MS. Epidemiology of primary brain tumors: current concepts and review of the literature. Neuro-oncology 2002;4(4): 278–299.

3. Hesselager G, Uhrbom L, Westermark B, Nister M. Complementary effects of platelet-derived growth factor autocrine stimulation and p53 or Ink4a-Arf deletion in a mouse glioma model. Cancer Res 2003;63(15):4305–4309.

4. Navas-Acien A, Pollan M, Gustavsson P, Floderus B, Plato N, Dosemeci M. Interactive effect of chemical substances and occupational electromagnetic field exposure on the risk of gliomas and meningiomas in Swedish men. Cancer Epidemiol Biomarkers Prev 2002;11(12):1678–1683.

5. Lonn S, Klaeboe L, Hall P, et al. Incidence trends of adult primary intracerebral tumors in four Nordic countries. Int J Cancer 2004;108(3):450–455.

6. Kleihues P, Louis DN, Scheithauer BW, et al. The WHO classification of tumors of the nervous system. J Neuropathol Exp Neurol 2002;61(3):215–225; discussion 226–229.

7. Behin A, Hoang-Xuan K, Carpentier AF, Delattre JY. Primary brain tumours in adults. Lancet 2003;361(9354):323–331.

8. Wong T, van der Westhuizen GJ, Coleman RE. Brain tumors. In: Oehr P, Biersack HJ, Coleman RE, editors. PET and PET/CT in Oncology. Heidelberg: Springer; 2004: 113–125.

9. Nelson SJ. Imaging of brain tumors after therapy. Neuroimaging Clin N Am 1999;9(4):801–819.

10. Delbeke D, Meyerowitz C, Lapidus RL, et al. Optimal cutoff levels of F-18 fluorodeoxyglucose uptake in the differentiation of low-grade from high-grade brain tumors with PET. Radiology 1995;195(1):47–52.

11. Paulus W, Peiffer J. Intratumoral histologic heterogeneity of gliomas. A quantitative study. Cancer 1989;64(2):442–447.

12. Hanson MW, Glantz MJ, Hoffman JM, et al. FDG-PET in the selection of brain lesions for biopsy. J Comput Assist Tomogr 1991;15(5):796–801.

13. Pirotte B, Goldman S, Brucher JM, et al. PET in stereotactic conditions increases the diagnostic yield of brain biopsy. Stereotact Funct Neurosurg 1994;63(1–4):144–149.

14. Pirotte B, Goldman S, Bidaut LM, et al. Use of positron emission tomography (PET) in stereotactic conditions for brain biopsy. Acta Neurochir (Wien) 1995;134(1–2): 79–82.

15. Pirotte B, Goldman S, David P, et al. Stereotactic brain biopsy guided by positron emission tomography (PET) with [F-18]fluorodeoxyglucose and [C-11]methionine. Acta Neurochir Suppl (Wien) 1997;68:133–138.

16. Alavi JB, Alavi A, Chawluk J, et al. Positron emission tomography in patients with glioma. A predictor of prognosis. Cancer 1988;62(6):1074–1078.

17. Patronas NJ, Di Chiro G, Kufta C, et al. Prediction of survival in glioma patients by means of positron emission tomography. J Neurosurg 1985;62(6):816–822.

18. Francavilla TL, Miletich RS, Di Chiro G, Patronas NJ, Rizzoli HV, Wright DC. Positron emission tomography in the detection of malignant degeneration of low-grade gliomas. Neurosurgery 1989;24(1):1–5.

19. De Witte O, Levivier M, Violon P, et al. Prognostic value positron emission tomography with [18F]fluoro-2-deoxy-D-glucose in the low-grade glioma. Neurosurgery 1996;39(3):470–476; discussion 476–477.

20. Hanson MW, Hoffman JM, Glantz MJ. FDG PET in the early postoperative evaluation of patients with brain tumor (abstract). J Nucl Med 1990;31:799.

21. Barker FG, 2nd, Chang SM, Valk PE, Pounds TR, Prados MD. 18-Fluorodeoxyglucose uptake and survival of patients with suspected recurrent malignant glioma. Cancer 1997;79(1):115–126.

22. Chao ST, Suh JH, Raja S, Lee SY, Barnett G. The sensitivity and specificity of FDG PET in distinguishing recurrent brain tumor from radionecrosis in patients treated with stereotactic radiosurgery. Int J Cancer 2001;96(3):191–197.

23. Coleman RE, Hoffman JM, Hanson MW, Sostman HD, Schold SC. Clinical application of PET for the evaluation of brain tumors. J Nucl Med 1991;32(4):616–622.

24. Reardon DA, Akabani G, Coleman RE, et al. Phase II trial of murine (131)I-labeled antitenascin monoclonal antibody 81C6 administered into surgically created resection cavities of patients with newly diagnosed malignant gliomas. J Clin Oncol 2002; 20(5):1389–1397.

25. Marriott CJ, Thorstad W, Akabani G, et al. Locally increased uptake of fluorine-18-fluorodeoxyglucose after intracavitary administration of iodine-131-labeled antibody for primary brain tumors. J Nucl Med 1998;39(8):1376–1380.

26. Di Chiro G, Hatazawa J, Katz DA, Rizzoli HV, De Michele DJ. Glucose utilization by intracranial meningiomas as an index of tumor aggressivity and probability of recurrence: a PET study. Radiology 1987;164(2):521–526.

27. Hoffman JM, Waskin HA, Schifter T, et al. FDG-PET in differentiating lymphoma from nonmalignant central nervous system lesions in patients with AIDS. J Nucl Med 1993;34(4):567–575.

28. Roelcke U, Radu EW, Hausmann O, Vontobel P, Maguire RP, Leenders KL. Tracer transport and metabolism in a patient with juvenile pilocytic astrocytoma. A PET study. J Neurooncol 1998;36(3):279–283.

29. Rohren EM, Provenzale JM, Barboriak DP, Coleman RE. Screening for cerebral metastases with FDG PET in patients undergoing whole-body staging of non-central nervous system malignancy. Radiology 2003;226(1):181–187.

30. Jager PL, Vaalburg W, Pruim J, de Vries EG, Langen KJ, Piers DA. Radiolabeled amino acids: basic aspects and clinical applications in oncology. J Nucl Med 2001; 42(3):432–445.

31. Weber WA, Avril N, Schwaiger M. Relevance of positron emission tomography (PET) in oncology. Strahlenther Onkol 1999;175(8):356–373.

32. Sasaki M, Kuwabara Y, Yoshida T, et al. A comparative study of thallium-201 SPET, carbon-11 methionine PET and fluorine-18 fluorodeoxyglucose PET for the differentiation of astrocytic tumours. Eur J Nucl Med 1998;25(9):1261–1269.

33. Chung JK, Kim YK, Kim SK, et al. Usefulness of 11C-methionine PET in the evaluation of brain lesions that are hypo- or isometabolic on 18F-FDG PET. Eur J Nucl Med Mol Imaging 2002;29(2):176–182.

34. Choi SJ, Kim JS, Kim JH, et al. [(18)F]3′-deoxy-3′-fluorothymidine PET for the diagnosis and grading of brain tumors. Eur J Nucl Med Mol Imaging 2005;32(6):653–659.

35. Sun H, Sloan A, Mangner TJ, et al. Imaging DNA synthesis with [(18)F]FMAU and positron emission tomography in patients with cancer. Eur J Nucl Med Mol Imaging 2005;32(1):15–22.

36. Sadato N, Yonekura Y, Senda M, et al. PET and the autoradiographic method with continuous inhalation of oxygen-15-gas: theoretical analysis and comparison with conventional steady-state methods. J Nucl Med 1993;34(10):1672–1680.

37. Okazawa H, Yamauchi H, Sugimoto K, et al. Quantitative comparison of the bolus and steady-state methods for measurement of cerebral perfusion and oxygen metabolism: positron emission tomography study using 15O-gas and water. J Cereb Blood Flow Metab 2001;21(7):793–803.

38. Bird TD, Sumi SM, Nemens EJ, et al. Phenotypic heterogeneity in familial Alzheimer's disease: a study of 24 kindreds. Ann Neurol 1989;25(1):12–25.

39. Hebert LE, Scherr PA, Bienias JL, Bennett DA, Evans DA. Alzheimer disease in the US population: prevalence estimates using the 2000 census. Arch Neurol 2003;60(8): 1119–1122.

40. Losing a million minds: confronting the tragedy of Alzheimer's disease and other dementias. US Congress Office of Technology Assessment; 1987.

41. Hay JW, Ernst RL. The economic costs of Alzheimer's disease. Am J Public Health 1987;77(9):1169–1175.

42. Ernst RL, Hay JW. The US economic and social costs of Alzheimer's disease revisited. Am J Public Health 1994;84(8):1261–1264.

43. Brookmeyer R, Gray S, Kawas C. Projections of Alzheimer's disease in the United States and the public health impact of delaying disease onset. Am J Public Health 1998;88(9):1337–1342.

44. Arnaiz E, Jelic V, Almkvist O, et al. Impaired cerebral glucose metabolism and cognitive functioning predict deterioration in mild cognitive impairment. Neuroreport 2001;12(4):851–855.

45. Berent S, Giordani B, Foster N, et al. Neuropsychological function and cerebral glucose utilization in isolated memory impairment and Alzheimer's disease. J Psychiatr Res 1999;33(1):7–16.

46. Chetelat G, Desgranges B, de la Sayette V, et al. Mild cognitive impairment: can FDG-PET predict who is to rapidly convert to Alzheimer's disease? Neurology 2003;60(8): 1374–1377.

47. Drzezga A, Lautenschlager N, Siebner H, et al. Cerebral metabolic changes accompanying conversion of mild cognitive impairment into Alzheimer's disease: a PET follow-up study. Eur J Nucl Med Mol Imaging 2003;30(8):1104–1113.

48. Silverman DH, Small GW, Chang CY, et al. Positron emission tomography in evaluation of dementia: regional brain metabolism and long-term outcome. JAMA 2001;286(17):2120–2127.

49. Minoshima S, Foster NL, Sima AA, Frey KA, Albin RL, Kuhl DE. Alzheimer's disease versus dementia with Lewy bodies: cerebral metabolic distinction with autopsy confirmation. Ann Neurol 2001;50(3):358–365.

50. Friedland RP, Koss E, Lerner A, et al. Functional imaging, the frontal lobes, and dementia. Dementia 1993;4(3–4):192–203.

51. Herholz K, Heiss WD. Positron emission tomography in clinical neurology. Mol Imaging Biol 2004;6(4):239–269.

52. Engler H, Lundberg PO, Ekbom K, et al. Multitracer study with positron emission tomography in Creutzfeldt–Jakob disease. Eur J Nucl Med Mol Imaging 2003;30(1): 85–95.

53. Epilepsy and seizure statistics. Epilepsy Foundation (www.epilepsyfoundation.org); 2003 Accessed February 2005.

54. Kim YK, Lee DS, Lee SK, et al. Differential features of metabolic abnormalities between medial and lateral temporal lobe epilepsy: quantitative analysis of (18)F-FDG PET using SPM. J Nucl Med 2003;44(7):1006–1112.

55. Henry TR, Mazziotta JC, Engel J, Jr. Interictal metabolic anatomy of mesial temporal lobe epilepsy. Arch Neurol 1993;50(6):582–589.

56. Blum DE, Ehsan T, Dungan D, Karis JP, Fisher RS. Bilateral temporal hypometabolism in epilepsy. Epilepsia 1998;39(6):651–659.

57. Kim DW, Lee SK, Yun CH, et al. Parietal lobe epilepsy: the semiology, yield of diagnostic workup, and surgical outcome. Epilepsia 2004;45(6):641–649.

58. Hwang SI, Kim JH, Park SW, et al. Comparative analysis of MR imaging, positron emission tomography, and ictal single-photon emission CT in patients with neocortical epilepsy. AJNR Am J Neuroradiol 2001;22(5):937–946.

59. Koepp MJ, Hammers A, Labbe C, Woermann FG, Brooks DJ, Duncan JS. 11C-flumazenil PET in patients with refractory temporal lobe epilepsy and normal MRI. Neurology 2000;54(2):332–339.

60. Padma MV, Simkins R, White P, et al. Clinical utility of 11C-flumazenil positron emission tomography in intractable temporal lobe epilepsy. Neurol India 2004;52(4):457–462.

61. Csaba J. Positron emission tomography in presurgical localization of epileptic foci. Ideggyogy Sz 2003;56(7–8):249–254.

62. Roelcke U, Blasberg RG, von Ammon K, et al. Dexamethasone treatment and plasma glucose levels: relevance for fluorine-18-fluorodeoxyglucose uptake measurements in gliomas. J Nucl Med 1998;39(5):879–884.

Glossary

Artifact: a general radiology and nuclear medicine term which refers to any feature present within an image that is not actually present within the object being imaged. Examples include respiratory motion artifact, attenuation artifact, and various other technical artifacts.

Attenuation: the number of photons reaching a detector is reduced by a patient's surrounding tissues. The photons emanating from an object of interest deep within a patient may not be sufficient to create an adequate image. Attenuation is a major source of image artifact; however, there are many computational and imaging techniques which have been devised to help lessen the impact of attenuation. In PET and PET/CT, a transmission scan creates an attenuation map of the patient to help offset this problem.

^{11}C: carbon-11. This is a positron-emitting radionuclide which has a half-life of approximately 20 minutes.

^{11}C methionine: a PET radiopharmaceutical which can be used as a marker of protein synthesis. Carbon-11 (^{11}C) is one of the positron-emitting radionuclides used in PET imaging.

Curie: a measure of radioactivity, abbreviated Ci. This term honors Marie Curie, a pioneer in the research of radioactivity and the discoverer of radium. 1 curie = 37 billion disintegrations per second. The typical FDG-PET dose for a whole-body scan is 10–15 mCi (140 µCi/kg).

Cyclotron: a type of particle accelerator. The cyclotron principle involves using an electric field to accelerate charged particles across a gap between two magnetic field regions. The magnetic field accelerates the particles in a semi-circle, during which time the electric field is reversed in polarity to accelerate the charged particle again as it moves across the gap in the opposite direction. ^{11}C, ^{18}F, ^{13}N, and ^{15}O are all produced in a cyclotron.

^{18}F: fluorine-18. This is the most widely used positron-emitting radionuclide in clinical medicine. It is most often in the form of the glucose analogue FDG. ^{18}F has a half-life of approximately 110 minutes.

FDG: fluorodeoxyglucose. The formal name is ^{18}F-2-fluoro-2-deoxy-D-glucose. This is an analogue of glucose and therefore a marker of metabolic activity. FDG is the most frequently used radiopharmaceutical in PET and PET/CT imaging.

Gamma camera: a nuclear medicine scanner. The gamma camera is the fundamental nuclear medicine imaging device. It is composed of a system of collimators, crystals, photomultiplier tubes, and computers arranged to collect, analyze, and create images based upon gamma photon emissions from a patient who has been injected with a radiopharmaceutical.

Gamma decay: a type of radioactive decay in which a nucleus in a high energy state changes to a lower energy state by emitting electromagnetic radiation in the form of a photon, or gamma ray. ^{99m}Technetium is an example of a radionuclide that undergoes gamma decay also called isomeric transition.

Gamma ray: a photon. A photon is a discrete packet of energy emitted by many substances as they undergo radioactive decay. This physical property is the basis behind nuclear medicine imaging. Gamma photons are collected by a gamma camera and then processed to generate an image. *See* photon.

G-code: nomenclature used by the Centers for Medicare and Medicaid Services when first covering PET scans. In PET imaging, a G-code can be thought of as an indication for the study, for example initial staging of lung cancer.

Glycolysis: an energy-generating process occurring inside mitochondria in which glucose is converted to pyruvic acid. The metabolic breakdown of glucose produces energy in the form of adenosine triphosphate (ATP) which has high energy phosphate bonds. FDG behaves similarly to glucose and is therefore a marker for metabolic activity.

Half-life: a physical property that refers to the time necessary for one half of a radioactive substance to decay. This is denoted as $t_{1/2}$. ^{18}F has a half-life of 110 minutes.

Image registration: a process of combining or fusing complementary but different image data. PET/CT provides both metabolic and anatomic information in one fusion image.

^{13}**N**: nitrogen-13. This is a positron-emitting radionuclide which has a half-life of approximately 10 minutes.

^{13}**N ammonia**: a PET radiopharmaceutical which is used primarily in cardiac imaging as a myocardial perfusion agent. Nitrogen-13 (^{13}N) is one of the positron-emitting radionuclides used in PET imaging.

Negative predictive value: the percentage of patients who test negative and truly do not have the disease.

Nuclide: a type of atom characterized by the constitution of its nucleus; that is, the number of protons, number of neutrons, and its energy state.

^{15}**O**: oxygen-15. This is a positron-emitting radionuclide which has a half-life of approximately 2 minutes.

PET: positron emission tomography. This is a type of nuclear medicine scan which uses positron-emitting radionuclides to generate images of various physiological and pathophysiological processes within the body. The most common type of PET scan is an FDG-PET scan.

PET/CT: positron emission tomography/computed tomography. A PET/CT scanner has both PET imaging and CT imaging capabilities. The PET scanner and the CT scanner are built in-line as one unit so that the functional information obtained from the PET scan can be correlated with the highly accurate anatomic information from the CT scan during the same imaging session. Most of the new PET scanners sold today are actually PET/CT scanners.

Photon: a packet of energy. All nuclear medicine images are created by photons, called gamma photons (sometimes denoted γ). Photons are generated in a variety of ways. In conventional nuclear medicine, they are released by radioactive nuclei when those nuclei undergo decay. In the case of FDG-PET, the photons do not come from the ^{18}F nucleus directly. ^{18}F emits a positron, which then annihilates with an electron a short distance away from the nucleus. This annihilation reaction produces two high energy photons which travel in opposite directions. Photon energy is measured in electron volts (eV), and the photons created by positron and electron annihilation are 511 keV.

Positive predictive value: the percentage of patients who test positive and truly have the disease.

Positron: a positively charged electron. Positrons are released from some radionuclides which are unstable due to an excess of protons within their nuclei. Positrons are often referred to as beta plus (or β^+) particles. *See* positron decay.

Positron decay: a type of radioactive decay in which a nucleus that has too many protons reaches a more stable state by emitting a positron. A positron is a positively charged electron. In positron decay, a proton is converted into a neutron, and a positron and a neutrino are emitted from the nucleus. A nucleus with too many protons undergoes positron decay when it does not have enough energy to emit an alpha particle.

Radionuclide: a nuclide that emits radioactivity; *see* nuclide.

Radiopharmaceutical: a combination of a radionuclide and a pharmaceutical agent; also referred to as radiotracer.

Radiotracer: another term for radiopharmaceutical. This term is sometimes used because the pharmaceutical portion of an administered radiopharmaceutical in a typical nuclear medicine study is in trace amounts and has negligible pharmacologic effect.

^{82}Rb: rubidium-82. This positron-emitting radionuclide is made by a generator rather than a cyclotron. It is an analogue of potassium and is used as a myocardial perfusion agent. ^{82}Rb has a half-life of approximately 1.3 minutes.

Scintigram: the formal term for a nuclear medicine scan (from the Latin *scintilla* meaning spark or glimmer). Scintillation refers to the creation of a minute flash of light when a photon emanating from the object being imaged interacts with a special crystal housed within a gamma camera.

Sensitivity: the percentage of patients who have a disease and test positive.

Spatial resolution: a description of how close two features can be within an image and still be resolved as unique. In other words, spatial resolution describes the ability to sharply and clearly define the size or shape of features within an image.

Specificity: the percentage of patients who do not have a disease and test negative.

SPECT: acronym for single photon emission computed tomography. This is a technique employed routinely in nuclear medicine in which the gamma camera rotates around the patient rather than remaining in a single plane. The collected data is then manipulated by a computer to generate cross-sectional images (tomograms).

Standardized uptake value (SUV): a semi-quantitative measurement of the FDG uptake within a region of interest on an FDG-PET scan. More specifically, it is the ratio of activity within tissue per milliliter to the activity in the injected dose per unit of patient body weight.

Uptake phase: the time between radiotracer injection and scanning. This time is necessary for adequate biodistribution of FDG. The uptake phase is usually 30–60 minutes and varies depending on scan type and facility guidelines.

Index